QUICK LOOK SERIES in Veterinary Medicine

METABOLIC AND ENDOCRINE PHYSIOLOGY

Larry R. Engelking, Ph.D.

Professor of Physiology
Department of Biomedical Sciences
Tufts University
School of Veterinary Medicine
North Grafton, MA

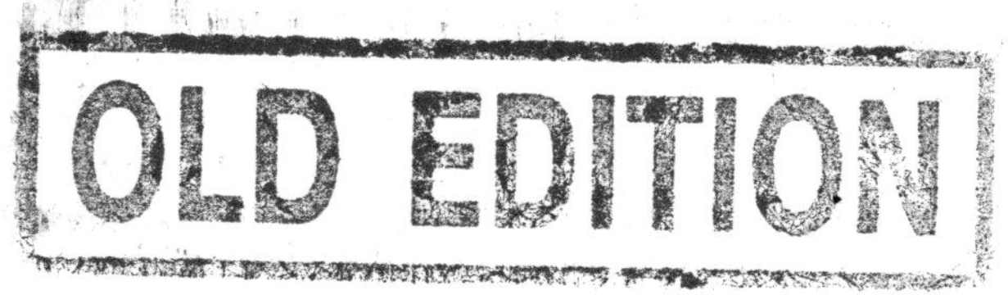

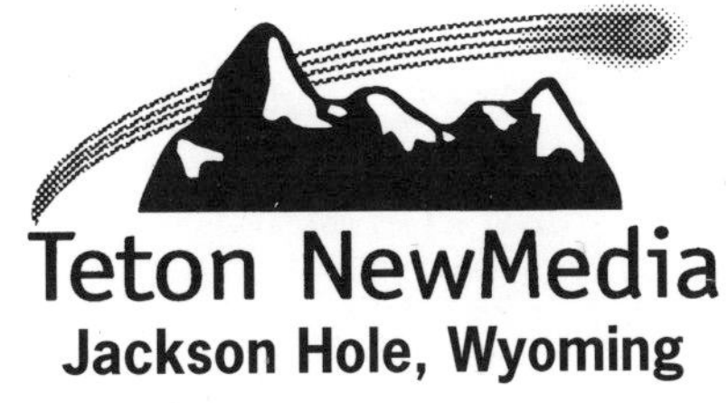

Teton NewMedia
Jackson Hole, Wyoming

Executive Editor: Carroll C. Cann
Development Editor: Susan L. Hunsberger
Editor: Cynthia J. Roantree
Production: Karen Feeney, Derra
Typeset by Achorn Graphics, Worcester, MA
Printed by McNaughton & Gunn, Saline, MI
Illustrations by Oxford Illustrators, Oxford, UK

Teton NewMedia
P.O. Box 4833
125 South King Street
Jackson, WY 83001
1-888-770-3165
http://www.tetonnm.com

The authors and publisher have made every effort to provide an accurate reference text. However, they shall not be held responsible for problems arising from errors or omissions, or from misunderstandings on the part of the reader.

Library of Congress Cataloging-in-Publication Data

Engelking, Larry R. (Larry Rex)
Metabolic and endocrine physiology / Larry R. Engelking.
p. cm. - - (Quick look series in veterinary medicine)
ISBN 1-893441-31-8
1. Veterinary endocrinology. 2. Endocrine glands- -Diseases. 3. Metabolism- -Disorders.
I. Title. II. Series.

SF768.3 .E55 2000
636.089'24- -dc21

00-059977

PRINTED IN THE UNITED STATES OF AMERICA

ISBN 1-893441-31-8

Print number 5 4 3 2 1

Table of Contents

Dedication

To my late father and mother, Rex and Ermalee, for setting high standards and instilling in me the desire to learn; to my wife, Rhonda, for her love and support; and to our children, Derek Rex, Jared Curtis and Kelly Lee, for making it all worthwhile.

Preface

Metabolic and Endocrine Physiology, the first published volume in the *QUICK LOOK SERIES in Veterinary Medicine* has been written primarily for veterinary students who wish to organize their thinking in endocrinology, interns and residents preparing for their specialty board exams, animal science and graduate students in physiology, and practicing veterinarians who wish to update their general knowledge of endocrinology. Emphasis has been placed on instructional figures, flow diagrams, and tables, while text material has been held to a minimum. Over 200 multiple choice questions have been included to gauge the reader's capacity to effectively deal with the subject matter.

This "quick look" is not intended to replace the excellent detailed manuscripts, reviews, and textbooks of endocrinology available, many of which were consulted during its preparation. Care has been taken to present relevant information in an up-to-date, accurate, and reliable fashion; however, all authors are fallible, this one being no exception, and if a reader detects errors or if clarity of presentation can be improved, feedback would be genuinely appreciated.

Only those who have tried to encompass the vast science of veterinary endocrinology into one instructional review know how difficult is the problem of organizing the material, and how impossible is the achievement of a complete, concise, consistent, and logical sequence. In general, the endocrine system is first defined and described, and then each endocrine gland is discussed separately. Where appropriate, common endocrine disorders have also been included.

The study of metabolism and endocrinology is distinguished from other basic health science disciplines by its steadfast concern with "integrative" mechanisms that control and fine tune virtually all tissues and organ systems. In the healthy animal, physiologic variables such as blood volume and pressure, body temperature, ionic composition of the extracellular fluid compartment, general anabolism vs. catabolism, metabolic rate, the onset of reproductive cycles, and the blood glucose concentration must be controlled and maintained within narrow limits, even in the face of significant environmental challenges. A primary goal in the preparation of this text has been to concisely elucidate the endocrine mechanisms responsible for maintaining homeostatic control of those and other important physiologic variables, and to assist the reader in understanding common pathophysiologic deviations from normal. I hope you will find this "quick look" at metabolic and endocrine physiology to be informative, inspirational, challenging, and relevant to your educational needs.

Larry Rex Engelking

Acknowledgments

I am grateful to Jim and Matt Harris for their support and encouragement during the planning and preparation of this text. I also wish to thank Karen Feeney, Kevin Sullivan, and Jan Cocker for their editorial assistance, patience, and attention to detail.

Thanks are also due to Carroll Cann, Cindy Roantree, and Susan Hunsberger of Teton NewMedia who have been instrumental in bringing this project to fruition.

QUICK LOOK SERIES IN VETERINARY MEDICINE

METABOLIC AND ENDOCRINE PHYSIOLOGY

1 The Endocrine System

A

Chemical class	*Hormone*	*Major source*
Amino acid derivatives		
Biogenic amines	Dopamine (DA)	CNS
	Norepinephrine (NE)	CNS, autonomic nervous system, adrenal medulla
	Epinephrine (Epi)	CNS, adrenal medulla
Iodothyronines	Melatonin	Pineal
	Thyroxine (T_4)	Thyroid
	Triiodothyronine (T_3)	Thyroid, peripheral tissues
	Reverse T_3 (rT_3)	Thyroid, liver
Small peptides (< 50 amino acids)	Vasopressin (ADH)	Posterior pituitary
	Oxytocin (Oxy)	Posterior pituitary
	Melanocyte-stimulating hormone (MSH)	Pars intermedia, anterior pituitary
	Thyrotropin-releasing hormone (TRH)	Hypothalamus, CNS
	Gonadotropin-releasing hormone (GnRH or LHRH)	Hypothalamus, CNS
	Somatocrinin (GHRH)	Hypothalamus, CNS
	Somatostatin (SS, GHIH or SRIH)	Hypothalamus, CNS, stomach, pancreas, intestine
	Adrenocorticotropic hormone (ACTH)	Anterior pituitary
	ACTH -releasing hormone (CRH)	Hypothalamus, CNS
	Angiotensins (A-II, A-III)	Plasma, CNS
	Opioid peptides (e.g., Enk, Endor)	CNS, other tissues
	Secretin	GI tract, CNS
	Cholecystokinin (CCK)	GI tract, CNS
	Gastrin (G)	GI tract, CNS, pancreas
	Gastric inhibitory polypeptide (GIP)	GI tract
	Vasoactive intestinal polypeptide (VIP)	GI tract, other tissues
	Glucagon	GI tract, pancreas
	Glucagon-like immunoreactivity (GLI)	GI tract
	Gastrin-releasing peptide (GRP)	GI tract, CNS
	Motilin	GI tract, CNS
	Neurotensin	GI tract, CNS
	Substance P	GI tract, CNS
	Guanylin	GI tract, CNS
	Pancreatic polypeptide (PP)	GI tract, pancreas, CNS
	Atrial natriuretic peptide (ANP)	Heart
Proteins (> 50 amino acids)	Calcitonin (TCT or CT)	Thyroid, other tissues
	Insulin	Pancreas
	Growth hormone (GH or somatotropin)	Anterior pituitary
	Thyroid-stimulating hormone (TSH)	Anterior pituitary
	Prolactin (PRL)	Anterior pituitary
	Follicle-stimulating hormone (FSH)	Anterior pituitary
	Luteinizing hormone (LH or ICSH)	Anterior pituitary
	Parathyroid hormone (PTH)	Parathyroids
	Erythropoietin (EPO)	Kidney
	Placental lactogen (PL)	Placenta
	Chorionic gonadotropin (CG)	Placenta
	Inhibin (I)	Gonads
	Activin	Gonads
	Relaxin	Gonads
	Somatomedins (e.g., IGF-1)	Liver
Steroids	Progesterone (Prog)	Corpus luteum, placenta, testes, adrenal cortex
	Testosterone (T)	Testes, ovaries, adrenal cortex, placenta
	Estrogens (E_1, E_2, E_3)	Ovaries, adrenal cortex, testes, placenta
	Dihydrotestosterone (DHT)	Testosterone-sensitive tissues
	Glucocorticoids (e.g., cortisol)	Adrenal cortex
	Mineralocorticoids (e.g., aldosterone)	Adrenal cortex
	Dihydrocholecalciferol (1,25-DHC or vitamin D_3)	Skin, liver, kidney
Fatty acid derivatives (Eicosanoids)	Prostaglandins (PGs)	Most tissues
	Leukotrienes (LTs)	White blood cells
	Thromboxanes (TXs)	Platelets, placenta

LHRH = leuteinizing hormone–releasing hormone; GHRH = GH-releasing hormone; GHIH = GH-release–inhibiting hormone; SRIH = somatotropin release–inhibiting hormone; ENK = enkephalin; Endor = endorphin; ICSH = interstitial cell–stimulating hormone; IGF-1 = insulin-like growth factor 1.

B

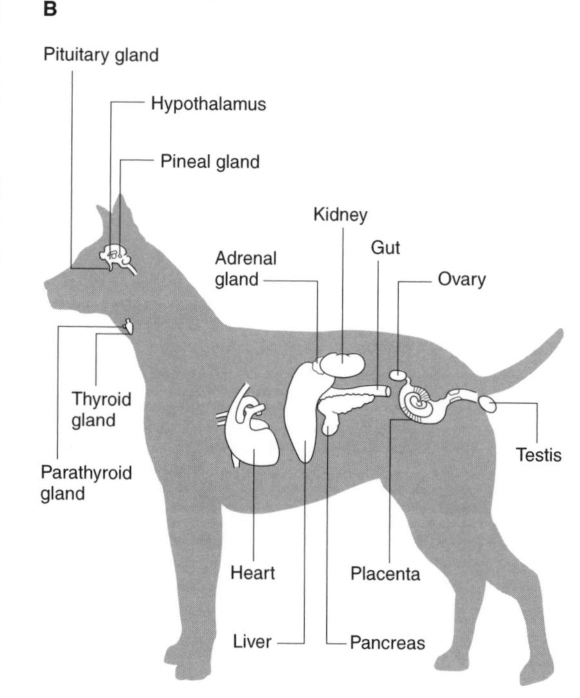

Overview

- Hormones regulate the rates of cellular reactions.
- Some hormones present in mammals have also been identified in single-cell organisms.
- Hormones can be steroids, amino acid derivatives, proteins, smaller peptides, or fatty acid derivatives.
- The CNS is a major component of the endocrine system.

The endocrine system can be described using two words of Greek origin: *endocrine* and *hormone.* The term *endocrine* means "to separate within," which refers to wide separation of endocrine tissues throughout the body, while the term *hormone* means "I excite."

Nonreproductive endocrinology in veterinary medicine has been based largely on studies in dogs; however, the increasing popularity of cats and other companion animals has resulted in studies that have increased awareness of their endocrine disorders as well. Endocrine disorders appear to be involved in about 10% to 20% of reported medical diseases in dogs and less than 5% in cats. *Reproductive veterinary endocrinology,* on the other hand, has primarily been based on studies in large animal species.

Hormones are synthesized in a variety of cell types and are secreted and transported to various target tissues, where they affect diverse metabolic functions by regulating rates of specific reactions without themselves contributing energy or initiating the process. Many hormones (e.g., insulin, adrenocorticotropic hormone, somatostatin, or their structurally similar progenitors) that were originally thought to have developed with complex multicellular and multitissue higher animals have been found in single-cell organisms, indicating an early role in intercellular communication.

Because many hormones are secreted into blood prior to use (endocrine action), circulating levels can give some indication of endocrine gland activity and target organ exposure. Because of the small amounts of hormones required, blood levels can be extremely low. For example, circulating levels of *protein hormones* normally range from 10^{-10} to 10^{-12} Mol, and circulating levels of *thyroid hormones* and *steroid hormones* normally range from 10^{-6} to 10^{-9} Mol. Hormones include *proteins* (often with molecular weights of 30 kd or less), *smaller polypeptides* (<50 amino acids), *amino acid derivatives* (the biogenic amines and iodothyronines), and *steroids;* sometimes *fatty acid derivatives* (the eicosanoids: prostaglandins, leukotrienes, and thromboxanes) are also classified as hormones (**Part A**).

Endocrine Glands

The **central nervous system (CNS)** is a major part of the endocrine system. Many hormones, particularly small polypeptides such as those found in the gut, are also important *CNS neurotransmitters* (see Chapters 59–63). Large amounts of these compounds and small amounts of insulin and adrenocorticotropic hormone (ACTH), as well as their respective receptors, have been found in the brain. There they appear to exhibit broad, although ill-defined, actions on pain sensitivity, as well as sexual, feeding, and other behavioral phenomena. Also, the synthesis, secretion, and action of neurotransmitters involve processes similar to those of hormones. Thus, the distinction between a hormone and a neurotransmitter is becoming increasingly difficult to make. Specialized nerve cells in a part of the brain known as the *hypothalamus* synthesize hormones that are either stored in the *posterior pituitary* (e.g., oxytocin and antidiuretic hormone, ADH) or transported by portal blood to the *anterior pituitary* (immediately below the hypothalamus; see Chapter 6). Through its ability to release additional hormones from the pituitary, the hypothalamus can control, for example, salt and water balance, sexual function, growth, skin darkening, lactation, and the body's response to stress. The *pineal gland* is also a part of the CNS and has been viewed historically as either the "seat of the soul" or "a third eye" (see Chapters 15 and 16). This gland produces *melatonin,* a biogenic amine that is involved with, among other things, photoperiodic regulation of reproductive events in seasonal breeders.

The **thyroid gland** produces iodothyronines (from iodine and the amino acid, tyrosine), namely *tetraiodothyronine (thyroxine, T_4), triiodothyronine (T_3),* and *reverse T_3 (rT_3)* (see Chapters 48–51). Triiodothyronine is the active metabolite of T_4 that increases oxygen utilization and therefore the basal metabolic rate of many tissues. Parafollicular cells of the thyroid produce *calcitonin (TCT or CT),* a protein hormone involved with calcium homeostasis (see Chapters 29 and 31).

The **parathyroid glands,** which are embedded in the thyroid just in front of the trachea (and behind the larynx), produce a protein hormone known as *parathyroid hormone (parathormone or PTH),* which plays an important role in maintaining optimal blood levels of calcium and phosphate (see Chapters 29 and 30).

The **adrenal glands** are situated immediately above the kidneys and are composed of an *outer cortex* and an *inner medulla.* The cortex produces *corticosteroids* (e.g., cortisol, aldosterone, and small amounts of the sex steroids), and the medulla produces *catecholamines* (e.g., epinephrine and norepinephrine). Cortisol is a *glucocorticoid* involved in glucose homeostasis, while aldosterone is a *mineralocorticoid* involved with electrolyte balance. The *catecholamines* help to produce the "fight or flight" response (see Chapters 32–41, 44–47).

The **gastrointestinal tract** is the largest endocrine organ and produces several *neurocrine, paracrine,* and *endocrine* mediators. Mediators such as cholecystokinin (CCK), secretin, and gastrin primarily regulate gastrointestinal physiology (i.e., motility, secretion, and digestive action). However, others may also be involved with the release of hormones such as insulin (e.g., gastric inhibitory polypeptide, GIP), and therefore become involved with energy balance (see Chapters 59–62).

The **endocrine pancreas** (which lies adjacent to the stomach) consists of islet tissue scattered throughout the larger exocrine portion of the gland. The endocrine pancreas produces insulin, glucagon, and somatostatin, and it is integrally involved with carbohydrate, protein, and lipid metabolism (see Chapters 54–58).

The **kidney** is a regulatory and excretory organ, filtering and secreting waste products and drugs from the circulation into urine. It also produces hormones involved in the control of blood pressure (renin), erythropoiesis (erythropoietin), and calcium/phosphate homeostasis (hydroxylation of vitamin D) (see Chapters 39–42).

The **gonads** (ovaries and testes) produce the sex steroids (e.g., progesterone, testosterone, and estrogen), as well as several protein hormones also involved with reproductive function (e.g., relaxin, inhibin, and activin; see Chapters 11–14).

The **placenta,** a primary organ of pregnancy serving the fetus, produces several hormones, many of which are also produced by other glands (see Chapter 17). Two hormones produced only by the placenta are *placental lactogen (PL)* and *chorionic gonadotropin (CG).*

Part B is a diagrammatic representation of all hormone-secreting tissues.

The action of a hormone at its target site is dependent on five general factors:

1. The rate of synthesis and/or secretion of the hormone from the endocrine gland of origin.
2. Specific (liver-derived) transport proteins in plasma (steroid and thyroid hormones).
3. Conversion to a more active form in target tissues (e.g., T_4 to T_3).
4. The number and/or activity of hormone-specific receptors on or in respective target cells.
5. Degradation, conjugation, and/or excretion of the hormone (by the liver and kidney).

2 Endocrine Secretory Control

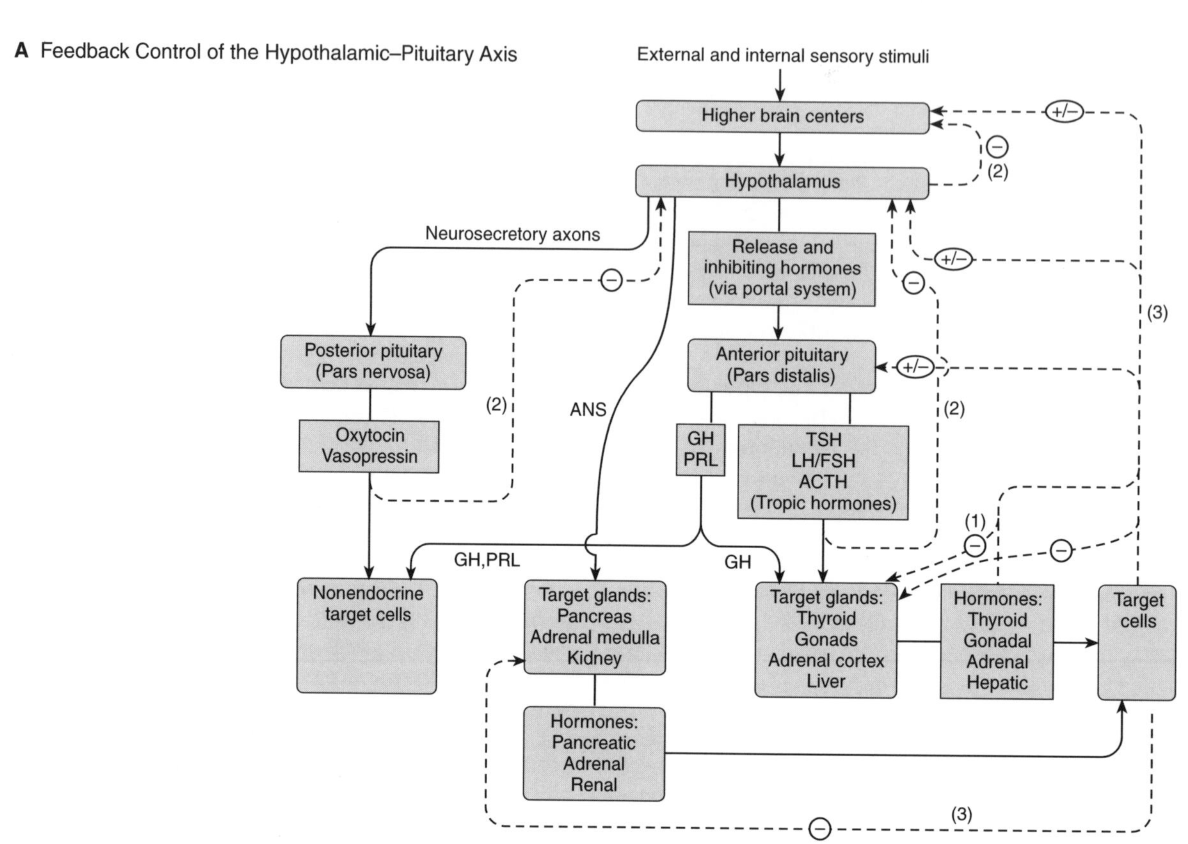

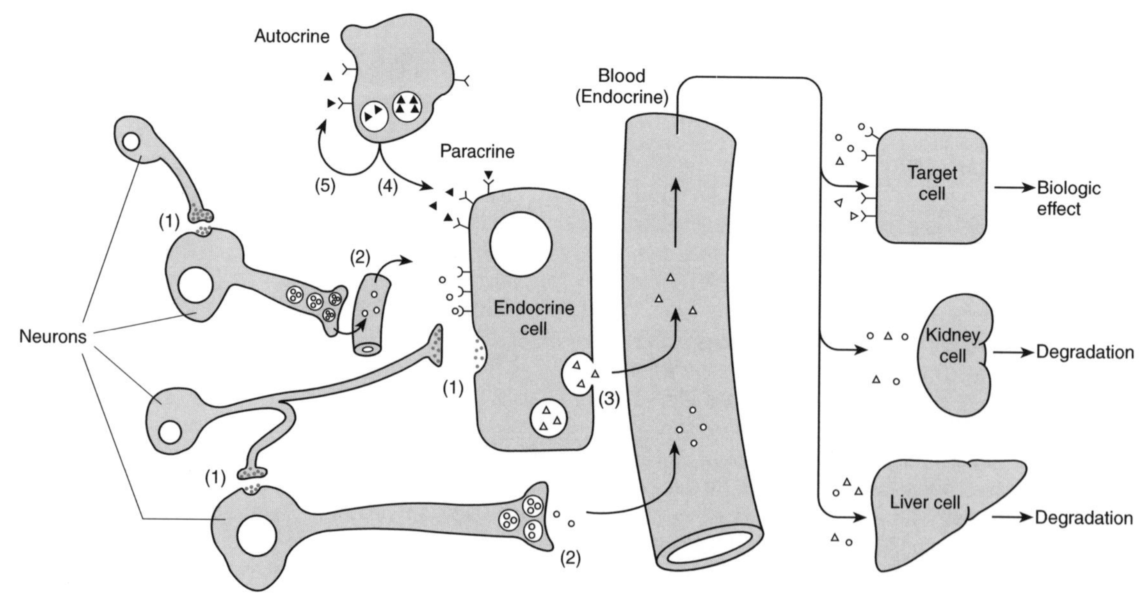

Overview

- Tropic hormones from the anterior pituitary promote secretion from target endocrine glands.
- The autonomic nervous system can control endocrine secretion.
- The hypothalamus is a neuroendocrine organ.
- Somatostatin in a paracrine mediator.
- There is structural conservation of chemical messengers across animal species.
- The endocrine system is slower than the nervous system.
- Some hormone metabolites are biologically active.
- Some hormones are eliminated unchanged into bile or urine.

It is characteristic of the endocrine system that a balanced state of feedback regulation be maintained among the various glands. This is particularly notable with respect to *release hormones* and *inhibiting hormones* (or factors) from the hypothalamus, which regulate synthesis and secretion of anterior pituitary hormones. *Tropic (or trophic) anterior pituitary hormones,* in turn, promote hormone secretion from various target endocrine glands. Characteristically, elevated hormone concentrations result in both *direct* and *indirect feedback control* of their production by the originating gland (autocrine control), anterior pituitary, hypothalamus, and higher brain centers. **Part A** depicts control via ultra-short-loop negative feedback (process *1* in **Part A**), short-loop feedback (process *2* in **Part A**), and long-loop feedback (process *3* in **Part A**). Target tissues may also produce nonendocrine products that either inhibit or stimulate further endocrine secretion, and sensory input (i.e., sight, sound, touch, taste, and smell) may also stimulate or inhibit hypothalamic activity, and thus endocrine secretion (see **Part A**). The *autonomic nervous system (ANS),* also controlled by the hypothalamus, influences certain endocrine gland secretions as well (e.g., pancreatic insulin and glucagon release, adrenal medullary catecholamine release, and renal renin release).

Categories of Chemical Regulators

Both classic endocrine and nerve cells synthesize and release chemical messengers. These messengers may then act on the same cell in which they are produced (autocrine) (process 5 in **Part B**), on other target cells in their vicinity without entering the circulation (paracrine) (process 4 in **Part B**), or they may go to distant target cells through the circulation (endocrine) (process 3 in **Part B**). Nerve cells produce neurotransmitters that are released at nerve terminals. These neurotransmitters can be released into blood to act as endocrine agents (neurocrine or neuroendocrine) (process 2 in **Part B**), or they can be released to act directly on a target cell in a paracrine fashion (e.g., another nerve, muscle, or endocrine cell) (process 1 in **Part B**).

Prostaglandins sometimes act in an autocrine fashion, and somatostatin acts in the stomach and endocrine pancreas as a paracrine agent (see Chapters 54, 59, and 60). Entrance of insulin into the circulation in search of its distant target cells (e.g., muscle and adipose tissue) is an example of endocrine secretion.

Exocrine glands, on the other hand, secrete their products into ducts through which they are conveyed to their sites of action in such places as the digestive tract or the body's surface. Exocrine secretions include saliva, sweat, milk, and pancreatic and biliary secretions. *Pheromones* are specialized chemical agents secreted through exocrine glands to the body surface for interorganismal communication, namely to other members of the same species.

Evolutionary Considerations

Chemical regulation of the internal environment is thought to have evolved from paracrine- and autocrine-type secretions as seen in primitive multicellular organisms. As more sophisticated cardiovascular and nervous systems evolved, the same primitive messengers continued to appear in endocrine, neural, and neuroendocrine secretions. Indeed, there is considerable structural conservation of chemical messengers across animal species. There are profound differences, however, in target organ responses to these messengers. For example, prolactin causes milk secretion in mammals, yet in fish and amphibians it is involved with water balance. It is generally believed that the functional adaptation of hormones evolved to fit the nutritional uniqueness of each animal species. Although chemical messengers and physiologic functions may not have changed throughout evolution, the means of fulfilling those functions did.

Higher animals (i.e., mammalian vertebrates) have well-developed nervous systems for immediate physiologic responses. Although their endocrine systems are slower acting, the physiologic responses they provoke generally last longer. Mammalian vertebrates also have well-integrated neural and endocrine regulatory systems, and in many cases these two systems are difficult to separate (e.g., the adrenal medulla, hypothalamic nuclei, the posterior pituitary, and neurocrine regulation of gut function). In contrast, invertebrates are more dependent on paracrine and autocrine regulation because they possess primitive nervous systems.

Degradation and Elimination of Hormones

Hormones may or may not be degraded before being eliminated from the body. Some metabolites of degraded hormones are biologically active, others inactive. Degradation of hormones may be carried out by serum proteases, by peripheral target cells, or more frequently by the liver or kidneys (**Part B**). Some hormones are eliminated unchanged into bile or urine.

There are also differences in a hormone's degradation and elimination in different animal species. Glucocorticoids, for example, are usually degraded by the liver to inactive metabolites that can eventually be eliminated in urine; however, dogs reduce these metabolites to a greater extent than do primates, and cats are thought to eliminate glucocorticoids primarily in bile.

3 Mechanisms of Catecholamine and Polypeptide Hormone Action: I

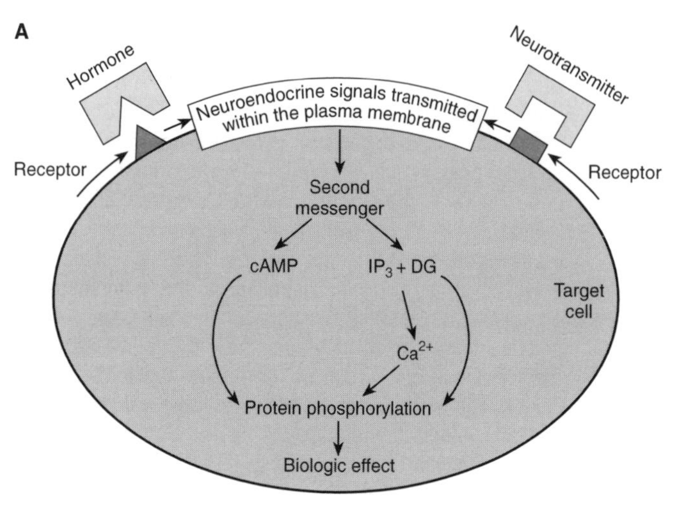

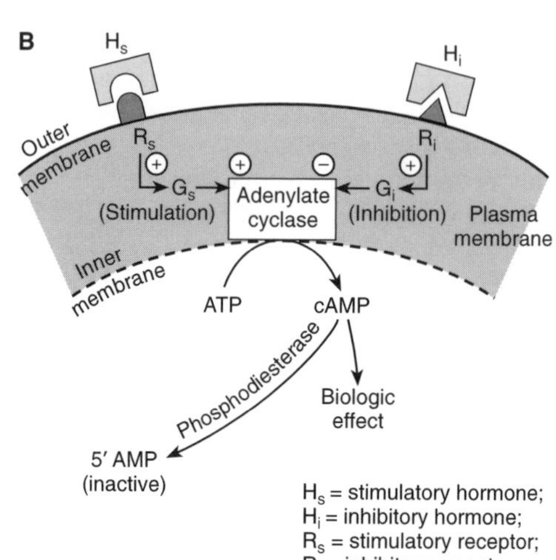

C

Hormones Capable of Stimulating Adenylate Cyclase	***Hormones Incapable of Stimulating Adenylate Cyclase***
Secretin	Angiotensin II
Calcitonin (CT)	α-Adrenergic catecholamines (NE more capable than Epi)
β-Adrenergic catecholamines (NE and Epi equally capable)	Placental lactogen (PL)
Glucagon	Growth hormone (GH)
Follicle-stimulating hormone (FSH)	Insulin
Chorionic gonadotropin (CG)	Oxytocin
Luteinizing hormone (LH)	Prolactin (PRL)
Melanocyte-stimulating hormone (MSH)	Somatomedins (e.g., IGF-1)
Parathormone (PTH)	Somatostatin (SS, GHIH)
Thyroid-stimulating hormone (TSH)	Gastrin
TSH-releasing hormone (TRH)	Cholecystokinin (CCK)
Antidiuretic hormone (ADH)	
Adrenocorticotropic hormone (ACTH)	

D Biologic Effects of cAMP

Process (and Hormones)	***Target Cells***
Membrane permeability, ions (PTH, CT)	Kidney tubules, intestine, bone
Membrane permeability, water (ADH)	Kidney (collecting ducts)
Steroid hormone synthesis (ACTH, LH, FSH)	Adrenal cortex, testes, ovaries
Secretory responses (Secretin, TRH, TSH)	Pancreas, pituitary, thyroid
Lipolysis (NE, Epi)	Adipocytes
Glycogenolysis (NE, Epi, Glucagon)	Muscle, liver
Gluconeogenesis (NE, Epi, Glucagon)	Liver, kidney
Vasodilation (Epi)	Arterioles (β-receptors)

Overview

- Only cells with appropriate receptors can respond to the presence of a hormone.
- Receptors for catecholamine and polypeptide hormones are found on the target cell surface.
- The number of receptors on a target cell can range from about 2000 to 100,000 depending on the physiologic conditions.
- The affinity of a hormone for its receptor also changes.
- The cAMP second messenger system is linked to G proteins attached to the cell membrane.
- Phosphodiesterase inactivates cAMP.

Target cells have *hormone-specific receptors* capable of recognizing and binding hormones; therefore, only these cells respond to the presence of the hormones. This binding, in turn, initiates intracellular events leading to the final physiologic effect. Generally, receptors are hormone specific, but to a limited extent other hormones or drugs with similar structure may bind to them.

Receptors

Hormone receptors occur in different cell locations depending on the class of hormone they bind. Receptors for catecholamine and polypeptide hormones are found on the surface of target cells, while those for steroid and thyroid hormones are found in the cytoplasm and/or nucleus. The number of receptors per target cell ranges from about 2000 to 100,000, varying under different physiologic conditions.

The affinity of a hormone for its receptor and the number of receptors are not static. Receptor concentration is affected by genetics, the stage of growth, the stage of the target cell's cycle, and the degree of its differentiation. Receptor concentration and affinity for its hormone are affected by ionic balance and temperature, by concentration of the homologous hormone and heterologous hormones, and by antibodies against the receptor.

Second Messengers

The two primary *intracellular second messenger systems* that respond to the presence of nervous stimulation or catecholamine/polypeptide hormone binding on the cell surface are the *cyclic adenosine monophosphate (cAMP)* and *calcium/diacylglycerol messenger systems* (**Part A**). These two systems are not totally unrelated.

The cAMP Messenger System

Hormones or neurotransmitters that affect cell metabolism via cAMP are bound on the cell surface to receptors specific for those substances. This binding results in either activation or inhibition of the enzyme *adenylate cyclase* (or adenyl cyclase), which is responsible for the formation of cAMP from adenosine triphosphate (ATP) (**Part B**). Transfer of the signal from the occupied receptor on the membrane's outer face to adenylate cyclase, located on the cytoplasmic side of the membrane, occurs via guanosine triphosphate–binding proteins [G_s (stimulatory) or G_i (inhibitory) proteins]. Some hormones that activate adenylate cyclase (**Part C**) have a sequence of five amino acids in common, with which they bind to gangliosides on the plasma membrane. This same amino acid sequence is found on the structures of the plant toxins abrin and ricin and on cholera and diphtheria toxins, all of which have gangliosides as their membrane receptors. Peptide hormones that do not activate cAMP may activate other enzymes, such as guanylate cyclase, or regulate the intracellular concentration of Ca^{2+}.

Cyclic AMP is often referred to as the second messenger, with the hormone stimulating its production being the first. It stimulates activation of cAMP-dependent protein kinase, which facilitates phosphorylation of some protein products of the target cell. Phosphodiesterase, which inactivates cAMP to 5′AMP, can be stimulated by insulin (in adipocytes and liver cells). Examples of some biologic effects of cAMP are listed in **Part D.**

Protein kinase A is the enzyme activated intracellularly by cAMP. This enzyme, in turn, is capable of activating a number of other intracellular enzymes by phosphorylating their kinases (see **Part A**), thus leading to a biologic effect specific for the cell type involved. Alternatively, cAMP-stimulated phosphorylation can deactivate other enzymes. Thus, after a hormone binds to its receptor, (e.g., epinephrine binding to β-adrenergic receptors), the cAMP messenger system generates a cascade of effects that ultimately alters the flux of metabolites within the cell. Activation or inactivation of reciprocal pathways within a responsive cell can inhibit metabolite release on the one hand, while stimulating storage on the other.

Cyclic-AMP can also act as a hormone second messenger by altering gene expression. Target DNA molecules are known to possess a **cAMP regulatory element (CRE)** that binds a protein transcription factor known as **cAMP response element binding protein (CREB).** Cyclic-AMP activates protein kinase A; the catalytic subunit of the enzyme is then free to be translocated into the nucleus where it phosphorylates CREB. Phosphorylated CREB now becomes capable of complexing with CRE and another transcription protein, such as activated transcription factor-1. The final result of this rather complex series of reactions is the stimulation or inhibition of RNA polymerase and transcription of the target gene, and hence stimulation or inhibition of synthesis of a specific protein.

The actions of cAMP are terminated when it is hydrolyzed by phosphodiesterase, as discussed above. Because the activity of phosphodiesterase is also modulated by hormones via a G protein, cAMP levels inside cells are under dual regulation. Two hormones can function antagonistically if one stimulates adenyl cyclase and the other stimulates phosphodiesterase (e.g., glucagon and insulin, respectively).

4 Mechanisms of Catecholamine and Polypeptide Hormone Action: II

E

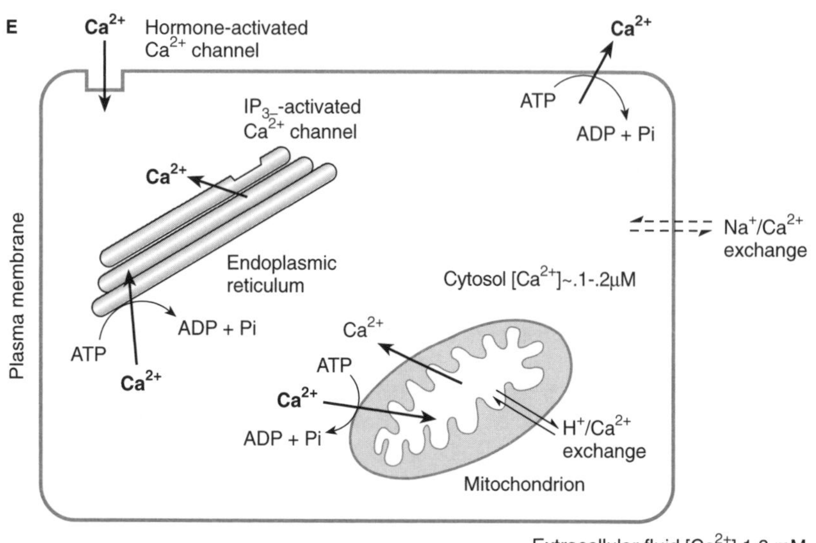

F

Spatial Aspects of Calcium Signaling

Elementary events
- Membrane excitability
- Mitochondrial metabolism
- Vesicle secretion
- Smooth muscle relaxation
- Mitosis

Global events (intracellular)
- Fertilization
- Muscle contraction (smooth, cardiac, and skeletal)
- Liver metabolism
- Gene transcription
- Cell proliferation

Global events (intercellular)
- Wound healing
- Ciliary beating
- Glial cell function
- Insulin secretion
- Bile flow
- Endothelial nitric oxide synthesis (blood vessels)

G

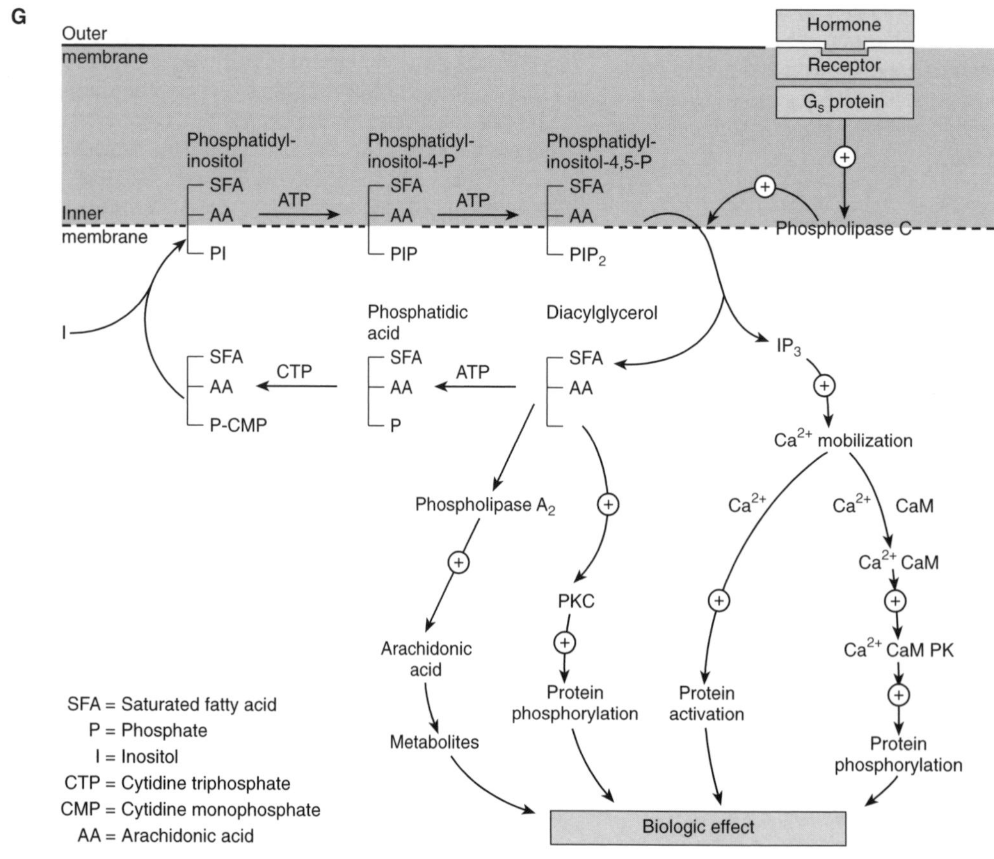

Overview

- The Ca^{2+}/DG second messenger system is a nearly universal means by which extracellular messengers regulate cell function.
- The Ca^{2+}/DG second messenger system is intimately related to both the arachidonic cascade and the cAMP messenger system.
- IP_3 induces Ca^{2+} release from mitochondria and the ER.
- DG activates PKC.
- Calmodulin binds cytoplasmic Ca^{2+}.
- The Ca^{2+}/DG second messenger system is inherently faster than the cAMP system.

The Calcium/Diacylglycerol Messenger System

The intracellular calcium/diacylglycerol (Ca^{2+}/DG) messenger system has a central role in mediating secretion of exocrine, endocrine, and neurocrine products, the metabolic processes of glycogenolysis and gluconeogenesis, the transport and secretion of fluids and electrolytes, the contraction of all forms of smooth muscle, and the birth, growth, and death (apoptosis) of cells (to name a few of its functions). It is a nearly universal means by which extracellular messengers (i.e., neurotransmitters and hormones) regulate cell function, and it is intimately related to both the arachidonic cascade and the cAMP messenger system.

Calcium is derived at the cellular level from both external and internal sources (**Part E**). It can enter from outside the cell by passing through Ca^{2+}-specific channels that span the plasma membrane, or it can be released from internal Ca^{2+} stores in mitochondria and the endoplasmic reticulum (ER) (or sarcoplasmic reticulum; SR). When a Ca^{2+} channel opens, a concentrated plume of Ca^{2+} forms around its mouth, then dissipates rapidly by diffusion after the channel closes. Such localized signals, which can originate from channels in the plasma membrane or on the internal stores, represent the *elementary events* that occur in Ca^{2+} signaling (**Part F**). These elementary signals have two basic functions: they can activate highly localized cellular processes in the immediate vicinity of the channels primarily through enzyme phosphorylation, or, by recruiting channels throughout the cell, they can activate processes at a more global level. In smooth muscle, for example, Ca^{2+} increases that arise locally near the plasma membrane activate potassium (K^+) channels, thus causing muscle to relax. Yet when elementary release events deeper in the cell are coordinated to create a *global Ca^{2+} signal,* the muscle contracts. This is an example of how spatial organization enables Ca^{2+} to activate opposing cellular responses in the same cell. For sites of elementary Ca^{2+} release to produce global responses, individual channels must communicate with each other to set up *Ca^{2+} waves.* If cells are connected, such intracellular waves can spread into neighboring cells and become intercellular waves to cause responses within tissues.

Elementary calcium signaling begins when certain hormones or neurotransmitters interact with their plasma membrane receptors (e.g., catecholamines interacting with α_1-adrenergic receptors, or acetylcholine interacting with muscarinic receptors). Activation of membrane-bound phospholipase C (through G_s protein) then catalyzes hydrolysis of phosphatidylinositol 4,5-bisphosphate (PIP_2) from the plasma membrane to produce DG and inositol triphosphate (IP_3) (**Part G**). Both DG and IP_3 act as intracellular messengers: DG acts as a membrane-associated activator of protein kinase C (PKC), and IP_3 acts as a water-soluble inducer of Ca^{2+} release from mitochondria and the ER, thereby causing a transient rise in the calcium/calmodulin (Ca^{2+}/CaM) concentration of the cytosol. (Calmodulin is a protein that binds Ca^{2+} within the cytosol). These two events initiate further biologic effects specific for the cells in which they occur. The IP_3 and DG may next be converted sequentially into intermediates that can be successively phosphorylated back into phospholipid (i.e., PIP_2) in the plasma membrane. The DG may be converted to phosphatidic acid, which can then enter the rephosphorylation pathway, or its unsaturated fatty acid in the 2 position (most likely arachidonic acid, AA) can be hydrolyzed by phospholipase A_2 and then used in the synthesis of eicosanoids (i.e., prostaglandins, thromboxanes, or leukotrienes). The eicosanoids are also capable of eliciting a biologic effect.

Summary

The cAMP and Ca^{2+}/DG second messenger systems are two major intracellular systems that are closely interwoven and, therefore, difficult to separate. The cAMP nucleotides may exert their effects in concert with or in opposition to those of Ca^{2+}/CaM and DG. Moreover, cAMP- and Ca^{2+}/CaM-dependent protein kinases may act on the same substrate that serves as a common effector of certain cellular processes. In controlling the metabolism and function of cAMP and Ca^{2+}, CaM integrates the two messenger systems on a molecular basis. Because the two systems are intertwined, cAMP may sometimes serve as a second messenger, and Ca^{2+} as the third messenger. At other times these roles may be reversed. Between the two systems, the response of the Ca^{2+} pathway appears to be inherently faster, partly because the availability of Ca^{2+} does not require enzymatic synthesis (as cAMP does). The Ca^{2+} system is also more diversified. Calmodulin is endowed with many receptor enzymes, including several protein kinases with different substrate specificities.

5 Mechanisms of Steroid and Thyroid Hormone Action

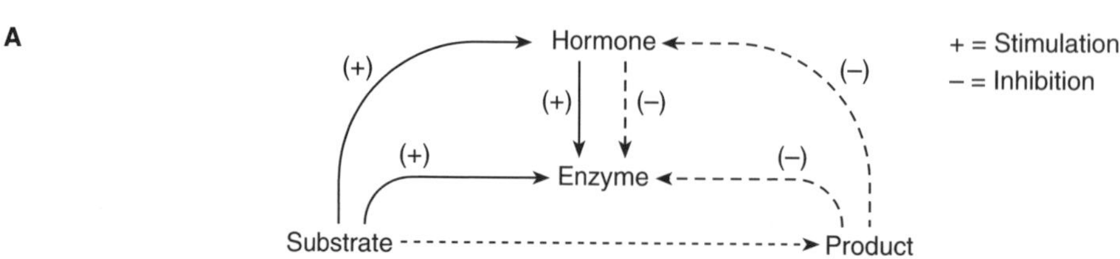

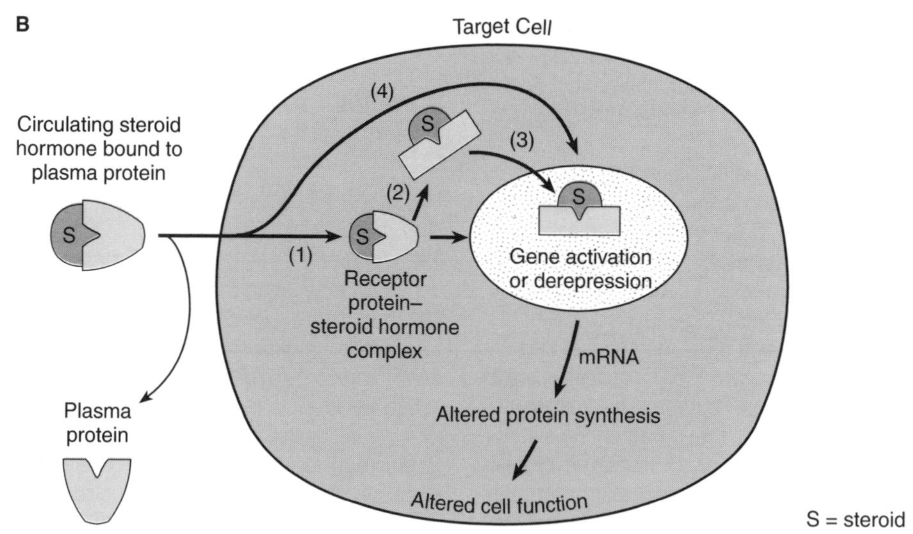

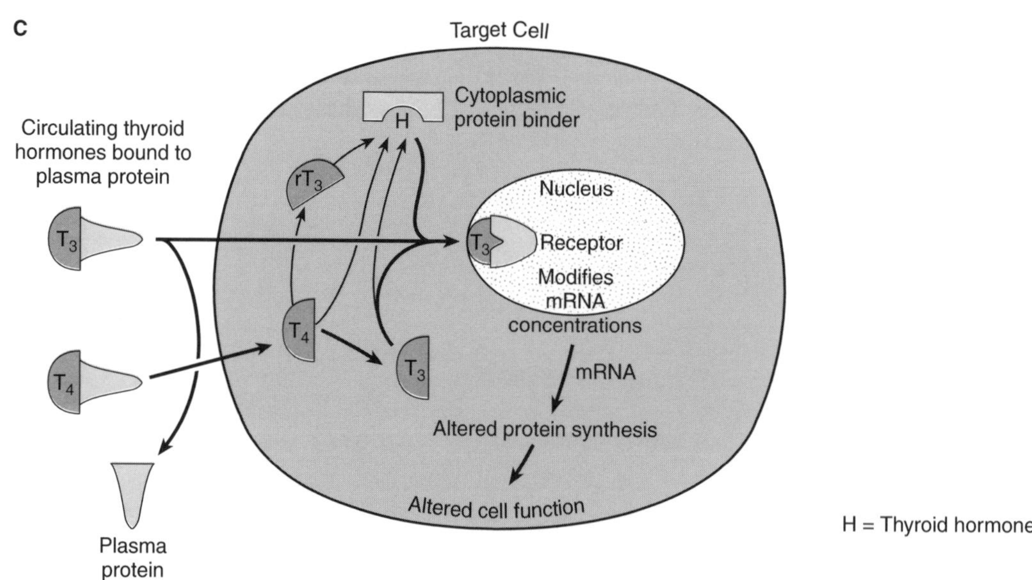

Overview

- Steroid and thyroid hormone receptors are found in the cytoplasm of target cells.
- Steroid and thyroid hormones act by influencing protein synthesis.
- Steroid, thyroid, catecholamine, and/or polypeptide hormones sometimes work synergistically in stimulating the metabolism of specific target cells.
- T_3 is the most metabolically active thyroid hormone.
- Steroid and thyroid hormones regulate about 1% of all genes expressed by responsive cells.
- Hours are generally required for the effects of steroid and thyroid hormones to become evident (compared to seconds to minutes for catecholamine and polypeptide hormones).

Hormones act by either increasing or decreasing protein (namely enzyme) activity and/or synthesis within target cells. Enzymes controlled by hormones are also generally under the influence of substrate induction and/or product negative feedback inhibition. Products produced by target cells can also return to further inhibit hormone secretion (e.g., glucose output by the liver feeds back negatively on glucagon secretion from the pancreas) (**Part A**). Other metabolites within target cells exert influences on the activity of specific enzymes (e.g., citrate inhibition of phosphofructokinase and the resulting anaerobic glycolysis, or second messengers generated in response to the presence of specific hormones on the outer plasma membrane).

Steroid Hormone Action

Unlike catecholamine and polypeptide hormones, steroids, which are lipophilic, are transported in plasma bound to carrier proteins (produced by the liver) and act in their target cells by either increasing or decreasing synthesis of specific proteins (e.g., enzymes). Steroids enter virtually all cells of the body, but they bind only to specific receptor proteins in the cytoplasm and/or nucleus of their target cells (which theoretically changes conformation of the receptor). For example, in the case of glucocorticoids, a receptor protein–steroid complex is first formed in the cytoplasm (process *1* in **Part B**). The receptor changes conformation once the cytoplasmic receptor complex has formed (process *2*). Then the entire complex is translocated into the nucleus (process *3*), where it binds reversibly to DNA. This classic view of the action of steroid hormones has recently been challenged by investigators who argue that, at least in some instances (e.g., sex steroids), the receptors may indeed be in the nucleus rather than in the cytoplasm from the beginning (process *4*), and that cytosolic forms of the receptor may be artifacts of preparation. In any case, the receptor–steroid complex binds to DNA in a region adjacent to a promoter of responsive genes known as the **hormone response element (HRE).** This binding stimulates *gene transcription,* resulting in increased formation of specific protein molecules, most with enzymatic activity.

Hormone receptors located in the target cell cytoplasm are thought, in general, to be inactive by themselves. One mode of inactivation (which is characteristic of adrenal steroid receptors), involves complexing the unoccupied receptor (via its C-terminus domain) with a blocking molecule, such as **heat shock protein.** The steroid hormone is thought to displace the blocking protein when it binds to its receptor, thus permitting the complex to be activated and translocated into the nucleus where it undergoes dimerization, and binds to a specific site on a target DNA molecule (sometimes with the help of another acceptor protein). As stated above, the DNA site, usually only 8 to 15 base pairs long, is known as the HRE. Each half of an HRE site binds one of the two hormone-receptor monomers in the dimeric complex. The HRE is thought to be upstream from the basal promoter site at the 5′ end of the gene. With the gene now fixed to the nuclear matrix, transactivating elements in both the N- and C-terminal domains of the receptor stimulate RNA polymerase activity, and the gene is transcribed. Negative regulatory elements also exist in DNA molecules. Occupancy of a negative regulatory HRE by the hormone-receptor complex suppresses basal rates of transcription. In addition to these direct effects of hormone receptors of the steroid, another mechanism that has been described involves the proto-oncogenes, **cJun** and **cFos.**

It should be noted that in some instances steroid, catecholamine, and/or polypeptide hormones work together, with the steroid increasing synthesis of the enzymes that catecholamine and/or polypeptide hormones activate, thus creating a longer-lasting effect of greater metabolic magnitude. For example, cortisol (a glucocorticoid) increases synthesis of hepatic gluconeogenic enzymes that are stimulated by epinephrine and/or glucagon. This coupling is an example of metabolic (endocrine) *synergism.*

Thyroid Hormone Action

Major effects of thyroid hormones, like those of steroid hormones, are produced via changes in the synthesis and/or activity of regulatory proteins in target cells, including key metabolic enzymes and receptors. Thyroid hormones, also being lipophilic, readily pass into a target cell's cytoplasm and nucleus to bind with receptors in the chromatin. The predominant nuclear receptor for thyroid hormones is specific for triiodothyronine (T_3), the most active form. Following binding, regulation of gene expression occurs with subsequent induction of RNA synthesis (**Part C**).

Most tetraiodothyronine (T_4) presented to its target cell is converted to T_3 (or in some cases reverse T_3 [rT_3], the inactive form) before nuclear binding. The thyroid hormone pool (T_4, T_3, and rT_3) within the cytoplasm of target cells is complexed with cytoplasmic protein binders.

Specific responses to thyroid hormones may be quite individual, and vary between species and tissues. The cell functions affected are often under multihormonal regulation, and therefore the direction metabolic pathways take under thyroid hormone stimulation may depend on the presence or absence of other hormones. In general, thyroid hormones (i.e., T_4 and T_3) increase the metabolic rate of their target cells by increasing oxygen consumption.

Binding sites for T_3 have also been identified on mitochondria and on the plasma membranes of erythrocytes, thymocytes, placenta, carcinoma cells, and several cell lines. After binding, T_3 is apparently internalized by endocytic vesicles (similar to peptides). The physiologic importance of this binding is not clearly understood, but may be associated with carbohydrate and amino acid uptake.

In summary, steroid and thyroid hormones are thought to regulate about 1% of all genes expressed by responsive cells. The proteins whose synthesis is either increased or decreased by these hormones may be enzymes, structural proteins, receptor proteins, transcriptional proteins that regulate expression of other genes, or proteins that are exported by cells (e.g., liver cells). Through this mode of action the response of metabolic pathways is either retarded or accelerated. Other consequences of steroid and thyroid hormone action include alterations in the processing of the primary RNA product, in the turnover of messenger RNA molecules, or in post-translational modification of proteins. This explains why hours are usually required for the biological effects of these hormones to become evident.

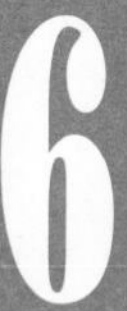

The Hypothalamus and Pituitary

A

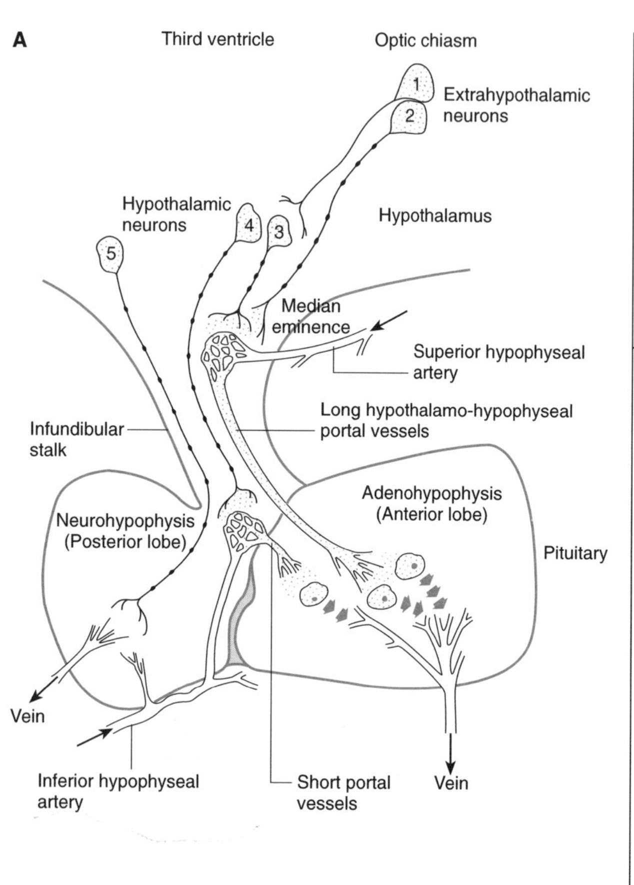

B

Agonist	*GH*	*TSH*	*LH and FSH*	*ACTH*	*PRL*	*α-MSH*
Norepinephrine	+	+	+	–	–	–
Acetylcholine	?	?	+	+	+	?
Dopamine	+	–	+	–	–	–
Serotonin	+	–/+	–	+	+	–
γ-Aminobutyric acid	+	–	+	–	–	?
Endorphin	+	?	–	?	+	?

+ =stimulatory; – = inhibitory

C

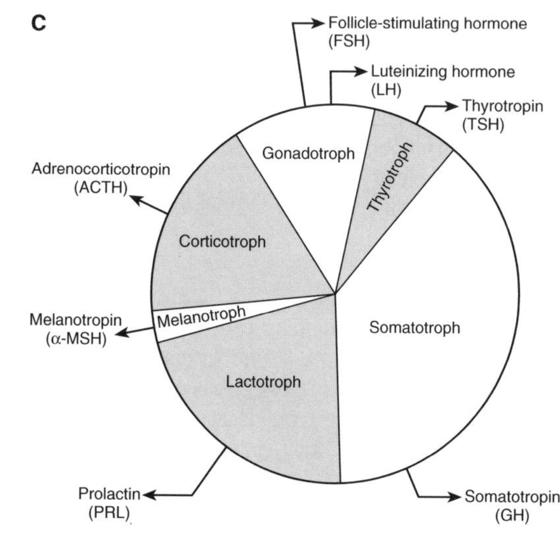

D

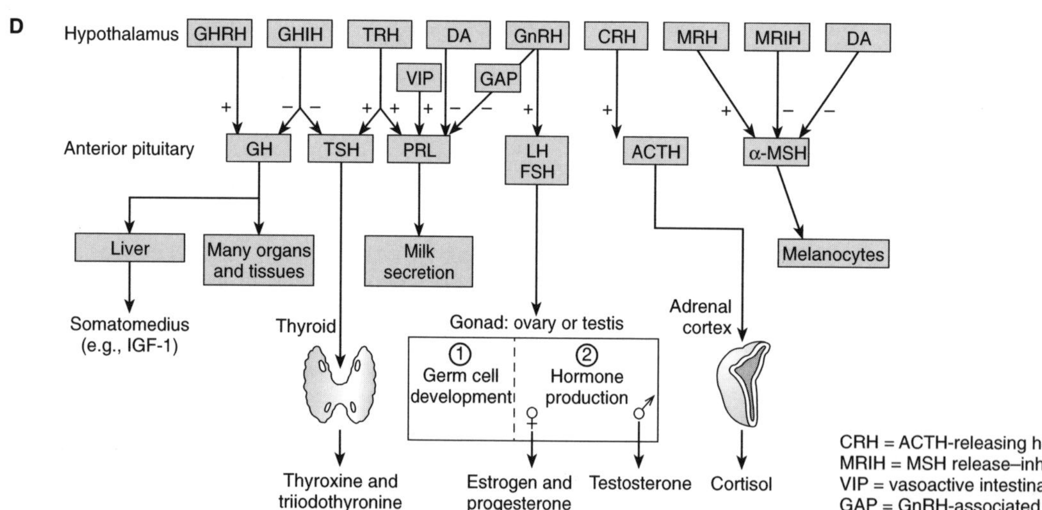

Source: **Part A** modified and redrawn from Gay VL. Fertil Steril 1972; 23:50. **Part C** modified from Berne RM, Levy MN. Principles of Physiology, 1st ed. St Louis: Mosby, 1990:537.

Overview

- The anterior pituitary and the posterior pituitary are anatomically and functionally distinct from each other.
- The hypothalamus controls the activity of the pituitary gland.
- The pituitary directs the endocrine orchestra.
- The hypothalamo-hypophyseal portal system carries release and inhibiting factors from the hypothalamus to the anterior pituitary.

Removal of the canine pituitary (*hypophysectomy*) was proven to be nonfatal earlier this century. Nonetheless, the pituitary gland (particularly the anterior lobe) has proved to be important in regulating secretory activity of other endocrine glands (with the notable exceptions of the pancreas and parathyroids). Only the outermost portion of the adrenal gland (i.e., the cortex) can match the complexity of the pituitary in the number of hormones produced. The primary difference between the two is that the adrenal cortex secretes closely related steroid hormones, whereas the pituitary secretes numerous polypeptide hormones, many being quite different in chemical structure and size. These vary from *octapeptides,* which are produced by the *neurohypophysis* (posterior pituitary), to ACTH, which is composed of 39 amino acids and produced by the *adenohypophysis* (anterior pituitary). Other polypeptides are actually larger than ACTH (e.g., GH, TSH, LH, and FSH) and are considered to be true proteins (>50 amino acids).

The pituitary gland is formed by the confluence of two primary embryonic rudiments, one of which originates from an outpouching of neural tissue from the brain's third ventricle (the neurohypophysis), the other from the ectoderm of the oral cavity (the adenohypophysis). The anterior lobe comprises about 80% of pituitary weight in most species. The pituitary stalk extends to the hypothalamus through a dural reflection, and an intermediate lobe located between the anterior and posterior lobes is present in certain species and during fetal development, but is vestigial in primates. Because surrounding structures are vital, expansion of the pituitary gland due to tumor formation can result in superior extension with compression of the optic chiasm and loss of vision.

Anatomic connections between the hypothalamus and pituitary are shown schematically in **Part A.** Note that neurosecretory cells are present in certain *hypothalamic nuclei* (neurons *3, 4, and 5* in **Part A**). Some secretory axons from these nuclei pass down the infundibular stalk and terminate near blood vessels in the neurohypophysis (neurons *4 and 5*), while others terminate near capillary loops of the *median eminence* (neuron *3*). Hormones of the neurohypophysis (ADH and oxytocin) are products of *hypothalamic neurosecretory cells* [supraoptic (neuron 5) and paraventricular (neuron 4) nuclei, respectively] and are stored and released from the pars nervosa. The *hypothalamo-hypophyseal portal system* starts as a primary plexus in the median eminence and conveys blood downward to sinusoids (i.e., capillaries) of the anterior lobe. This anatomical arrangement fits the true classification of a portal system (i.e., one that begins and ends in capillaries). Hypothalamic axons of the median eminence (e.g., neuron *3*) liberate multiple release and/or inhibiting factors (or hormones) into the portal system, and these short neural peptides in turn become involved with regulation of anterior pituitary function (by either stimulating or inhibiting release of anterior pituitary hormones). Although the anterior lobe does not appear to have nerve fibers (unlike the posterior lobe), it does have limited vasoregulatory sympathetic innervation. It is generally believed, however, that there are no direct regulatory nerve fibers to the anterior lobe that involve selective endocrine secretory function.

Part A also depicts a somewhat hypothetical relationship between the hypothalamic area and the pituitary. Both long portal vessels (originating from the superior hypophyseal artery) and short portal vessels (originating from the inferior hypophyseal artery) may provide means for communication between hypothalamic neurons and hormone-secreting cells of the adenohypophysis. Several types of neural stimuli are thought to bring about secretion of releasing hormones:

- Extrahypothalamic neurons (neuron *1*) may stimulate hypothalamic neurons (neuron *3*) to secrete releasing hormones. For example, norepinephrine (from neuron *1*) may stimulate secretion of gonadotropin-releasing hormone (GnRH) from neuron *3.*
- Neurons that have cell bodies located in higher brain centers (neuron *2*) may also secrete releasing hormones. For example, dopamine (DA), secreted from neuron *2* and subsequently entering the hypothalamo-hypophyseal portal system, may inhibit secretion of prolactin (PRL) from the adenohypophysis.
- The pathway depicted by neuron 4 indicates transport of hormones (e.g., oxytocin from paraventricular nuclei) into a capillary bed that drains into the short portal vascular network servicing the periphery of the adenohypophysis. In this way, oxytocin could promote secretion of PRL from the adenohypophysis, for example. Both oxytocin and PRL are needed to initiate and maintain lactation (see Chapters 18 and 19).

In addition, it should be noted that neurotransmitters from higher brain centers (neuron *2*) may also be exerting control over the secretion of pituitary hormones (**Part B**).

Anterior Pituitary Cell Types

The adenohypophysis contains six major *endocrine-secreting cell types,* as well as some *null cells* that have all the cytoplasmic organelles needed for protein hormone synthesis but contain few secretory granules. Their products, if any, have yet to be identified. The six major mammalian endocrine-secreting cell types, their relative proportions, and their major secretory products are depicted in **Part C.** Although they are known to aggregate to some extent, they do not form enclaves but rather are interspersed among each other. They vary somewhat in size and in the characteristics of their secretory granules, but they can be identified with certainty by immunohistochemical staining of the hormones within.

Each anterior pituitary cell is regulated by one or more hypothalamic neurohormones that reach them through the hypothalamo-hypophyseal portal system (**Part D**). Three cell types produce classic tropic hormones that stimulate hormone secretion from the thyroid gland (thyroid-stimulating hormone, TSH), the adrenal cortex (ACTH), or the gonads (follicle-stimulating hormone, FSH, and luteinizing hormone, LH). Growth hormone (GH), melanocyte-stimulating hormone (melanotropin, α-MSH), and PRL are not true tropic hormones because they do not directly stimulate secretion of other hormones (unless one recognizes somatomedin secretion from the liver as such in response to GH). Although α-MSH is found in the adenohypophyses of all vertebrates examined, in some mammalian species (e.g., rat, rabbit, sheep, and cattle) the pars intermedia is a well-defined structure and contains large amounts of α-MSH (hence the other name for α-MSH, intermedin).

7 Proopiomelanocortin and Related Peptides: I

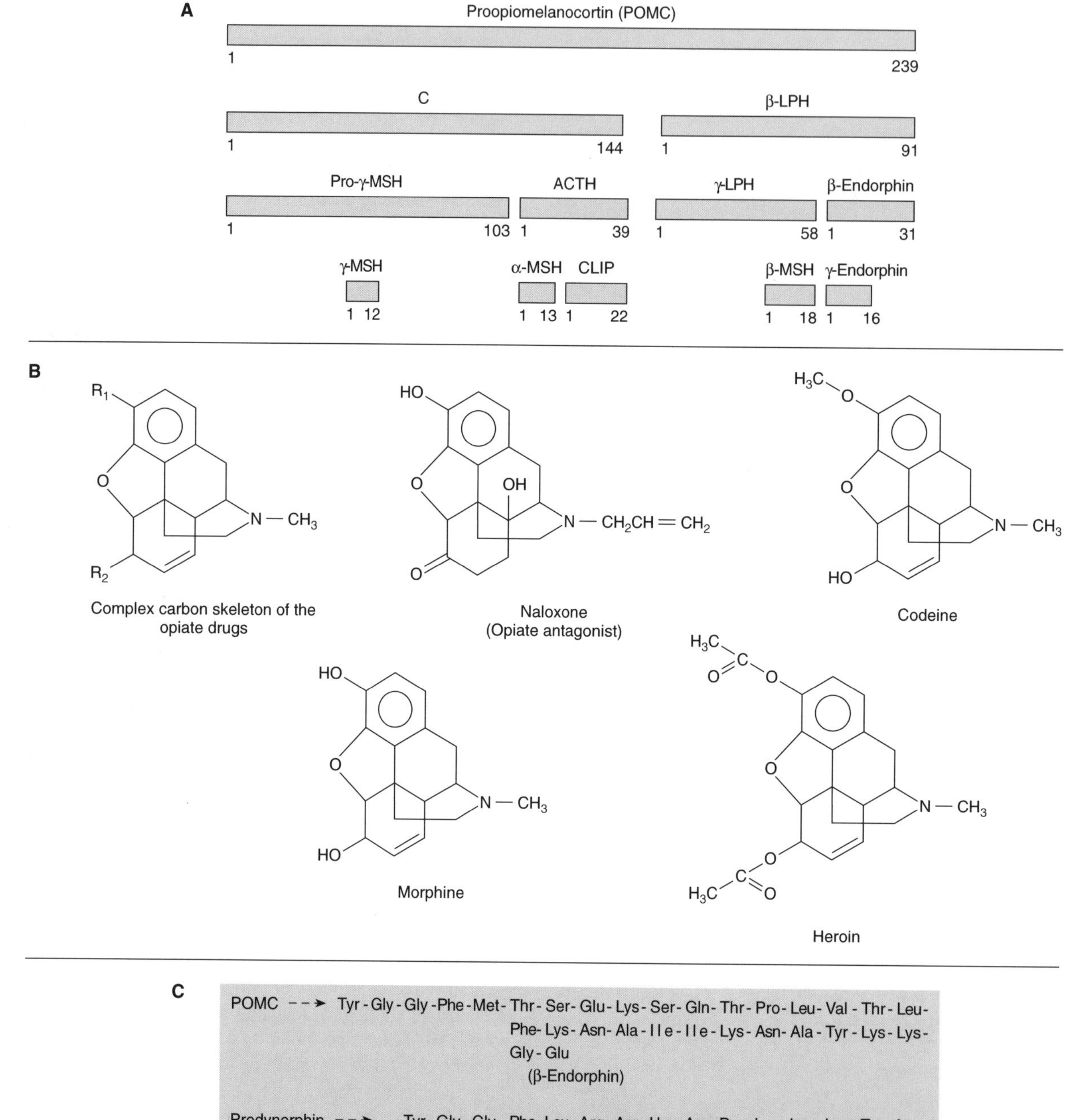

C

POMC ⇢ Tyr-Gly-Gly-Phe-Met-Thr-Ser-Glu-Lys-Ser-Gln-Thr-Pro-Leu-Val-Thr-Leu-Phe-Lys-Asn-Ala-Ile-Ile-Lys-Asn-Ala-Tyr-Lys-Lys-Gly-Glu
(β-Endorphin)

Prodynorphin ⇢ Tyr-Gly-Gly-Phe-Leu-Arg-Arg-Ile-Arg-Pro-Lys-Leu-Lys-Trp-Asp-Asn-Gln
(Dynorphin A)

Proenkephalin ⇢ Tyr-Gly-Gly-Phe-Met (Met-Enkephalin)
⇢ Tyr-Gly-Gly-Phe-Leu (Leu-Enkephalin)

Source: Part A modified from Ganong WF. Review of medical physiology. 17th ed. Stamford, CT: Appleton & Lange, 1995: 368.

Overview

- POMC is the precursor of several important polypeptides.
- Endogenous opiate-like peptides stimulate the same receptors as their exogenous non-peptide cousins (morphine, codeine and heroin).
- Endogenous opiate-like peptides are analgesic.
- Naloxone blocks opiate receptors.
- The opiate peptides are involved with GH, PRL, GnRH (and therefore LH and FSH) release.

A large precursor glycoprotein of 239 amino acid residues and a molecular weight of 31 kd is synthesized by specialized basophils in both the mammalian and the nonmammalian adenohypophysis. This prohormone, known as *proopiomelanocortin (POMC),* is the precursor of several important polypeptides, including ACTH, α-MSH, and the opioid peptide, *β-endorphin* (**Part A**). Polypeptides derived from POMC may themselves be precursors to other substances with important physiologic actions, as they are found in not only the adenohypophysis (pars distalis) but also the pars intermedia (where present) and areas of the CNS where electrical stimulation can relieve pain. The persistence of these peptides following hypophysectomy indicates they are synthesized in the brain.

In basophils of the adenohypophysis, POMC is cleaved to produce ACTH (39 amino acids), an *N*-terminal 103-amino-acid fragment with little known biologic activity (pro-γ-MSH), and a *C*-terminal 91-amino-acid fragment known as β-lipotropin (β-LPH). In turn, β-LPH may be cleaved to a 58-amino-acid fragment known as γ-LPH and the 31-amino-acid fragment, β-endorphin (residues 61–91). In melanotropes of the adenohypophysis and pars intermedia, ACTH is further cleaved to yield α-MSH (residues 1–13 of ACTH) and a 22-amino-acid fragment called *corticotropin-like intermediate peptide* (*CLIP*, residues 18–39), which has little if any biologic activity.

Endogenous Opiate-Like Peptides

Morphine is a nonpeptide exogenous opiate analgesic (pain-killing) drug that binds specific receptors in the CNS (μ, κ, and δ receptors). Three common opiate drugs, *morphine, heroin,* and *codeine,* differ according to the groups attached to their complex carbon skeleton at R_1 and R_2 (**Part B**). The action of morphine is blocked by closely related molecules such as naloxone.

Researchers postulated that there are endogenous compounds that produce analgesic opiate-like properties, and, although their structures may differ from those of morphine, three distinct families of endogenous opiate-like peptides have been identified: *endorphins, dynorphins, and enkephalins.* All three have the same *N*-terminal 4- or 5-amino-acid sequence that allows them to bind the same receptors (**Part C**). Opiate effects of these peptides are also blocked by naloxone, indicating that exogenous opiate drugs and the endogenous opiate-like peptides bind the same μ, κ, and δ receptors. Endorphins arise from POMC, and dynorphins from prodynorphin. Although β-endorphin contains the 5-amino-acid sequence for metenkephalin at its amino terminus, it is **not** converted to this peptide. Instead, enkephalins are derived from proenkephalin (see **Part B**).

Endorphins are found in the pituitary, pancreatic islets, and CNS, with high levels in the arcuate nucleus. Peptides from proenkephalin (meaning "in the head") and prodynorphin are distributed widely throughout the CNS. Although each peptide family is usually located in different groups of neurons, occasionally more than one family is found within the same neuron. Proenkephalin peptides are present in areas of the CNS related to pain perception, modulation of affective behavior (e.g., eating, drinking, and sexual behavior), motor control, and regulation of the ANS and neuroendocrine system (i.e., the median eminence). Peptides from proenkephalin are also found in the adrenal medulla and in nerve plexuses and exocrine glands of the stomach and intestine.

In addition to peptides, it now appears that morphine, codeine, and related compounds might occur naturally in mammalian tissues, as hepatic metabolic pathways that could synthesize these drugs have been described.

The opiate-like peptides are, mole for mole, as potent analgesics as morphine, and β-endorphin is actually five to ten times more potent. Since these compounds do not easily penetrate the blood–brain barrier, their effects in animals have been described only following injection into the CNS. Discovery of these compounds led to a new theory of the mechanism of pain perception in which "nonpain" is perceived as an equilibrium between incoming pain signals, and tonic "antipain" signals generated by mechanisms involving the endogenous opiate-like peptides. It is interesting, for example, that the analgesic, "antipain" effect of acupuncture can apparently be blocked by naloxone.

The opiate-like peptides also modulate secretion of certain pituitary hormones. For example, they are involved with decreasing GnRH output, and therefore with LH and FSH release from the pituitary, yet they facilitate GH and PRL release (probably at the hypothalamic level).

8 Proopiomelanocortin and Related Peptides: II

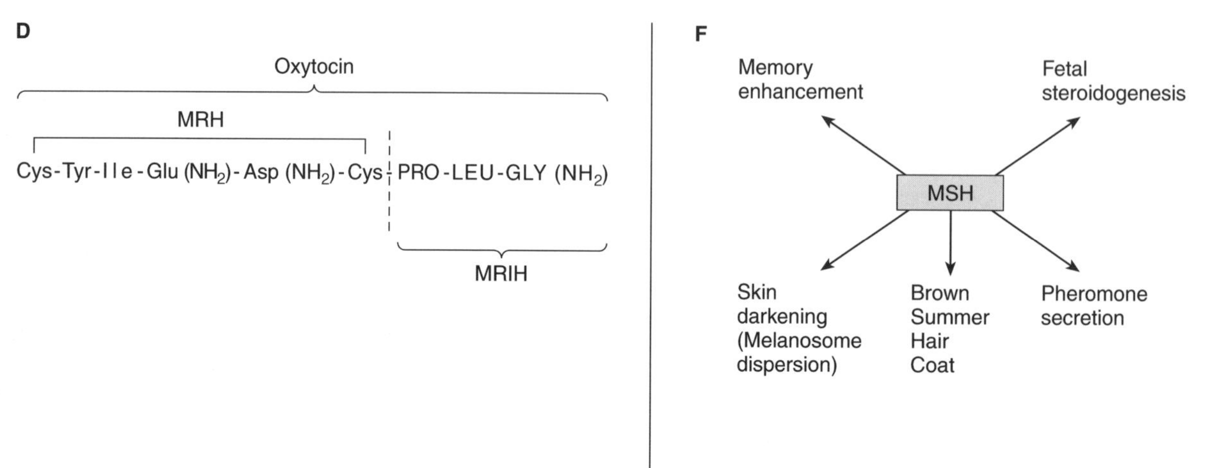

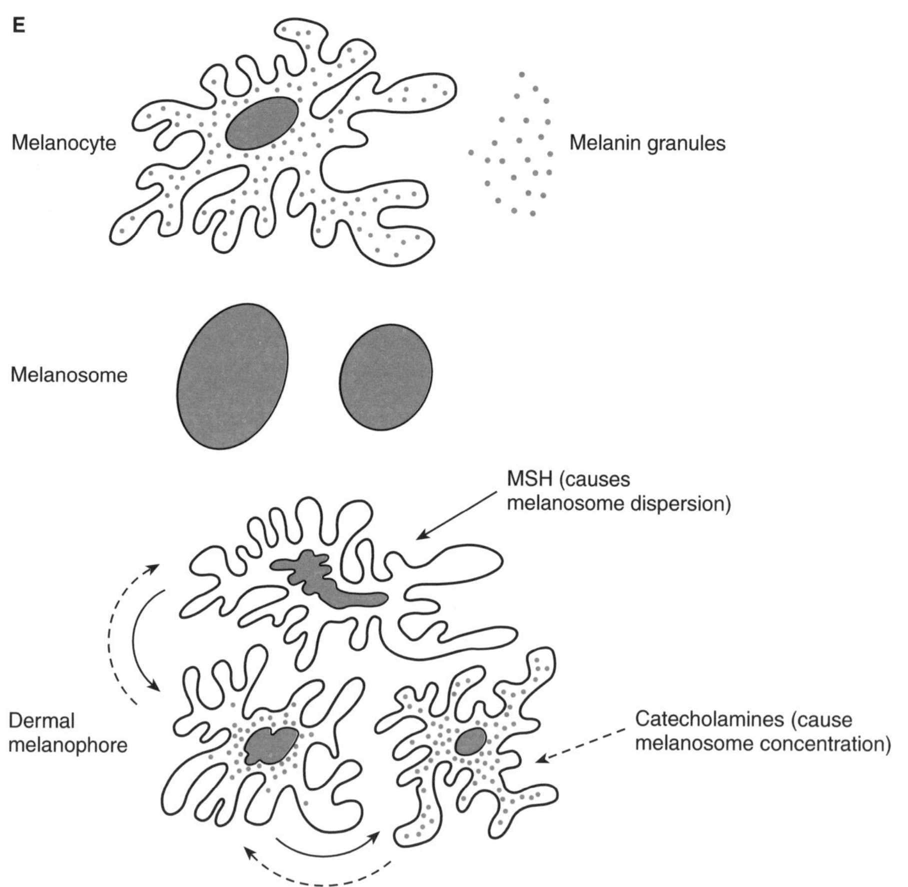

Source: Part E modified from Norris DO: Vertebrate endocrinology. 3rd ed. San Diego, CA: Academic Press, 1997:200.

Overview

- MSH has both a release and a release-inhibiting hormone that controls its secretion.
- All endogenous substances with MSH activity are derived from POMC.
- ACTH shares a common amino acid sequence with α-MSH, and therefore can promote skin darkening.
- Catecholamines cause melanosome concentration (and, therefore, skin pallor), whereas MSH causes melanosome dispersion (and, therefore, skin darkening).
- MSH may have a fetal steroidogenic effect.
- MSH may stimulate sebaceous gland activity.

Melanocyte-Stimulating Hormone

The darkening effect in amphibian skin caused by extracts of the pars intermedia was described *earlier this century,* with the putative causative agent called *intermedin.* Today, this agent is called *melanocyte-stimulating hormone (MSH).* In some mammalian species (rat, rabbit, ox, etc) the pars intermedia is well defined and contains large amounts of α-MSH, but in other mammals (and birds) it is practically vestigial, and so α-MSH is thought to originate from the adenohypophysis.

The release of MSH from the pars intermedia or the anterior pituitary is controlled by *MSH-releasing hormone (MRH), MSH release–inhibiting hormone (MRIH),* and dopamine. The ring structure of oxytocin, which is produced by paraventricular nuclei in the hypothalamus and stored in the neurohypophysis, may be the source of MRH, and the tripeptide side chain the source of MRIH (**Part D**). There does not appear to be any direct feedback effect on MSH release from target tissues. Stimulation of melanocytes by α-MSH does not release any possible feedback candidates into the circulation. Perhaps the strong two- or three-way control of MSH release precludes a biologic requirement for negative feedback.

There are five known substances with MSH activity: α-MSH, β-MSH, γ-MSH, ACTH, and β-LPH. All are derived from POMC. The following *heptapeptide,* which appears in the five substances enumerated above, is apparently responsible for MSH activity: Met-Glu(or Gly)-His-Phe-Arg-Trp-Gly.

While α-MSH is a major peptide in species possessing a distinct pars intermedia, it is found in low levels in the adenohypophysis of other species. β-Melanocyte-stimulating hormone is believed to be an artifactual breakdown product of γ-LPH (see **Part A**). While MSH is approximately 30 times more potent than ACTH as a skin-darkening agent, sufficient amounts of ACTH can account for *hyperpigmentation* (e.g., Cushing's-like and Addison's-like diseases). Whether γ-MSH is physiologically significant is unknown.

At one stage of evolution, MSH apparently mediated a protective adaptation (i.e., camouflage in the dark). The major bioassay for MSH, which is capable of detecting MSH with great precision over a range of 20 to 50 pg, is based on the darkening of amphibian skin under standardized conditions.

Vertebrates possess a variety of specialized, pigmented cells known as *chromatophores,* with the *dermal melanophore* being perhaps the most important. Melanin granules are concentrated in special organelles of the melanophore called *melanosomes* (**Part E**). Melanophores differ from *melanocytes,* which deposit their melanin products extracellularly. When melanosomes are concentrated around the nucleus of the melanophore, the skin appears lighter than when they are dispersed throughout the cytoplasm. **The degree of concentration of melanosomes is inversely related to the darkness of the skin.** Coloration patterns in some vertebrates may be determined by the distribution of different types of chromatophores and by the relationship of dermal melanophores to other chromatophores. The major target of MSH is the dermal melanophore, and in a few cases other chromatophores may be affected. MSH causes melanosome dispersion, while catecholamines and melatonin cause skin pallor (melanosome concentration).

Since MSH plays only a minor camouflage role in mammals, it is possible that this highly conserved peptide was put to different uses as the evolutionary process continued. Animals that change from a white "winter coat" to a brown "summer coat" employ the services of MSH to stimulate melanin production for the summer coat (**Part F**). Hypophysectomy of the short-tailed weasel during the winter causes the summer coat to be white, and treatment with either MSH or ACTH is sufficient to cause regrowth of the normal brown summer coat. It has been postulated that, in hairy mammals, MSH may stimulate modified sebaceous gland activity containing pheromones (i.e., sexual attractants secreted to the outside of the body). This function may be important in species that rely heavily on olfaction when participating in reproductive activities.

The prominence of a pars intermedia in the primate fetus, coupled with the observation that the *N*-terminal pro-MSH peptide stimulates release of glucocorticoids and aldosterone, indicates to some that the hormone may have a *fetal steroidogenic effect.* Finally, MSH, which is distributed in the brain, has figured prominently in studies on the enhancement of memory.

The physiologic roles of α-MSH are not known in fishes, where most pigmentary changes apparently are under ANS control. In birds, the fact that feather pigments (including melanin) are under the control of gonadal, thyroidal, and gonadotropic hormones seems to be related to the loss of the pars intermedia. Black feathers, however, reportedly develop in birds treated with either MSH or ACTH.

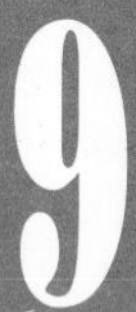

9 Growth Hormone: I

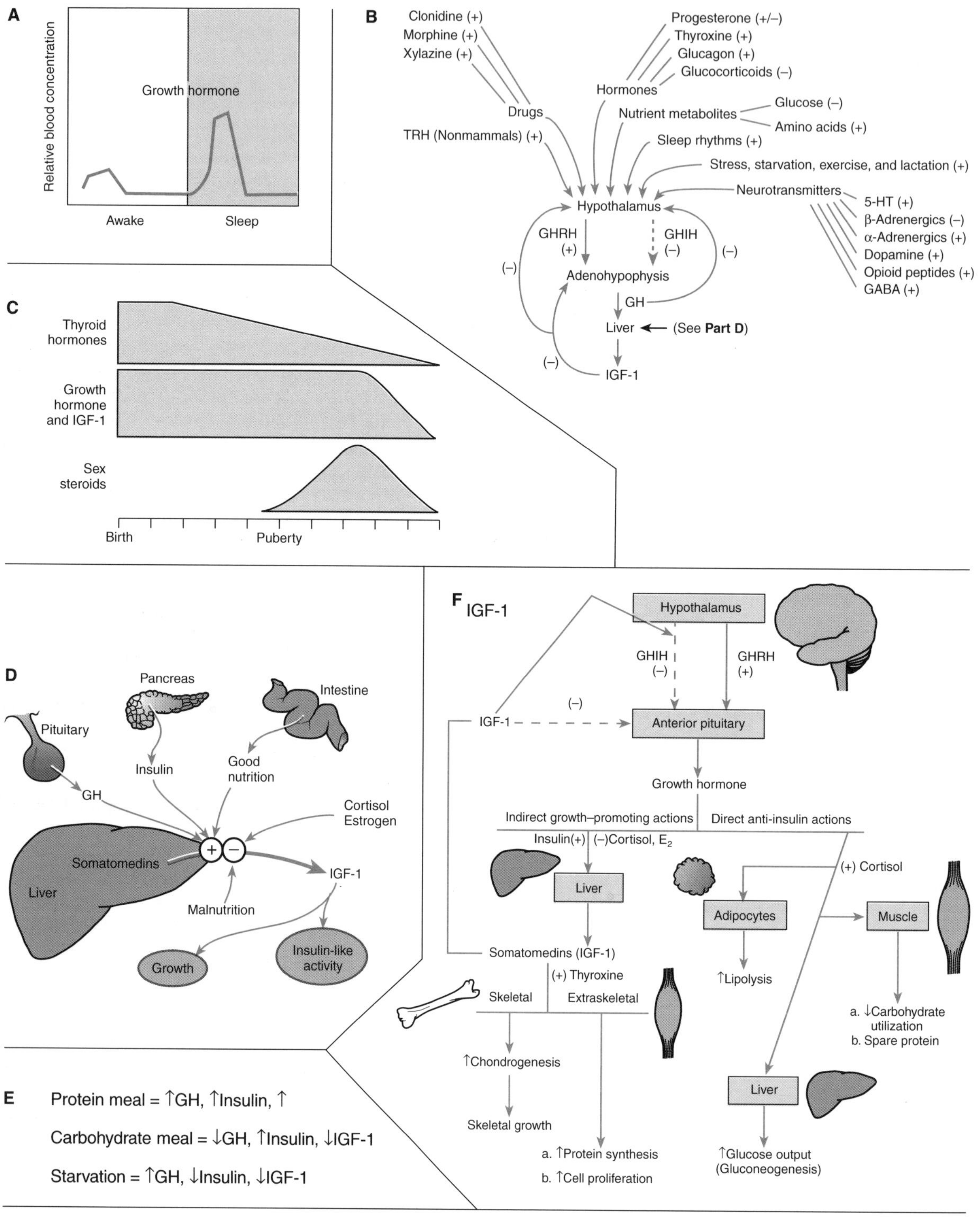

E

Protein meal = ↑GH, ↑Insulin, ↑

Carbohydrate meal = ↓GH, ↑Insulin, ↓IGF-1

Starvation = ↑GH, ↓Insulin, ↓IGF-1

Source: Part C modified from Ganong WF. Review of medical physiology. 18th ed. Stamford, CT: Appleton & Lange, 1997: 382.

Overview

- GH is related structurally and functionally to both PRL and PL.
- GH has both anabolic and catabolic properties.
- The anabolic properties of GH are exerted indirectly through the action of somatomedins.
- GH exerts its catabolic action by virtue of its direct anti-insulin activity.

Produced by somatotropes of the adenohypophysis (see Chapter 6), *growth hormone (GH)* is a protein hormone of 191 amino acids, with two to four disulfide bridges. Its structure, which is similar to that of prolactin and placental lactogen, varies enough among different animal species that GH from one species may not have GH-like effects in another. The primary physiologic actions of GH are promoting growth in young, well-fed animals and providing a ready source of energy (e.g., glucose and long-chain fatty acids) during starvation. Its indirect *anabolic actions* are mediated via other polypeptides known as *somatomedins* (namely insulin-like growth factor 1, IGF-1), whereas the anti-insulin, *catabolic actions* of GH are a result of its direct effects on target cells. The somatomedins were so named because they mediate the anabolic actions of somatotropin (GH).

Control of GH Secretion

Growth hormone is secreted from the adenohypophysis in a pulsatile fashion that is regulated by a hypothalamic *GH-releasing hormone (GHRH or somatocrinin)* and a hypothalamic *GH release–inhibiting hormone (GHIH or somatostatin).* Somatostatin is distributed throughout the nervous system and is also found in extraneural tissues of the stomach, pancreas, and intestine. These two hypothalamic peptides act together to precisely regulate GH secretion during fetal, adolescent, and adult life. At the onset of puberty, secretion continues at levels that are not dissimilar from those recorded before puberty.

Approximately one-half of GH secretion occurs during deep sleep (**Part A**), with timing during the day and night hours shifted accordingly in nocturnal animals. The episodic pattern of GH release is important in modulating its metabolic actions, because the nearly complete absence of GH effects during trough periods is vital in maintaining its anabolic versus its catabolic actions on peripheral tissues. The plasma half-life of GH is about 20 minutes, and it is cleared from the circulation by the liver and kidney.

Factors known to stimulate GHRH and therefore GH secretion include various neurotransmitters and drugs; the hormones progesterone (in dogs), glucagon, and thyroxine; stress; exercise; lactation; sleep rhythms; certain amino acids (e.g., arginine); and thyrotropin-releasing hormone (TRH; in nonmammals). Factors associated with a decrease in GH output include hypothalamic β-adrenergics, glucose, cortisol, synthetic progestins (in primates), and GH and IGF-1 (negative feedback). **Part B** shows both stimulatory and inhibitory factors involved in GH secretion.

Differences regarding the effects of the various stimuli above have been reported to exist between species. For example, stress, which is associated with elevating glucocorticoid levels, generally increases GH secretion in primates, inhibits GH secretion in rodents, and has no effect in domestic ungulates (hoofed mammals). Starvation and lactation increase GH output in primates and domestic ungulates, whereas moderate exercise, amino acids (e.g., arginine), and hypoglycemia give inconsistent results in dogs. Synthetic progestins such as megestrol acetate stimulate GH output in dogs, yet decrease it in primates. Megestrol acetate does not affect GH output in cats, but continued use may lead to diabetes mellitus because of its glucocorticoid activity.

Indirect Growth-Promoting Effects

During fetal and adolescent life, thyroxine, GH, and the somatomedins exert profound synergistic effects on growth and development (**Part C**). Insulin-like growth factor 2 (IGF-2) may be the most important fetal somatomedin, with IGF-1 assuming this role after birth. Animals with hyposomatotropism are born as *pituitary dwarfs,* while those with inadequate fetal thyroxine are born as *cretins.* Pituitary dwarfism is usually recognizable in dogs 2 to 3 months following birth. After the onset of puberty, the sex steroids (androgens and estrogens, which are secreted in low amounts throughout adolescence) assume a larger role in modulating growth and development than does thyroxine. Although sex steroids initially stimulate pubertal growth, they ultimately terminate it by causing the epiphyses to fuse to the long bones, thus stopping linear body growth.

Secretion of IGF-1 (also known as somatomedin C) from the liver of young animals is increased by good nutrition, GH, and insulin (**Part D**). The IGF-1 peptide structurally resembles proinsulin and binds to both insulin and IGF-1 receptors. Interestingly, mean IGF-1 (but not GH) concentrations in dogs are reported to vary according to breed, with smaller breeds having lower concentrations of IGF-1 than larger breeds. **A close correlation exists between body size and IGF-1 levels.** Factors inhibiting release of IGF-1 include the steroid hormones cortisol and estrogen, as well as malnutrition (see **Part D**). In animals fed a protein meal (e.g., felines), blood levels of GH, insulin, and IGF-1 all rise (**Part E**). In animals fed a carbohydrate meal only, GH and IGF-1 levels fall, yet insulin levels rise. During starvation, GH levels rise, yet insulin and IGF-1 levels fall.

The growth-promoting actions of GH (mediated through the somatomedins) include enhanced amino acid entry into cells, enhanced Ca^{2+} absorption from the intestinal tract, K^+, Ca^{2+}, and PO_4^{3-} retention by tissues, proliferation of lymphoid tissue, enhanced skeletal growth, and generalized extraskeletal cell proliferation (**Part F**). All of these anabolic effects are enhanced by the concurrent presence of thyroid hormones (T_4 and T_3). As chondrogenesis is stimulated, the cartilaginous epiphyseal plates widen and lay down more bone matrix at the ends of long bones. In this manner stature is increased. Hypersecretion or prolonged treatment with synthetic GH in adolescent animals leads to *gigantism* (see Chapter 10).

Direct Catabolic Effects

The direct anti-insulin actions of GH are manifested primarily through carbohydrate and lipid metabolism and through interference with insulin's action on peripheral tissues. Cortisol and GH (in the absence of insulin) directly stimulate hepatic gluconeogenesis, lipolysis (via activation of hormone-sensitive lipase in adipocytes), and decreased carbohydrate utilization by muscle tissue (see **Part F**). They also spare breakdown of muscle protein (while encouraging muscle to extract free fatty acids from the circulation for metabolic purposes). Direct catabolic actions of GH are most profound during starvation (or hibernation, when insulin levels are low). In abnormal situations, the net effect (if GH levels remain high) could be hyperglycemia, ketonemia, and insulin antagonism. Diabetes mellitus may develop following prolonged increases in serum GH levels in adult animals (e.g., acromegaly or over-use of GH obtained from recombinant DNA technology).

10 Growth Hormone: II

G

Signs of Hyposomatotropism

Small (proportional) stature
Soft puppy haircoat
Symmertric alopecia
Hyperpigmentation
Aggression (e.g., fear biting)
Delayed dental eruption
Short mandible
Suppressed immune responses
Cardiac disorders
Cryptorchidism
Megaesophagus
Testicular atrophy
Estrual abnormalities
Delayed epiphyseal closure
Normal to subnormal mentality

H

Signs of Hypersomatotropism

Exercise intolerant
Enlargement of:
- Pharyngeal and laryngeal soft tissues
- Head
- Extremities
- Viscera (cardiomyopathy)

Hyperglycemia
Hypercholesterolemia
Myxedema and excessive skin folds
Broad face
Prominent jowls
Increased interdental spaces
Rapid toenail growth
PU/PD
Diabetes mellitus (secondary)
Cardiomyopathy/congestive heart failure

I

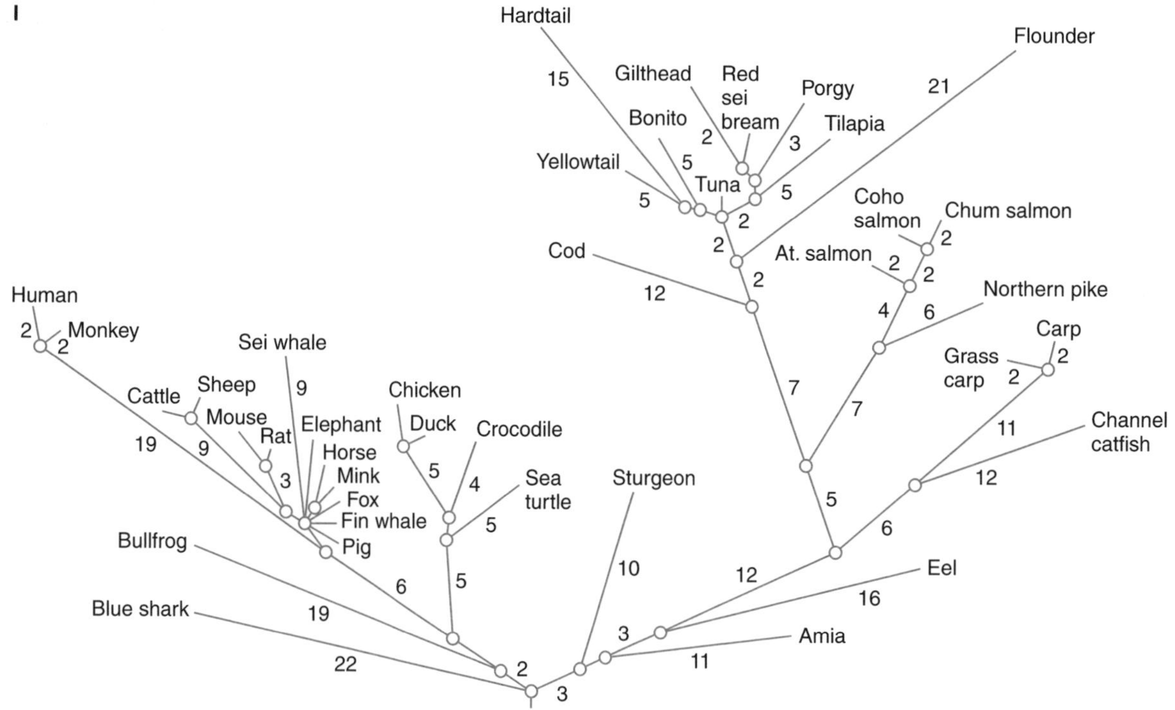

Source: **Part I** modified from Noso T, Lance VA, Kawauchi H. Complete amino acid sequence of crocodile growth hormone. Gen Comp Endocrinol 1995;98:244–252.

Overview

- Pituitary dwarfism is largely a result of hyposomatotropism.
- Excess GH causes gigantism, acromegaly, and sometimes diabetes mellitus.
- Synthetic human GH (hGH) is used to treat hyposomatotropism in dogs.
- Recombinant bovine somatotropin (rbST) increases milk production in dairy cows.

Various abnormalities are associated with small stature in domestic animals. These include malnutrition and gastrointestinal disease, portosystemic shunt, glycogen storage disease, renal and cardiovascular abnormalities, hydrocephalus, skeletal dysplasia, hypothyroidism, hypo- or hyperadrenocorticism, diabetes mellitus, and hyposomatotropism. This discussion will be limited to the pathophysiologic effects of *hyposomatotropism* and *hypersomatotropism.*

Pituitary Dwarfism

Pituitary dwarfism is largely a result of hyposomatotropism, and may be an inherited condition in some dogs and cats. Additional deficiencies in other adenohypophyseal hormones may lead to various degrees of secondary hypogonadism, hypoadrenocorticism, and hypothyroidism (which also limit growth). The most commonly reported cause of pituitary dwarfism in prepubertal dogs is a *cystic Rathke's pouch,* a condition first reported in Germany around 1940. Most domestic animals with primary hyposomatotropism are reportedly detected by 2 to 3 months of age, and are found to grow slowly with near-normal body proportions.

Insensitivity to GH, as seen in the pygmies of Central Africa, may also cause pituitary dwarfism. Circulating levels of GH are apparently increased; however, IGF-1 levels are deficient. This disorder is reportedly associated with absent or defective GH receptors. Insensitivity to GH may also arise from abnormalities in GH structure or lack of responsiveness to IGF-1. Although these secondary causes of pituitary dwarfism may well exist in domestic animals, they have yet to be convincingly described. All cases of pituitary dwarfism described in dogs show low to undetectable GH and IGF-1 concentrations.

Part G lists several abnormalities associated with pituitary dwarfism. Significant growth takes place only if treatment with GH occurs before epiphyseal closure. Otherwise, response to therapy is limited. The long-term prognosis for pituitary dwarfism is poor in domestic animals.

Acquired Hyposomatotropism

Hyposomatotropism may also develop in the adult dog or cat following destruction of the pituitary by inflammatory, traumatic, vascular, or neoplastic conditions. *Panhypopituitarism,* a deficiency of all pituitary hormones, may also occur.

Because glucocorticoids suppress GH secretion, prolonged or excessive administration of glucocorticoids, or Cushing's-like syndrome, may cause hyposomatotropism. Signs of acquired hyposomatotropism in dogs include alopecia and hyperpigmentation (i.e., adult-onset, GH-responsive dermatosis).

Gigantism and Acromegaly (Hypersomatotropism)

Excess GH causes *gigantism* if it is present before the epiphyses of the long bones close at puberty. *Acromegaly* is caused by high circulating titers of GH in the adult, and is commonly associated with pituitary adenoma in older cats, excessive exogenous or endogenous progesterone in female dogs, and GH-induced diabetes mellitus (DM).

Saucerotte first described acromegaly in 1772 as a condition where patients exhibited excessive growth and where body proportions became distorted because linear growth had ceased and could not be reinitiated. Cartilage tends to proliferate in the joints of patients with acromegaly, resulting in abnormally proportioned extremities and an elongated jaw.

Cats reportedly manifest hypersomatotropism and acromegaly at 8 to 14 years of age and exhibit many of the signs listed in **Part H.** Polyuria and polydipsia (PU/PD) may result from renal hypertrophy or glucouria (i.e., GH-induced DM). Acromegaly in dogs reportedly develops following prolonged administration of progestins for estrus suppression (megestrol or medroxyprogesterone acetate), which may cause hypertrophy and hyperplasia of pituitary somatotrophs. This condition may also evolve in untreated dogs during the diestrual phase of the estrous cycle, particularly in intact, older bitches. Pregnancy, which is also associated with prolonged, elevated progesterone levels, is not associated with hypersomatotropism, and progesterone-induced acromegaly has not been described in cats. Progesterone-induced acromegaly has also been associated with the development of canine mammary tumors.

Since GH is a strong *diabetogenic hormone,* promoting hepatic gluconeogenesis and insulin resistance in peripheral tissues, patients with gigantism or acromegaly are susceptible to GH-induced DM.

Synthetic GH

Mammalian nonprimate GH, previously used to treat dwarfism in young animals and acquired hyposomatotropism in adult dogs and cats, has been replaced by synthetic *human GH (hGH)* manufactured by recombinant DNA technology. Human GH is similar to mammalian nonprimate GH immunologically, and it appears to be active in the dog and possibly the cat. *Recombinant bovine somatotropin (bST or rbST)* also appears to be biologically active in dogs.

Recombinant bovine somatotropin has made possible the manipulation of bovine lactational physiology. It appears that bST (working through IGF-1) can increase milk production in dairy cows by 5% to 25% after the first two to three months of lactation, with feed efficiency increasing from 5% to 15%. Given daily injections of bST (or use of sustained-release preparations), this increased yield has been reported to persist throughout the remainder of lactation. An increase in the average number of services (from about 2.0 to 2.5), however, is required to achieve conception, which causes cows to remain open (unbred) for about 21 days longer. Growth hormone, IGF-1, PTH-related peptide (PTH_{rp}), and PRL have all been detected in milk.

The Phylogenetic Tree of Somatotropin

Soon after GH release was demonstrated in goldfish following intraperitoneal injection of synthetic human GHRH (hGHRH), immunologically and chromatographically similar molecules were isolated from several different animal species. **Part I** relates the scheme of GH molecules from different animal species on the basis of their amino acid composition. Numbers indicate the inferred number of amino acid changes per 100 aligned residues that characterize each branch of this phylogenetic tree.

Species variation in GH structure implies that its physiologic actions may not be transferable across some species. For example, porcine and primate GHs have only transient effects in the guinea pig, probably due to rapid anti-GH antibody formation, and bovine and porcine GHs are thought to have insignificant growth effects in primates.

11 Gonadotropins: I

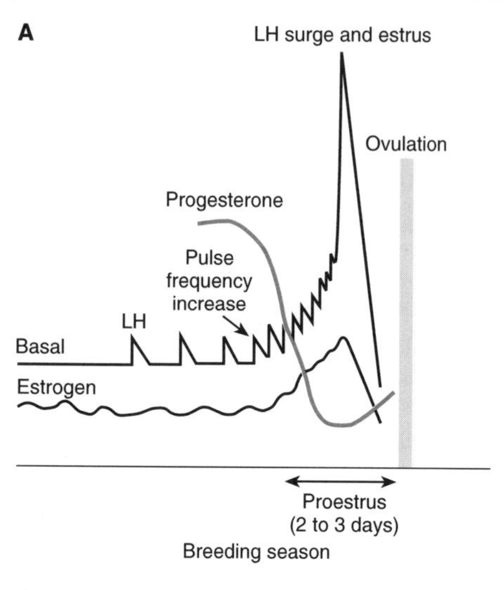

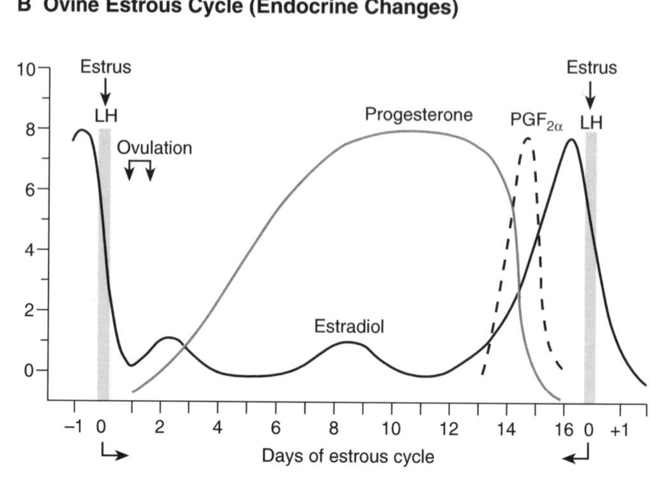

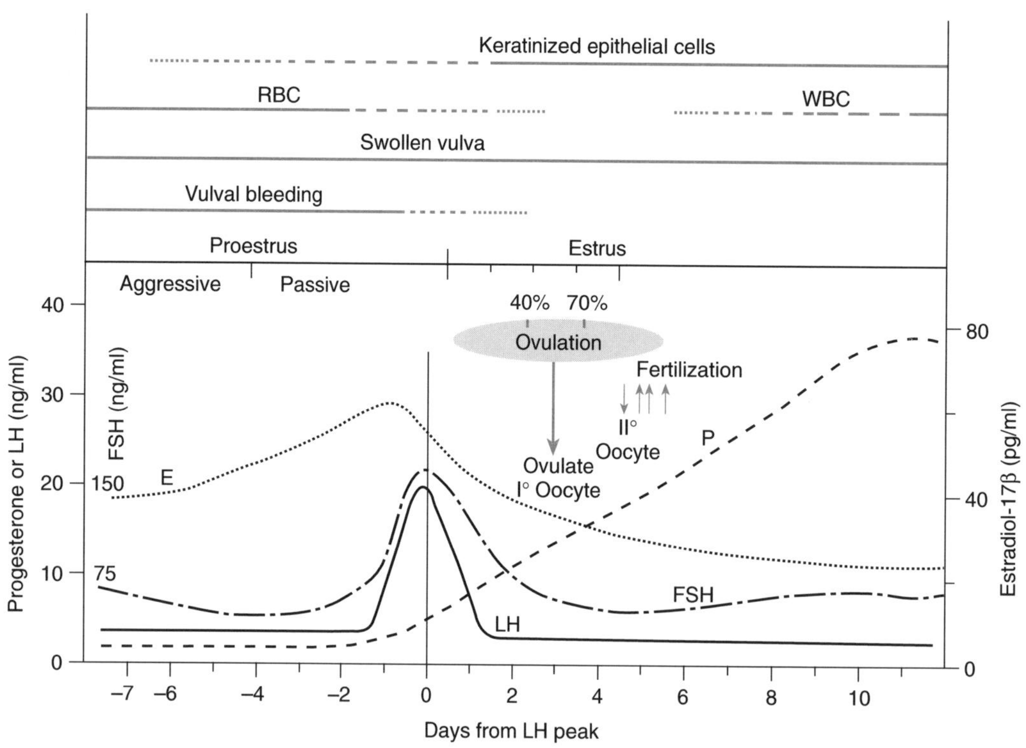

Source: Part B modified from Caldwell BV, Tillson SA, Brock WA, Speroff L. The effects of exogenous progesterone and estradiol on prostaglandin F levels in ovariectomized ewes. Prostaglandins 1972;1:217. **Part C** modified from McDonald LE. Veterinary endocrinology and reproduction. 4th ed. Philadelphia: Lea & Febiger, 1989:465.

Overview

- The pattern of gonadotropin release from the anterior pituitary takes three forms—basal, pulses, and surges.
- Progesterone inhibits gonadotropin release.
- $PGF_{2\alpha}$ causes CL regression in the ewe but perhaps not in the bitch.
- Ovulation occurs after behavioral estrus in the ewe.
- Most bitches ovulate during estrus.

Two hormones from the adenohypophysis that most affect the gonads of mammals are the gonadotropins *luteinizing hormone (LH)*, sometimes called *interstitial cell-stimulating hormone (ICSH)* in males, and *follicle-stimulating hormone (FSH)*. *Prolactin* exerts luteotropic effects in certain species, including the mouse, rat, and ferret.

Mammalian ovaries are dependent on FSH for follicular growth and maturation, and on LH for estrogen synthesis, ovulation, and initial growth of the corpus luteum (CL). Both gonadotropins are continuously synthesized and stored in the pituitary, from which they are released throughout the estrous cycle. The pattern of their release takes three forms: basal, pulses, and surges (**Part A**). *Basal* release refers to low and relatively constant concentrations of gonadotropins in blood; *pulses* are sharp, increased concentrations above basal levels; and a *surge* is a large increase in concentration significantly above basal levels lasting for more than one hour (see Chapter 12). The LH surge is associated with estrus (i.e., mating) behavior, with ovulation generally occurring a few hours later.

Examination of the ovine estrous cycle (**Part B**) shows the following:

1. The CL is the main source of progesterone. Blood levels of progesterone are low during estrus, then increase rapidly from day 2 following estrus. High levels of progesterone from the CL inhibit gonadotropin release.
2. If embryos are not present in the uterus, progesterone levels decline rapidly due to prostaglandin (PG)$F_{2\alpha}$-induced CL regression about two weeks following estrus.
3. As progesterone declines, estrogen increases due to FSH-stimulated follicular growth and maturation.
4. Estrogen peaks on day 16, followed by an LH surge 12 hours later. Behavioral estrus begins.
5. Ovulation occurs 10 hours after the end of estrus.
6. The CL develops and progesterone rises.

Although hormonal patterns during the estrous cycle may differ somewhat between animal species, those occurring in the ewe are not atypical.

During the nonbreeding season, the ovaries of the ewe undergo some follicular development, but ovulation does not occur and the ewe does not express behavioral estrus. However, as the breeding season approaches, gonadotropic hormones stimulate ovarian follicles to mature, secrete estrogen, and ovulate (**Part A**). Estrogen secreted by maturing follicles also stimulates changes in the oviducts, uterus, and vagina that help prepare them for copulation and pregnancy.

Although spermatozoa are thought to survive within the reproductive tract of the ewe for about 48 hours, the fertilizable life of the ovulated ewe oocyte is considered to be only about 10–12 hours. However, ovulation in ewes usually occurs at the end of estrus and matings are most likely to occur during estrus.

Comparative examination of the canine estrous cycle (**Part C**) reveals the following:

1. As preovulatory blood levels of estrogen increase, the bitch develops a few external signs associated with estrogenic stimulation, such as edema of the vulva, bloody discharge, and increased receptivity to the male. Red blood cells and cornified epithelial cells appear in vaginal smears early in proestrus. Toward the end of estrus, a few white blood cells appear.
2. Near the end of proestrus, increasing blood levels of LH stimulate follicular luteinization, as in the ewe, which results in increasing blood levels of progesterone.
3. About 40% of bitches spontaneously ovulate within two days, and 70% within three days, following the onset of estrus.
4. The bitch, unlike farm animals, continues to accept the male for mating several days after ovulation.
5. Estrogen waves are not seen in the bitch during the luteal phase as are seen in the ewe.
6. Corpora lutea continue to survive and secrete progesterone for 50 to 70 days from ovulation in the bitch, whether she is pregnant or not. Luteotropic factors during nonpregnancy, such as $PGF_{2\alpha}$ in the ewe, may be lacking in the bitch, or she may be highly resistant. Unlike the ewe, corpora lutea regression in the bitch appears to be due to aging.

Each oocyte is released from the follicle of the bitch before completion of meiosis. However, completion is thought to occur during oviductal transport with oocytes remaining viable for several days following ovulation. Pregnancy and conception rates are not reported to be different when bitches are mated only once, either on the 1st or 7th day following the onset of estrus. Canine spermatozoa are also thought to retain their viability for over 1 week within the genital tract of the bitch.

12 Gonadotropins: II

D Timing of Human Menstrual Cycle Versus Porcine Estrous Cycle

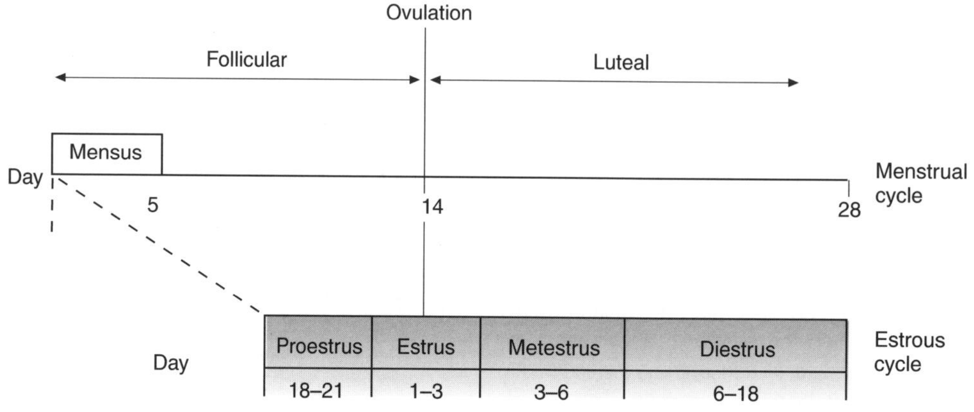

E

END
5-HT
ACh
GABA
?
NE
DA
(–)
(+)
GnRH
Preoptic area
Hypothalamus
Hypothalamo-hypophyseal portal system
GnRH
Gonadotropes
Anterior pituitary
Estrogen positive feedback leads to LH surge
Progesterone negative feedback inhibits further gonadotropin secretion
Activin
Inhibin
FSH
LH
Ovaries
Estrogen:
Follicles grow in response to FSH and produce estrogen
Progesterone:
After LH surge triggers ovulation, CL produces progesterone
Uterus
Estrogen stimulates endometrial proliferation
Progesterone stimulates endometrial secretion

Overview

- Domestic animals and New World monkeys do not menstruate. They have a short pre-ovulatory period following the luteal phase of their estrous cycles.
- Day 1 of the estrous cycle is the first day of "heat," whereas day 1 of the menstrual cycle is the first day of "menstruation."
- High levels of estrogen (in the absence of progesterone) stimulate activity of the hypothalamic pulse generator.
- Inhibin decreases while activin increases FSH release.
- Serotonin (5HT) and the opioid peptides reduce the hypothalamic GnRH pulse frequency, while catecholamines, GABA, and ACh increase it.

Menstrual Versus Estrous Cycles

The reaction of the uterus to gonadotropins in domestic animals with an estrous cycle is similar to that in primates with a menstrual cycle (such as women and Old World monkeys like macaques, mandrills, chimpanzees, and baboons). Although some animals may shed minor amounts of blood from the uterus during the estrous cycle, domestic animals and New World monkeys, such as the squirrel monkey, do not menstruate. Cows may shed some blood from the uterus during metestrus (about 48 hours after the onset of heat), due largely to intensive endometrial stimulation by estrogen during proestrus and estrus. A similar condition occurs in the bitch, but usually blood is shed earlier in proestrus. Again, the cause is thought to be overstimulation of the endometrium by estrogen from growing follicles. There may also be some shedding of the endometrial epithelial lining in domestic animals at the end of the estrous cycle. These patches of epithelium, sometimes referred to as *casts*, are shed because of a failing gonadal hormone supply that is unable to maintain the highly developed endometrium. In other words, it is the reaction of a steroid-deficient endometrium when pregnancy does not occur. However, the physiologic shedding of blood or epithelial casts from the uterus of domestic animals is relatively unimportant and should not be confused with menstruation.

The primary difference between menstruating and nonmenstruating species is the anatomy of the endometrial arterial supply (i.e., the menstruating species have coiling arteries supplying the endometrium). It should also be noted that in nonmenstruating species, the endometrium does not degenerate following the decline of the CL (to the same extent as in menstruating species). Therefore, the preovulatory (or follicular) phase of the estrous cycle (*proestrus*) is generally quite short (two to three days) because there is no need to fully regenerate the endometrium (**Part D**). Timing of the menstrual and estrous cycles also differs. Day 1 of the estrous cycle is the first day of "heat" (i.e., estrus, the most obvious behavioral event), while day 1 of the menstrual cycle is the first day of menstruation (i.e., the most obvious physical event).

Regulation of Gonadotropin Release

Hypothalamic control of gonadotropin release is exerted by GnRH (also called LHRH), which is secreted into portal hypophyseal blood (**Part E**). GnRH stimulates release of FSH as well as LH, and it is uncertain whether there is an additional separate FSH-releasing hormone (FRH).

GnRH is normally secreted in a pulsatile fashion, which is essential for normal LH and FSH release. If large amounts are administered by constant infusion, GnRH receptors in the adenohypophysis downregulate and LH secretion ceases. However, if GnRH is administered in small amounts episodically at the rate of approximately 1 pulse/hr, LH and FSH release is stimulated. It is clear that fluctuations in both frequency and amplitude of GnRH bursts are important in generating other hormonal changes responsible for the estrous cycle. Frequency is increased and amplitude decreased by high levels of estrogen in the absence of progesterone (preovulatory, follicular phase), yet frequency decreases with high levels of progesterone (luteal phase) or testosterone. Frequency increases late in the follicular stage, culminating in the LH surge and ovulation (see **Part A**). Duration of the gonadotropin surge is relatively short (usually 12 to 24 hours). During the luteal phase, frequency decreases due in large part to high levels of progesterone and inhibin. When estrogen and progesterone secretion decrease at the end of the cycle, frequency once again increases (due to lack of progesterone and inhibin). Activin modulates the effects of inhibin by promoting FSH release (see Chapter 13).

Although the precise location and nature of the "GnRH pulse generator" in the preoptic area of hypothalamus are still undefined, it is generally recognized that catecholamines, GABA, and acetylcholine (ACh) increase GnRH pulse frequencies, while serotonin (5-HT) and opioid peptides reduce them.

13 Gonadotropins: III

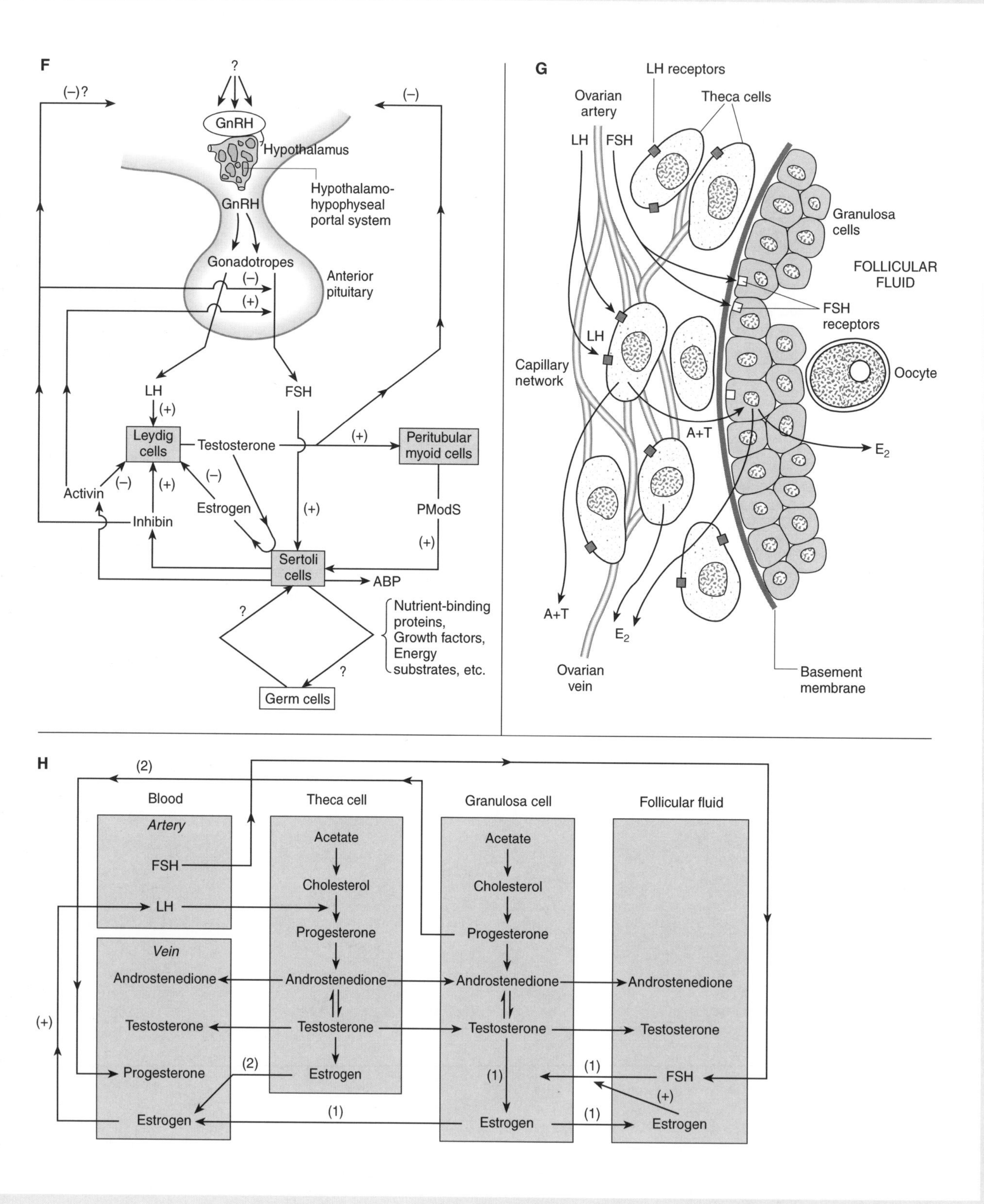

Overview

- LH (ICSH) stimulates testicular Leydig cells while FSH stimulates Sertoli cells.
- Sertoli cells produce ABP (which binds testosterone).
- Ovarian theca cells are biochemically similar to testicular Leydig cells, while ovarian granulosa cells are similar to testicular Sertoli cells.
- The processes of spermatogenesis and ovulation appear to have some biochemical similarities.

Male Gonadotropins

The release of *gonadotropin-releasing hormone (GnRH),* and subsequently of gonadotropins, is thought to proceed in a more continuous fashion in males, compared with the typical cyclic pattern described for females. The *preoptic area* of the hypothalamus, which contains neurons responsible for regulating the ovulatory surge of gonadotropins in females (see Chapter 11, **Part E**), does not appear to be as functional in males. However, some seasonal variation in male gonadotropin release does occur, indicating that sensory input to the hypothalamus from higher centers in the CNS is involved in male GnRH output. In general, the frequency, quality, and fertility of ejaculates are reportedly improved during the breeding season.

As in females, GnRH stimulates *luteinizing hormone (LH)* release from the anterior pituitary (**Part F**). Luteinizing hormone binds to specific membrane receptors on *Leydig cells* (interstitial cells) of the testes, which leads to generation of cAMP and other messengers that ultimately cause the secretion of androgens (i.e., testosterone). Elevation of testosterone in turn inhibits further LH secretion. This inhibitory effect on the hypothalamus is mediated principally by estrogen, which is formed locally in hypothalamic cells from testosterone.

After stimulation by GnRH, the gonadotropes also secrete FSH into the circulation. This glycoprotein hormone binds to specific receptors on *Sertoli cells* of the testes, stimulating production of *androgen-binding protein (ABP).* FSH is necessary for the initiation of spermatogenesis. However, full maturation of spermatozoa also appears to require testosterone. Indeed, the major action of FSH on spermatogenesis may be stimulation of ABP production, which allows a high intratubular concentration of testosterone to be maintained. In addition to ABP, there is substantial evidence that other compounds are synthesized and secreted by the gonads. For example, testicular Sertoli cells (like ovarian granulosa cells) secrete peptide and protein products that act in endocrine, paracrine, and even autocrine fashion to modulate the processes of gametogenesis. *Inhibin* and *activin* are members of the same superfamily of growth-regulating factors as discussed in Chapter 9. Inhibin is a glycoprotein that circulates in plasma and inhibits GnRH-stimulated FSH release by the pituitary. It is not known whether inhibin also exerts a significant negative feedback at a hypothalamic locus. Activin, another gonadal glycoprotein, has the opposite action, stimulating FSH release. At the gonadal level, inhibin increases whereas activin decreases testosterone secretion; thus, FSH can influence Leydig cell function indirectly by modulating production of inhibin and activin. Other paracrine interactions may also be important in maintaining a proper testicular environment for spermatogenesis. Testosterone from Leydig cells further stimulates differentiation and proliferation of *peritubular myoid cells.* The latter secrete a protein known as *PModS* that stimulates Sertoli cell function. Each of these pathways may vary in functional activity and significance at different points in the cycle of spermatogenesis. **Part A** is an overall diagram of pituitary and testicular control of Leydig cell, peritubular myoid cell, and Sertoli cell secretion, as well as spermatogenesis.

Not depicted in **Part A** are other testicular-derived factors that also appear to play important roles in spermatogenesis. *Follistatin* is another FSH-suppressing protein that is produced by the gonads. It may act by binding activin. Insulin-like growth factor 1 is also synthesized by this cell line and appears to modulate cell growth and hormonal responses within the gonads. Leydig cells are also known to synthesize and secrete proopiomelanocortin products and oxytocin. A peptide functionally resembling GnRH (but structurally dissimilar to it) is also produced by Sertoli cells. Intragonadal GnRH has been hypothesized to function in modulating the effects of LH on interstitial cell testosterone secretion. However, a specific role for locally produced GnRH has not yet been established. In addition, a variety of trace metal–binding proteins, steroid-binding proteins, proteases, prostaglandins, lymphokines, and extracellular matrix molecules such as laminin, collagen types I and IV, and proteoglycans are also produced. These compounds are thought to exert local actions in the nurturance and development of germ cells, as well as in the exodus of these cells from the gonadal enclave.

Female Gonadotropins

During the early follicular phase of the estrous cycle, ovarian *theca cells* (similar to testicular Leydig cells) produce androgens [androstenedione (A) + testosterone (T)] and some estrogen (estradiol, E_2) in response to LH (see **Parts F** and **G**). During this time, *granulosa cells* (similar to testicular Sertoli cells) proliferate, and they aromatize the androgens to estrogen under the effect of FSH (see **Parts G** and **H**). The estrogen so produced also synergizes with FSH to promote replication of granulosa cells (positive feedback; **Part H,** process [1]). During the midfollicular phase, theca cells continue producing androgens, and granulosa cells estrogen. Also during this time, granulosa cells initiate production of inhibin, which inhibits further FSH secretion (see Chapter 11, **Part E**). During the late follicular phase, extensive aromatization of androgens to estrogen occurs in granulosa cells (see **Part H,** process [1]), causing a positive feedback demand on the hypothalamic–pituitary axis, which results in an LH surge. During the very late follicular phase (just before ovulation), granulosa cells begin secreting progesterone (see **Part H,** process [2]), and theca cells enhance their production of estrogen (see Chapter 11, **Parts B** and **C**). During the luteal phase (following ovulation), granulosa cells of the CL produce mainly progesterone, with theca cells continuing their production of estrogen (albeit at decreased levels; see **Part H,** process [2]).

As in testicular Sertoli cells, FSH also stimulates production of a variety of nonsteroidal compounds by granulosa cells that likely have paracrine effects. As previously mentioned, inhibin, whose secretion parallels that of progesterone, inhibits FSH secretion, which is thought to keep competitor follicles (with fewer FSH receptors) from developing. Inhibin also increases androgen secretion from theca cells. Activin (also produced by granulosa cells) modulates the effects of inhibin by increasing pituitary FSH secretion and decreasing androgen secretion by theca cells (see Chapter 11, **Part E**). However, because there is a greater production of inhibin than activin around the time of ovulation, the supply of precursor androgens from theca cells is increased. Inhibin is also produced by the CL.

Other paracrine agents from granulosa cells include *transferrin* and *ceruloplasmin* (which pick up iron and copper, respectively, from their plasma-binding analogues and transfer these vital elements to the oocyte). Various *granulosa growth factors* (such as IGF-1) modulate growth and steroid hormone secretion by neighboring endocrine cells and conceivably by the oocyte itself. For example, IGF-1 is thought to potentiate FSH action on granulosa cell differentiation and progesterone synthesis, and also to potentiate LH stimulation of androgen production by theca cells. Other agents thought to play a role in ovulation (because of their strong presence in follicular fluid) include $PGF_{2\alpha}$, oxytocin, proteolytic enzymes, plasminogen activator, renin, and angiotensin, as well as some GnRH-like peptides. Indeed, the ovulation processes in females appear to utilize the same biochemical factors as the spermatogenesis processes in males.

14 Estrous Cycles

A

Spontaneous (Silent) Ovulators	*Induced (Reflex) Ovulators*
Seasonal	**Seasonal**
Horse	Mink
Sheep	Cat
Goat	Ferret
Donkey	Skunk
Dog	Wild rabbit
Nonseasonal (continuous breeders)	**Nonseasonal**
Cow	Lab rabbit
Pig	Llama
Human	
Mouse	
Monkey	
Rat	
Guinea pig	

B

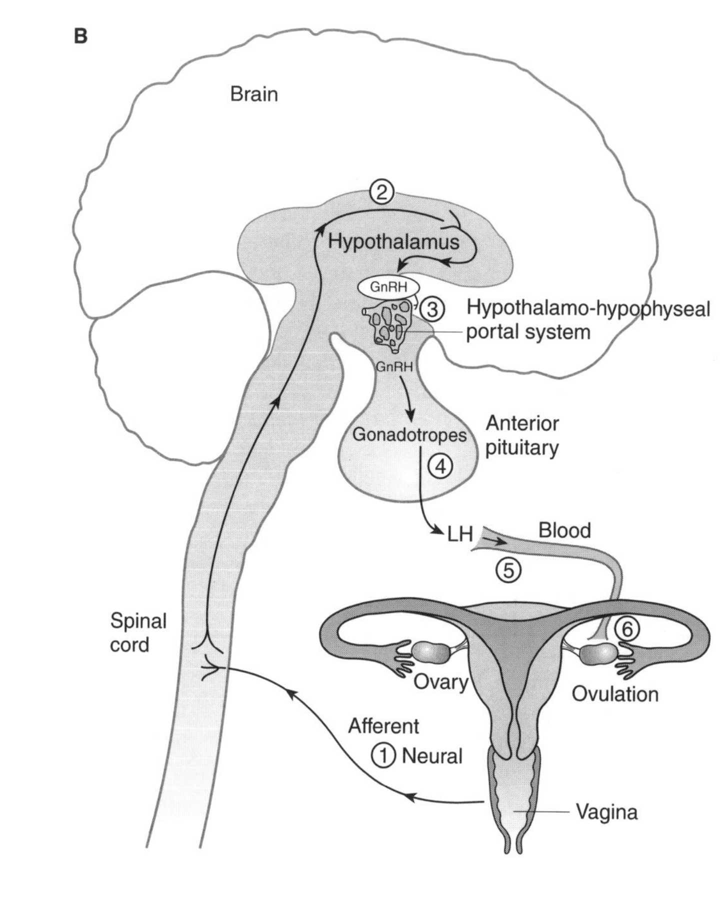

C

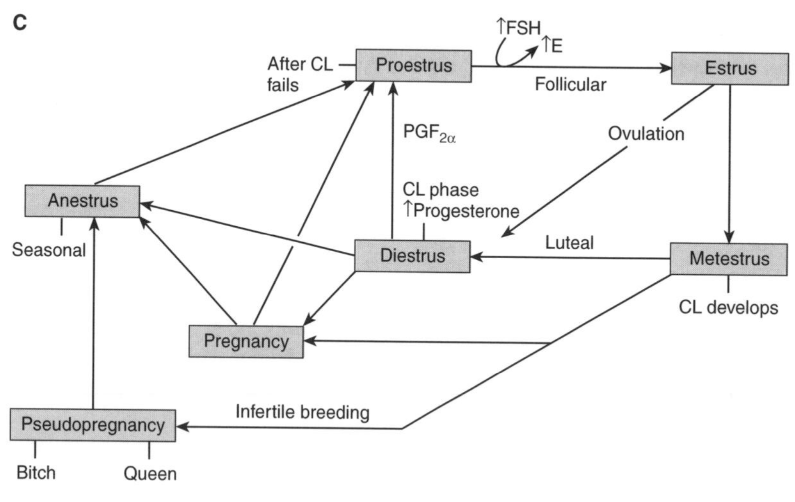

Overview

- Domestic female animals are classified as being either spontaneous or induced ovulators.
- Metestrus is not recognized in animals that produce progesterone quickly following ovulation.
- Proestrus precedes estrus.
- Pseudopregnancy is an exaggerated diestrual response of the bitch and queen.
- Anestrus is a stage of sexual quiescence.

Two types of estrous cycles are commonly observed in domestic animals (**Part A**). One type is exemplified in nonseasonal breeders, such as the cow and sow, and in the bitch, mare, and ewe during the breeding season. The infertile cycle of these species culminates in *spontaneous (silent) ovulation* of mature follicles; CLs automatically form, become functional, and exist for a defined period of time. Species such as the rat and mouse are also included in this type of estrous cycle in which ovulation is spontaneous, but CLs that form in these species are dysfunctional unless mating occurs. The estrous cycles are short (5 days) when rats are not mated, and longer (12 days) if cervical stimulation occurs. Some of these animals are polyestrous (exhibit more than one estrous cycle in sequence), while others are monestrous (come into heat once, then exhibit an anestrus period). Examples include the following:

- Nonseasonal polyestrous: cow and sow
- Seasonal polyestrous: mare, ewe, and goat
- Monestrous: bitch

In the second type of estrous cycle, maturation and ovulation of follicles fail unless the male copulates with the female. The rabbit, cat, and mink are examples of this type, commonly referred to as *reflex ovulators* or *induced ovulators*. Successive groups of follicles mature and degenerate rhythmically in these animals during the breeding season, and at any time there are a number of follicles capable of being ovulated if copulation occurs. The cat and mink could therefore be considered seasonally pseudopolyestrous, because if mating does not occur in these animals, follicles regress and subsequent periods of follicular growth and estrus recur several times during the breeding season. Copulation in these species is thought to stimulate afferent neural pathways to the hypothalamus (processes *1* and *2* in **Part B**), causing release of GnRH (process *3*), which stimulates the adenohypophysis (process *4*) to release LH into blood (process *5*). Luteinizing hormone in turn, promotes the ovulatory process (process *6*).

Phases of the Estrous Cycle

The estrous cycles of domestic animals are generally divided into four phases (plus alternates) (**Part C**). These are called *estrus, metestrus, diestrus,* and *proestrus.* The duration of each varies with species, but in the sow are 2 to 3 days, 3 days, 11 to 13 days, and 3 days, respectively.

Estrus is the period of sexual receptivity (i.e., heat), during which ovulation occurs in most species and CLs begin to form. At the end of estrus circulating estrogen and LH decline. In cows, ovulation occurs 12 to 16 hours after estrus.

Metestrus is the immediate postovulatory phase, in which CLs develop before producing significant amounts of progesterone. In some species CLs produce progesterone quickly, and in others the follicular wall initiates progesterone production before ovulation. Therefore, in these species metestrus is not recognized, and animals proceed from estrus directly into diestrus. In the cow and sow, metestrus lasts two to three days from ovulation until significant quantities of progesterone are produced.

Diestrus is the period during which the influence of luteal progesterone on accessory sex structures predominates. Together, metestrus and/or diestrus are referred to as the phase of the CL. Generally, diestrus is identified as the first day the female refuses to mate with the male, an effect thought to be due to high circulating levels of progesterone (see Chapter 11). This negative effect of progesterone on sexual behavior may not be exhibited in dogs.

Pregnancy may occur during metestrus or diestrus as a result of a fertile mating. Gestation length varies with species, from 31 days in the Western chipmunk to 660 days in the African elephant.

Proestrus is the period after the CL fails (due to $PGF_{2\alpha}$) when progesterone levels drop, FSH release stimulates follicular growth, and rising estrogen levels lead to estrus. Proestrus and early estrus are referred to as the follicular phase (before ovulation). Proestrus is short (two to three days) in domestic animals compared to the follicular phase of menstruating primates (14 days), due largely to the fact that regeneration of the endometrial stratum functionale is unnecessary in domestic animals because it does not fully degenerate when the CL fails.

Pseudopregnancy, or false pregnancy, is an exaggerated diestrual response of the bitch and queen. It may be related to the extreme sensitivity of the canine endometrium and mammary glands to progesterone, in synergy with prolactin. The CL of the nonpregnant bitch remains functional for an extended period of time after ovulation. In *overt pseudopregnancy* (which may sometimes last as long as pregnancy), mammary glands develop, the uterus enlarges, the abdomen may relax, the pelvis and external genitalia may change as they would during pregnancy, and the bitch may develop a whelping nest. In fact, some pseudopregnant bitches have been reported to adopt and effectively nurse puppies from other bitches. Queens that are induced to ovulate by mechanical stimulation of the vagina, exogenous hormones, or matings with sterile males may also become pseudopregnant. Pseudopregnancy lasts from 30 to 70 days in the queen, yet it is not associated with the profound organic and behavioral changes seen in the bitch and seldom leads to lactation and nesting behavior. However, pseudopregnant queens undergo vaginal, uterine, and oviductal changes induced by progesterone secreted by CLs.

Anestrus is a stage of sexual quiescence characterized by the lack of estrus behavior. It is a normal stage of reproductive function in prepubertal and aged animals and in pregnant animals of all species. In fact, pregnancy is the most common cause of anestrus in polyestrous species. After puberty, anestrus in nonpregnant animals is normal for monoestrous species such as dogs, for seasonally polyestrous species during the nonbreeding season, and for lactating females of most species.

15 The Pineal Gland: I

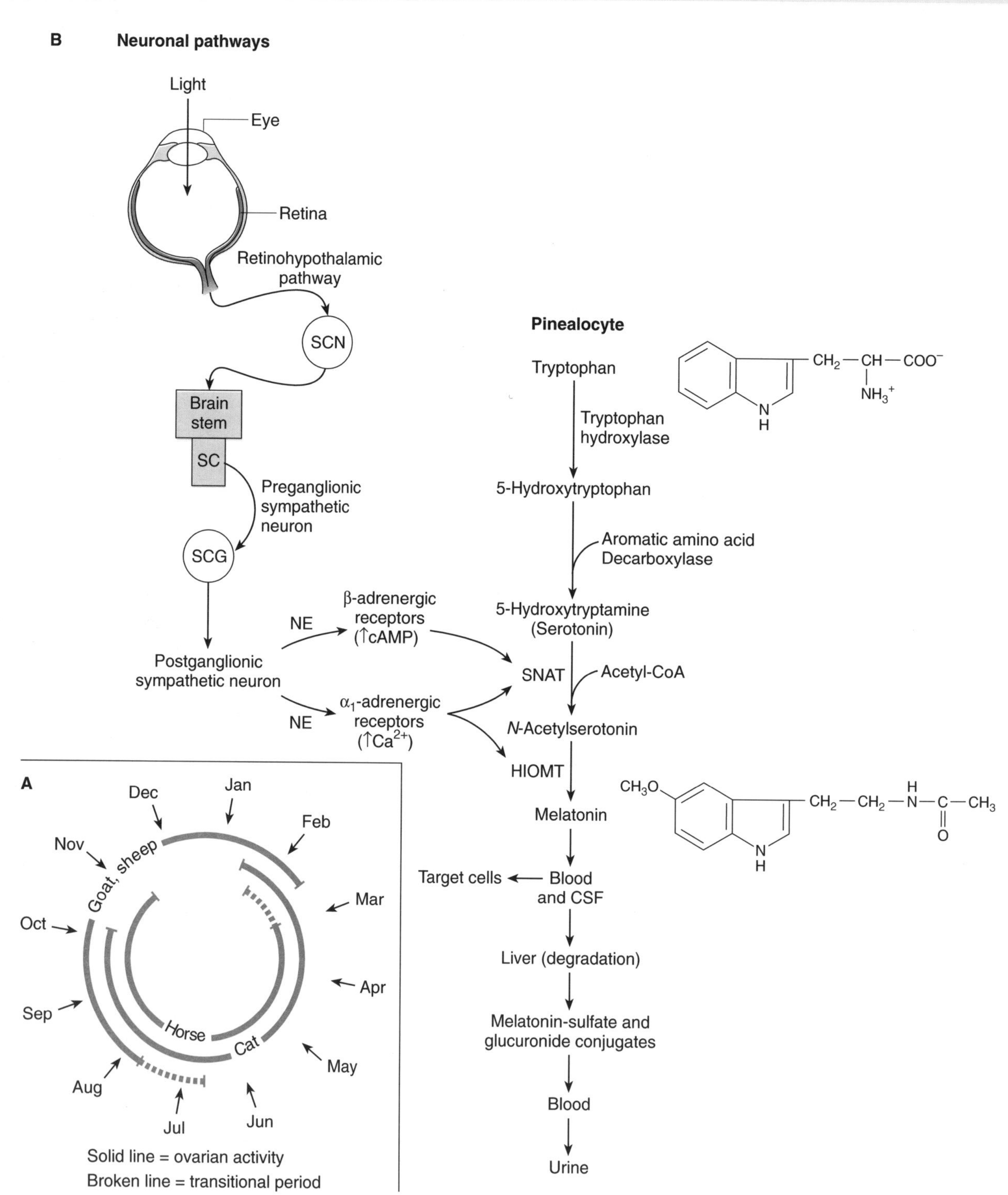

Source: Part A modified from Stabenfeldt GH, Edqvist L-E: Female reproductive processes. In Swenson MJ, Reece WO [eds]: Dukes' physiology of domestic animals. 11th ed. Ithaca, NY: Cornell University Press, 1993:691.

Overview

- The pineal gland is a neurotransducer organ that influences the reproductive cycles of a number of seasonal breeders.
- The SCN and the pineal gland are the primary translators of photoperiod.
- Melatonin is antigonadal in a number of species, but not in sheep and goats.
- Melatonin is derived from serotonin by the action of the enzymes SNAT and HIOMT.
- The sympathetic nervous system is involved in melatonin formation.
- Hypothalamic peptides like AVT, oxytocin, TRH, PRL, and somatostatin have also been found in the pineal gland.

The pineal gland, viewed historically as "a third eye," as "the seat of the soul," and at one time as a "sphincter to control the flow of thought," is viewed by pinealogists today as a *neuroendocrine transducer organ.* Since the discovery of melatonin in 1958, the study of the pineal gland and its hormones has significantly advanced our understanding of the "biological clocks" that are thought to help synchronize various physiologic events.

Photoperiodic Regulation of Reproductive Events

Photoperiodism is known to influence the reproductive cycles of a number of seasonal breeders, including cats, goats, horses, and sheep, resulting in periods of continuous (cyclic) ovarian activity followed by periods of anestrus (**Part A**). However, the response to photoperiod changes is different among species. For example, horses and cats appear to be positively affected by increasing day-length, whereas goats and sheep are positively affected by decreasing day-length. The primary translators of photoperiod appear to be the suprachiasmatic nucleus (SCN; reported to control a number of circadian rhythms in mammals), and the pineal gland, which produces melatonin in response to darkness (**Part B**). Although melatonin is antigonadal in some species, it apparently is not in sheep and goats, in which melatonin levels rise during the short-day-length breeding season. Administration of melatonin to sheep during the spring results in early onset of ovarian activity.

The cat is reported to be highly sensitive to changes in photoperiod, with a day-length increase of as little as 15 minutes in January perceived (presumably through the pineal gland) and translated by the hypothalamus into gonadotropin output and thus ovarian activity. Also, the suppressive effects of melatonin due to long periods of darkness are reportedly overcome by exposure to artificial lighting regimens in cats and horses. The customary time for placing mares, for example, under lights is December 1 (Northern Hemisphere), with cyclic ovarian activity anticipated early in February.

In mammals that experience reproductive suppressive effects from melatonin (e.g., cats and horses), data indicate that melatonin released from the pineal gland acts through either blood or cerebrospinal fluid (CSF) on the hypothalamus to lower GnRH output, thus lowering LH output from the pituitary. As indicated in **Part B,** light inhibits sympathetic input to the pineal, resulting in decreased melatonin synthesis followed by increased levels of GnRH and LH leading to estrus. Photolic signals that strike the retina pass via the retinohypothalamic tract to the SCN of the hypothalamus and then to the brain stem. From there, sympathetic preganglionic pathways leave thoracic segments of the spinal cord (SC) and terminate on the superior cervical ganglion (SCG). The postganglionic sympathetic fibers of the SCG travel along the tentorium cerebelli and enter the pineal gland via the conarian nerve. The SCN, operating through the brain stem and SC, reduces activity of sympathetic fibers to the SCG and pineal gland in the presence of light. In pinealocyte synthesis of melatonin, tryptophan is hydroxylated in position 5 to hydroxytryptophan by the enzyme tryptophan 5-hydroxylase. 5-Hydroxytryptophan is next decarboxylated to 5-hydroxytryptamine (serotonin) by L-aromatic amino acid decarboxylase. The concentration of serotonin undergoes circadian variation: during daylight hours it increases, while at night it decreases due to increased activity of serotonin *N*-acetyltransferase (SNAT) and the dark-adapted enzyme hydroxyindole-*O*-methyltransferase (HIOMT). Both β- and α_1-adrenergic receptor agonists seem to increase activity of SNAT in rats, whereas melatonin synthesis in sheep may be controlled more by α_1-adrenergic receptor stimulation of HIOMT. β-Adrenergic receptor agonists work through cAMP, whereas α-receptor agonists work primarily through the Ca^{2+}-CaM second messenger system.

The morphology of the pineal gland reportedly differs between pregnant and nonpregnant sows, implying that functional modifications occur in this gland to meet physiologic requirements during pregnancy. Evidence from human studies indicates that the pineal gland may help control the onset of puberty. Circulating melatonin decreases by 75% between the ages of 7 and 12 years, when LH levels are observed to rise (Chapter 16, **Part D**). The pineal glands of the rat and human also synthesize *arginine vasotocin (AVT).* If AVT is administered to neonatal mice during the period when the brain is undergoing sexual differentiation, increased growth of reproductive organs occurs. In contrast, if AVT is administered after the brain has undergone sexual differentiation, growth of accessory organs (and in some cases the gonads themselves) is reduced. The presence of other hypothalamic peptides, including oxytocin, TRH, prolactin, and somatostatin, has also been demonstrated in human pineals.

16 The Pineal Gland: II

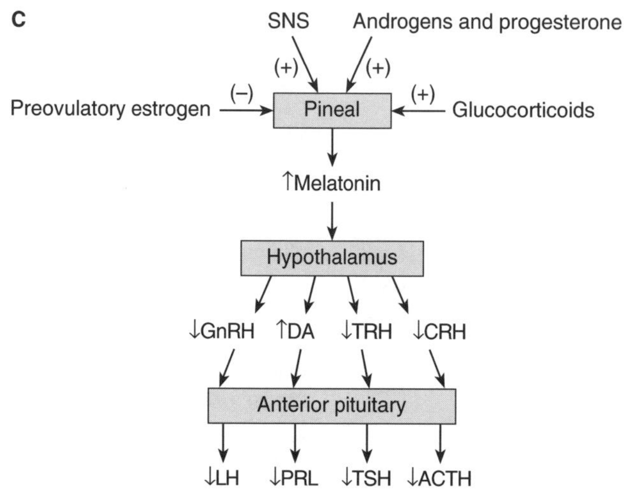

D

Melatonin Targets in Mammals	*Actions*
Photoperiodic regulation of reproduction	Melatonin, released from the pineal gland according to light/dark cycles, acts on the hypothalamus to reduce GnRH secretion. Major effects of the pineal gland are seen in seasonal breeders. Preovulatory estrogen decreases melatonin output, helping to promote a GnRH and thus LH surge.
Puberty	Circulating melatonin decreases by 75% between the ages of 7 and 12 years in humans.
Stress response	Both acute and chronic stress affect pineal function through the sympathetic nervous system and glucocorticoids, respectively (See **Part C**)
Hibernation	Melatonin has a pronounced effect on sleep–awake and arousal cycles.
Immune response	Melatonin enhances and 5-HT impairs immune function.
Free radicals	Melatonin reduces and 5-HT enhances free radical formation.
Hair	Melatonin inhibits hair growth of mice.
Melanophores (melanocytes)	Melatonin implants in weasels (*Mustela erminea*), cause them to grow white winter coats in the spring instead of brown coats.
Adrenal cortex	A pineal substance (e.g., adrenoglomerulotropin) may directly stimulate aldosterone release, and melatonin inhibits cortisol release (probably by reducing hypophyseal CRH release; see **Part C**). Excessive aldosterone release leads to hypertension.
Parathyroids	Pinealectomy causes parathyroid hypertrophy in rats.
Thyroid	Melatonin reduces thyroid function, probably by inhibiting hypophyseal TRH release (see **Part C**). Thyroid function is involved with thermoregulation and hibernation.
Lactation	Melatonin enhances hypothalamic DA release, thereby reducing adenohypophyseal PRL release (see **Part C**).
Cardiovascular system	Vasopressor activity has been reported for pineal extracts (probably AVT).

Overview

- Although preovulatory estrogen inhibits melatonin output, catecholamines, androgens, progesterone, and glucocorticoids facilitate its release.
- Pineal glands possess MAO activity.
- Melatonin appears to be involved in sleep-awake and arousal cycles (e.g., hibernation).
- The pineal gland may be involved in biological aging.
- Melatonin appears to enhance immune function.
- Melatonin decreases hypothalamic GnRH, TRH, and CRH output and increases DA release.

Androgens (e.g., testosterone and dihydrotestosterone) and progesterone inhibit *monoamine oxidase (MAO)* activity in the pineal, which in turn allows for increased melatonin synthesis (see **Part C**). Monoamine oxidase is a catecholamine-degrading (i.e., norepinephrine-degrading) enzyme. Increased melatonin can reduce LH release, which decreases testosterone synthesis in testicular Leydig cells. In contrast to androgen effects in males, the preovulatory estrogen surge in females reportedly increases MAO activity in the pineal and, therefore, decreases melatonin secretion (thus enhancing GnRH release and the LH surge).

Acute stress stimulates pineal melatonin synthesis, presumably through enhanced sympathetic stimulation. *Chronic stress* (e.g., starvation) is associated with elevated glucocorticoids, which reduce pineal MAO activity and allow for increased melatonin production (see **Part C**). Thus, stress, working through either or both pathways, can depress reproductive function via the pineal gland.

Nonreproductive Actions of the Pineal Gland

In addition to the inhibition of GnRH and therefore LH secretion, melatonin may influence the secretion of other adenohypophyseal hormones (see **Part C**). Thyroid function in some mammals is affected by photoperiod changes. This influence appears to be exerted through the control of melatonin release (see **Part D**). Melatonin treatment reduces thyroid function, presumably by limiting hypothalamic release of TRH. This would seem to be advantageous to hibernating animals, who have a need to reduce their basal metabolic rate during periods of hibernation. Melatonin is also directly involved in sleep–wake and arousal cycles.

Long photoperiods are correlated with increased prolactin secretion (and lactation) in ruminant ungulates (sheep, cattle, goats). Melatonin treatment decreases adenohypophyseal prolactin release in both sheep and goats, presumably through stimulating hypothalamic dopamine (DA) release. Exogenous glucocorticoids stimulate melatonin release, which in turn may be involved in reducing ACTH release as part of its negative feedback loop. A pineal substance known as *adrenoglomerulotropin* is also thought to stimulate aldosterone release, which in turn can cause hypertension if secreted in excess (see **Part D**). The vasopressor activity reported for pineal extracts could also be due to AVT.

Biologic aging may also involve the pineal gland. One popular theory of aging involves the formation and accumulation of *free radicals,* compounds that can interact with and damage certain proteins, carbohydrates, phospholipids, and nucleic acids. One of the most dangerous free radicals is produced during the breakdown of hydrogen peroxide. In a number of disorders (including Parkinson's disease, atherosclerosis, muscular dystrophy, multiple sclerosis, and rheumatoid arthritis), free radicals are responsible for cell damage. In certain in vitro systems, melatonin has been found to reduce free radical formation, whereas serotonin (5-HT), the precursor to melatonin, increases free radical formation. One theory of aging holds that as mammals age, the SCN, which sends important regulatory messages to the pineal, becomes dysfunctional, and the pineal reduces its production of melatonin while elevating that of 5-HT. Another influence of the pineal on aging may be related to effects of melatonin on the immune response. Melatonin appears to enhance immune function, and has been claimed to increase immune surveillance and decrease the risk of cancer. In contrast, 5-HT may impair immune function. As decreased immune function in general is associated with aging, melatonin may have a dual retarding effect on the aging process (by reducing free radicals and enhancing immune surveillance) (see **Part D**).

Biodegradation of Melatonin

Circulating melatonin is highly lipid-soluble, and therefore is taken up by virtually all tissues, including brain. It is rapidly metabolized by hydroxylation in the liver, followed by conjugation with either sulfate or glucuronic acid. Once returned to blood, these conjugates are filtered by the kidneys and excreted in urine.

Extrapineal Sources of Melatonin

The *harderian gland,* described by Harder in 1694 in the red deer, is located directly behind and around the eye of all vertebrates that possess nictitating membranes (reptiles, birds, and many mammals). In humans this gland is rudimentary. Melatonin has been demonstrated in the rat harderian gland, and continuous illumination causes enlargement of this gland and an increase in hydroxyindole-O-methyltransferase (HIOMT) activity. Harderian HIOMT apparently differs from that found in the pineal, where continuous illumination decreases pineal weight and HIOMT activity. The full significance of these observations remains to be determined.

17 Placental Hormones

A

Animal Species Known to Produce Chorionic Gonadotrophin (CG)

Humans (hCG)

Sheep (oCG)

Horses (eCG)

Nonhuman primates (e.g., Rhesus CG, RhCG)

B

Species Known to Produce Placental Lactogen (PL)

Rats	Cattle
Sheep	Goats
Primates	Mice
Voles	Guinea pigs
Chinchillas	Hamsters

D

Placental Hormones

Sex steroids (e.g., progesterone, estrogen)

Vitamin D

Chorionic gonadotropin

Chorionic thyrotropin

Chorionic corticotropin

Growth hormone variant

Relaxin

Placental lactogen

Gonadotropin-releasing hormone

Prolactin

Insulin-like growth factors I and II

C

Major Physiologic Actions of Placental Lactogen (PL) During Pregnancy)

GH-like effects:

Decreased use of glucose and amino acids by the mother and increased transport of these compounds across the placenta for fetal growth and development.

Increased use of free fatty acids by the mother.

Decreased maternal responsiveness to insulin.

Increased maternal erythropoietin production and therefore red blood cell mass.

PRL-like effects:

Stimulate growth and development of mammary tissue (along with estrogen and progesterone).

Overview

- Chorionic gonadotropin prolongs biosynthetic activity of the corpus luteum.
- The placenta produces several steroid and protein hormones that affect maternal physiology.
- The protein hormones produced by the placenta are similar in structure to the anterior pituitary hormones.
- The placenta produces an insulin-like hormone.
- Placental lactogen exerts both GH-like and PRL-like effects on maternal physiology.

Ovulation occurs either during or immediately after estrus, and estrus leads to mating. Sperm deposited in the vagina through copulation are transported mainly by *peristalsis* through the uterus and ascend into the oviduct, through which recently ovulated ova are descending. *Fertilization* typically occurs in the upper part of the oviduct, and cleavage begins soon after fertilization, giving rise to a small, multicellular *blastocyst.* The blastocyst is comprised of an *inner cell mass* that will develop into an *embryo,* and an outer *trophoblast* that will become the *chorion.* The trophoblast enables the blastocyst to erode the highly vascularized, secretory uterine endometrium (i.e., receive "uterine milk") and settle in (i.e., *implant*) for development. Gestation may last as long as 22 months in elephants (eutherians), or be as short as 12 days in the opossum (a marsupial).

In contrast to the mammalian norm, species such as bats, skunks, and mink evolved a mechanism of *delayed implantation,* whereby development of the blastocyst is arrested and the unimplanted blastocyst remains in the oviduct or uterus for an extended period of time. Delayed implantation appears to be an adaptation allowing copulation and fertilization to occur at a time that is advantageous to the parents, while ensuring that the young are born at a time more favorable to their survival. The biochemical basis for delayed implantation is unknown. A similar phenomenon occurs in marsupials, and its continuation is related to the presence of young that suckle at the teat. This is not, however, the eutherian mechanism.

Several animal species such as the dog, rat, mouse, hamster, rabbit, pig, and goat have CLs that produce progesterone throughout pregnancy. Other animals such as guinea pigs, sheep, cattle, horses, and primates maintain their CLs only during the early phase of pregnancy and allow the placenta to be the primary source of progesterone thereafter. The question remains: How do these animals "know" they are pregnant during the preplacentation phase, so that they can prolong CL progesterone production and thus prevent premature regression of the endometrium?

Rescue of the CL

The signal for prolongation of CL function in some species is the synthesis of LH-like *chorionic gonadotropin (CG)* by trophoblastic cells (*syncytiotrophoblasts*) (**Part A**). The trophoblast will eventually become the fetal component of the placenta, which will continue to secrete CG throughout pregnancy. In order for trophoblastic tissue to produce CG, it must have intimate contact with the interstitium of the endometrium. This contact occurs by *interstitial implantation* in primates, wherein the trophoblast penetrates the endometrium approximately 7 days following fertilization. Secretion of CG begins 24 to 48 hours after implantation, with immediate enhancement of luteal progesterone production. In horses and pigs, relatively minor trophoblastic invasion of the endometrium occurs, and in ruminants there is minor invasion of endometrial caruncles. Implantation, however, is less invasive with the *eccentric implantation* of the dog and cat.

Equine CG (eCG), formerly called *pregnant mare's serum gonadotropin (PMSG),* is similar in structure to LH in the mare and FSH in other species. An *ovine CG (oCG)* may also exist, and other species may secrete proteins that function similarly. Equine CG enhances progesterone production by the primary CL of pregnancy and aids in the formation of additional (secondary) CLs through the luteinization, or ovulation, or preformed follicles. Whether eCG is essential for pregnancy maintenance is unknown, because the primary CL seems to be adequate in this regard. Unlike human CG, eCG is not detectable in urine. However, it rises in plasma at 36 to 40 days following fertilization, peaks at 60 days, then declines at 120 to 150 days.

Other Placental Hormones

During the last third of pregnancy in several animal species, another pituitary-like hormone, *placental lactogen (PL)* (also called *chorionic somatomammotropin, CS,* or *chorionic growth hormone-prolactin, CGP),* is secreted by the placenta (**Part B**). Secretion of PL is in direct proportion to placental size and maturity. It is found in high concentration in the maternal circulation; however, little reaches the fetus. This hormone shares activity and a common 161-amino-acid sequence with GH (which has 191 amino acids), and it also has prolactin (PRL)-like activity. Antibodies to PL cross-react with both GH and PRL. Major roles for PL appear to involve effects on metabolism (GH-like) and stimulation of the mammary gland to initiate milk synthesis (PRL-like) (**Part C**). It has been postulated that secretion of PL may be influenced by blood glucose levels in the placenta.

The human placenta also secretes minor amounts of PRL identical to pituitary PRL. Placental PRL accumulates in amniotic fluid during pregnancy, where it is thought to help regulate both volume and ionic composition. Four additional hypothalamic/adenohypophyseal-like hormones have been identified in placental tissue: GnRH, chorionic thyrotropin, chorionic corticotropin, and GH variant (**Part D**). Although placental GnRH appears to increase CG production, functions of chorionic thyrotropin and chorionic corticotropin are not well established. Some speculate that they may help to replace their adenohypophyseal counterparts (i.e., TSH and ACTH), which are inhibited throughout pregnancy. The placental GH variant and the placental somatomedins (IGF-1 and IGF-2) are secreted into both maternal and fetal circulation, where they are thought to help modulate energy metabolism and fetal growth.

Relaxin, discovered in 1932, is an *insulin-like peptide* unique to pregnancy. It causes relaxation and softening of estrogen-primed pelvic ligaments, allowing the pelvis to stretch and expand (relax) during birth, and it increases myometrial oxytocin-receptor synthesis (as does estrogen). Relaxin reaches peak levels prior to birth and then rapidly disappears from the maternal circulation thereafter. The CL is the major source of relaxin in species where it is retained throughout gestation (e.g., the dog, pig, and rat). Relaxin is produced by the human CL during early gestation, and to some extent by the placenta. Some relaxin is found in the placentas of sheep, rats, cows, and rabbits, but in horses the placenta appears to be the major source of relaxin. In humans, ovarian interstitial cells are a major site for relaxin synthesis after the CL recedes.

Although relaxin may be important in several animal species during parturition, it has not been shown to be clinically useful in human patients with dysmenorrhea or premature labor, or during prolonged labor. Relaxin may be mammotropic in humans, and it may enhance myometrial glycogen content and decrease contractility (like progesterone). It is found in the semen of males, and it appears to be produced by the prostate.

18 Fetal Endocrine System: I

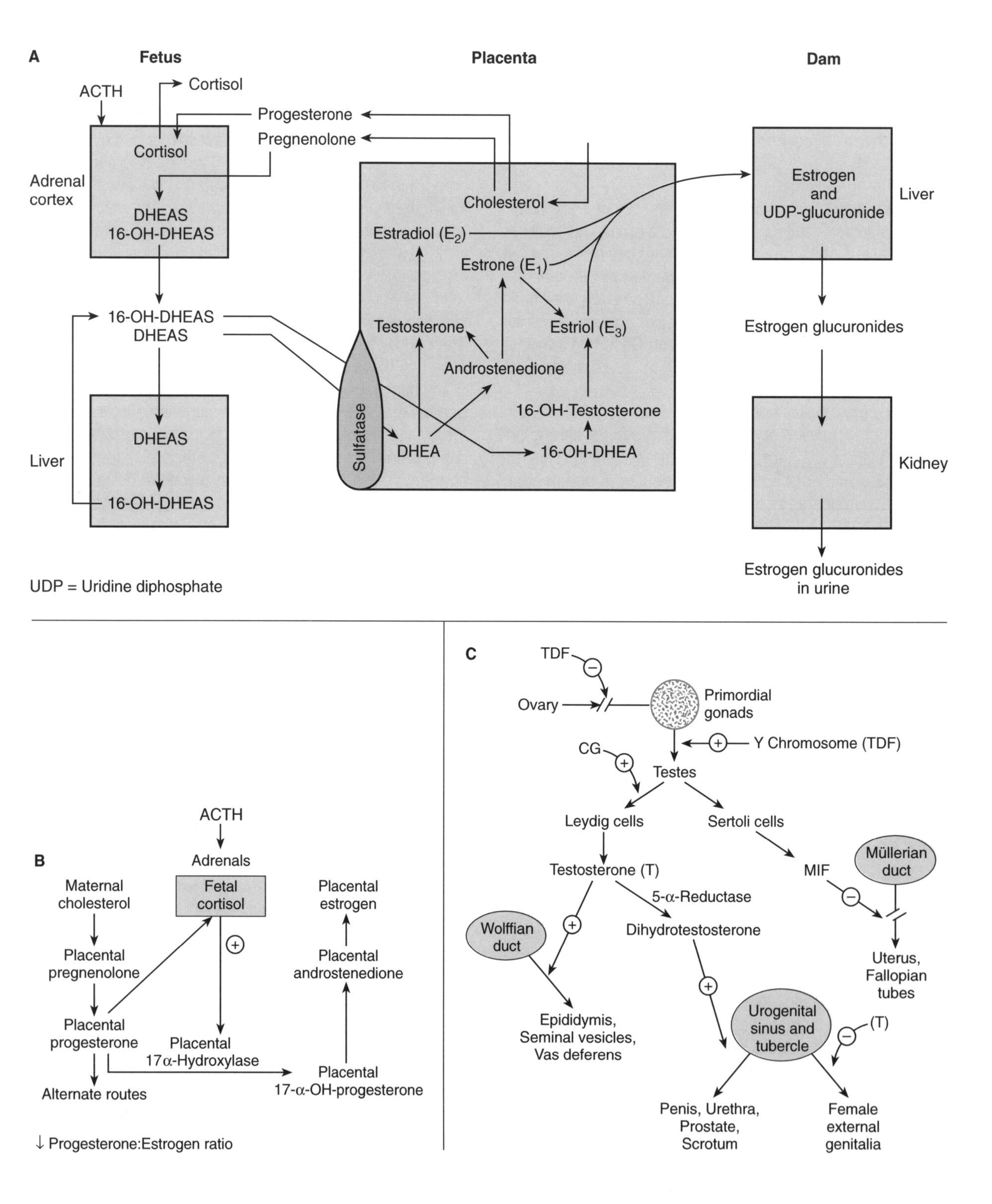
A
Fetus
Placenta
Dam
ACTH
Cortisol
Progesterone
Pregnenolone
Cortisol
Adrenal cortex
DHEAS
16-OH-DHEAS
Cholesterol
Estradiol (E_2)
Estrone (E_1)
Estrogen and UDP-glucuronide
Liver
16-OH-DHEAS
DHEAS
Testosterone
Estriol (E_3)
Androstenedione
Estrogen glucuronides
16-OH-Testosterone
DHEAS
Sulfatase
DHEA
16-OH-DHEA
Liver
16-OH-DHEAS
Kidney
UDP = Uridine diphosphate
Estrogen glucuronides in urine
B
ACTH
Adrenals
Maternal cholesterol
Fetal cortisol
Placental estrogen
Placental pregnenolone
Placental androstenedione
Placental progesterone
Placental 17α-Hydroxylase
Placental 17-α-OH-progesterone
Alternate routes
↓ Progesterone:Estrogen ratio
C
TDF
Ovary
Primordial gonads
Y Chromosome (TDF)
CG
Testes
Leydig cells
Sertoli cells
Testosterone (T)
MIF
Müllerian duct
5-α-Reductase
Wolffian duct
Dihydrotestosterone
Uterus, Fallopian tubes
Epididymis, Seminal vesicles, Vas deferens
Urogenital sinus and tubercle
(T)
Penis, Urethra, Prostate, Scrotum
Female external genitalia

Overview

- Estrogen is synthesized by the fetoplacental unit.
- Male sexual differentiation requires testicular evocators.

Physiologic function of most organ systems begins in the embryonic or early fetal period. Although inaccessibility makes the mammalian fetus difficult to study, investigators believe that the endocrine system is one of the first organ systems to develop.

The fertilized ovum generally implants within the endometrium soon after reaching the uterine cavity. Following progressive cell division and growth, the *embryonic stage* begins. The *fetal stage* follows sometime after the outline of most organ systems has been established and the placenta has developed sufficiently to provide needed nutrients. The *preplacentation period* is generally referred to as the "period of the embryo," with the *postplacentation period* being the "period of the fetus." Most intrauterine deaths are thought to occur during the preplacentation period.

Fetal Substrate Utilization

Studies using fetal sheep demonstrate that the fetus utilizes amino acids, glucose, and lactate as major metabolic substrates, with amino acids supplying 40% to 50% of required calories. Lactate is normally present in fetal plasma in concentrations higher than in the mother, and is derived from both fetal and placental glucose oxidation. Roughly half of the glucose, lactate, and amino acids are used to provide energy. Under normal circumstances, free fatty acids (bound to albumin) seem to be less utilized by the fetus, which may be due to a reduced capacity for transport across the placenta. However, their maternal hepatic products, *ketone bodies*, are water-soluble and, therefore, cross the placenta with ease. These are used by the fetus as energy substrates and building blocks for needed macromolecules.

Hormones That Cross the Placenta

Few maternal protein or peptide hormones effectively traverse the placenta (with the exception of TRH, ADH, and lesser amounts of PL and PRL). Although maternal thyroid hormones also have difficulty crossing the placenta because they are tightly bound to plasma proteins, catecholamines readily cross. Steroid hormones (and their precursors), particularly cortisol, progesterone, pregnenolone, dehydroepiandrosterone sulfate (DHEAS), and 16-OH-DHEAS, also cross the placenta to participate in the fetoplacental synthesis of estrogen.

The Fetoplacental Unit

The biosynthesis of estrogens during pregnancy is considerably more complicated than the biosynthesis of progesterone. Estrogens (e.g., estrone (E_1), estradiol (E_2), estriol (E_3), equilin, and equilenin) are synthesized in varying amounts throughout pregnancy in different mammalian species; however, the presence of estrogen conjugates in the urine of the pregnant animal is generally a reflection of the fetal state, because the complete synthesis of estrogen requires certain steps in the fetal adrenal glands, fetal liver, and/or fetal gonads. This interaction has been best described in primates (**Part A**).

Although the placenta has enzymes to synthesize cholesterol from acetate, it instead takes cholesterol from maternal blood for progesterone and pregnenolone synthesis. Because most mammalian placentas lack the 17-α-hydroxylase needed for further metabolism to estrogen, progesterone and pregnenolone are released into umbilical venous blood and carried to the fetal adrenal cortex, where progesterone is used to form glucocorticoids (e.g., cortisol) and pregnenolone is used to form DHEAS and 16-OH-DHEAS. Some 16-hydroxylation of DHEAS also occurs in the fetal liver. Then DHEAS and 16-OH-DHEAS are transported back to the placenta, where active sulfatases split the ester linkages, with the resulting DHEA converted to E_1 and E_2, and 16-OH-DHEA converted to E_3. While E_3 is the major maternal estrogen of primates, E_1 and E_2 are the major maternal estrogens of most domestic animals.

Estrogens finally produced by the placenta eventually travel to the maternal liver, where they are conjugated to glucuronides, returned to the circulation, filtered by the kidney, and excreted in urine. The measurement of urinary estrogen levels is thus an indirect indicator of fetal function. Depending on species, maternal estrogens (or estrogen precursors) may also be synthesized in the corpus luteum, ovarian follicles, adrenals, fetal gonads, or a combination of these tissues (in addition to the placenta).

The fetal adrenal cortex is well developed after the first trimester of gestation due to stimulation by fetal ACTH. It is proportionally larger than the adult gland and begins to involute some following parturition. As the fetus continues to mature, the fetal adrenals increase production of cortisol and estrogen precursors (from placental progesterone and pregnenolone, respectively), thus decreasing the progesterone-to-estrogen ratio (a biochemical cue for parturition). As this ratio declines, endometrial prostaglandin synthesis is increased, the inhibitory effects of progesterone on myometrial contraction are lessened, and the stimulatory effects of estrogen (and prostaglandin) on myometrial contraction are thus increased.

Not all species lack placental 17-α-hydroxylase. The placenta of the ewe (**Part B**), for example, possesses 17-α-hydroxylase and can complete the synthesis of estrogen from progesterone. Increased diversion of progesterone into fetal cortisol synthesis, however, serves a similar purpose in ewes as it does in other animals, because cortisol in turn stimulates activity of placental 17-α-hydroxylase. This, in turn, lowers the progesterone-to-estrogen ratio at the time of parturition (see **Part B**).

The equine fetoplacental unit produces two unique estrogens termed *equilin* and *equilenin* in addition to the more typical estrogens (E_1 and E_2). Equilin and equilenin appear after about the eighth week of gestation and are thought to be produced in the placenta by aromatization of precursors arriving from fetal gonads. It appears that equine fetal gonads, not fetal adrenals, are the key fetal endocrine organs involved in the cooperative synthesis of estrogens. Equine fetal gonads enlarge to a size greater than those of the mare during the latter part of gestation.

Male Sexual Differentiation

Fetal testicular development begins during the preplacentation phase. *Testicular differentiation factor (TDF)* on the Y chromosome directs differentiation of Sertoli cells, which are the sites of *Müllerian duct–inhibiting factor (MIF)* production (**Part C**). Production of MIF keeps the Müllerian duct from developing into a uterus and fallopian tubes. Embryonic androgen production begins in developing Leydig cells due to the presence of placental CG (or a similar protein). Fetal testosterone is needed for Wolffian duct development into an epididymis, vas deferens, and seminal vesicles, and also to inhibit the urogenital sinus and tubercle from developing into female external genitalia. Another important fetal testicular product is the reduced testosterone metabolite, *dihydrotestosterone (DHT)*, which is required for proper male differentiation of the urogenital sinus and tubercle into a prostate, penis, urethra, and scrotum. In contrast to the male fetus, ovarian steroid production is not considered essential for female phenotypic development.

An example of intersexuality in cattle is the freemartin heifer, produced when a (sterile) genetic female is modified in the male direction by masculinizing factors from a male co-twin. Placental fusion with vascular anastomosis is reported to occur in about 90% of bovine twins. Testicular evocators (i.e., TDF, MIF, testosterone, and DHT) from the male twin enter the vascular system of the female prior to development of the ovary and Müllerian system. Therefore, all degrees of masculinization are noted, and the gonads resemble testes to some degree. Similar intersexes have been reported less frequently in sheep, pigs, and goats.

19 Fetal Endocrine System: II

D

Physiologically relevant hormones in the fetal circulation	
Chorionic gonadotropins	Glucagon
Testosterone	ADH and oxytocin
Dihydrotestosterone	Thyroxine
Müllerian-inhibiting factor	PTH_{rp}
TRH and TSH	Calcitonin
GnRH	Catecholamines
Somatostatin	Cortisol
GH	Aldosterone
PRL and PL	DHEAS and 16-OH-DHEAS
ACTH	IGF-2
Insulin	

E

1. **Improves breathing**
   Increases lung surfactant
   Increases lung-liquid absorption
   Improves lung compliance
   Dilates bronchioles

2. **Protects heart and brain**
   Increases blood flow to vital organs

3. **Mobilizes fuel**
   Breaks down normal fat into fatty acids
   Breaks down glycogen (in liver) to glucose
   Stimulates new production of glucose by liver

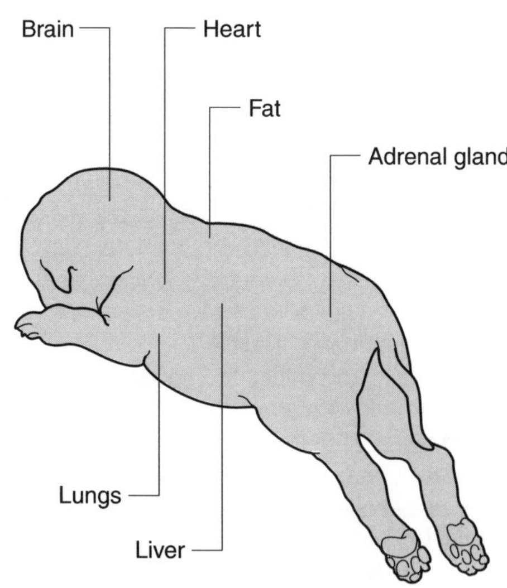

Overview

- Fetal endocrine glands become active early in fetal development.
- The third trimester is the time when the majority of fetal body development occurs.
- PTH_{rp} helps to stimulate the active transport of Ca^{2+} across the placenta.
- The fetal adrenal cortex increases to a mass that is considerably larger than its relative postnatal size.

Although a number of placental transport proteins help to regulate movement of substrates across the placenta, only calcium, iron, phosphate, water-soluble vitamins, and amino acids are thought to be transported actively from maternal to fetal blood, and no active transport mechanisms for the transfer of substances from the fetal to maternal circulation have been identified. Although the fetus is exposed to placental and some maternal hormones, it also produces hormones (discussed below) thought to be instrumental in influencing fetal growth and development, as well as potentially directing the transport of nutrients across the placenta (**Part D**).

Fetal Adenohypophysis

Characteristic anterior pituitary cell types are discernible during the first trimester, with all adenohypophyseal hormones being extractable at that time. Similarly, hypothalamic TRH, GnRH, and somatostatin are also present at this time, although the circulatory connection between the hypothalamus and pituitary develops somewhat later. The role of the fetal pituitary in organogenesis, however, appears to be negligible during the first trimester. As discussed in Chapter 18, development of the gonads during the first trimester appears to be directed more by chorionic gonadotropins than by fetal pituitary gonadotropins.

During the second trimester there is increased secretion of all anterior pituitary hormones, which coincides with maturation of the hypothalamo-hypophyseal portal vascular system. There is a rise in GH and TSH production, with an increase in thyroidal iodine uptake. Gonadotropin release also increases, with the female achieving higher FSH levels than the male. Although fetal pituitary gonadotropins do not apparently direct early gonadal development, they are thought to be important for continued development of differentiated gonads and external genitalia in the second and third trimesters. Fetal ACTH rises and helps direct maturation of the adrenal cortex (as previously discussed). Fetal PRL levels also rise in the second trimester and may exert some GH-like effects. Fetal and placental GH, PL, PRL, and insulin all stimulate hepatic production of somatomedins (e.g., IGF-1 and IGF-2, with IGF-2 likely being the most important growth factor in fetal life).

The third trimester is the period when most fetal development occurs, and all fetal pituitary hormones except PRL have been found to rise during this time.

Fetal Neurohypophysis

During the second trimester, ADH and oxytocin are demonstrable in fetal neurohypophyseal tissue. During parturition, the umbilical artery oxytocin level is higher than that in the umbilical vein. Therefore, the fetal posterior pituitary may be contributing to the onset and/or maintenance of labor.

Fetal Thyroid

The fetal thyroid gland has been reported to develop in the absence of detectable TSH, and it is capable of concentrating iodine early in fetal life. However, during the second trimester, TRH, TSH, and free thyroxine (T_4) all begin to rise. Triiodothyronine (T_3) and reverse T_3 (rT_3) only become detectable during the third trimester. Because very little placental transfer of thyroid hormones occurs, most thyroid hormones found in fetal blood are thought to have originated in the fetus. A relative hyperthyroid state exists in the fetus during the last half of gestation in order to assure proper growth and development, particularly neural development, and prepare the fetus for thermoregulatory adjustments needed in extrauterine life. Fetal hypothyroidism results in *cretinism* (and irreversible mental retardation).

Fetal Parathyroids

Although fetal parathyroids are capable of synthesizing PTH by the end of the first trimester, only low levels have been reported in umbilical blood. However, active transport of Ca^{2+} from maternal to fetal blood is probably stimulated by another protein hormone from the fetal parathyroids known as *PTH-related peptide* (PTH_{rp}). This hormone is a natural product of several additional tissue types including the amnion, squamous cell tumors (in which it was originally discovered), the uterus, and the lactating mammary gland. It relaxes uterine smooth muscle and is present in milk, where it may aid in the transport of Ca^{2+} across the neonatal intestinal mucosa. Although PTH_{rp} has a similar structure to PTH, a completely different segment of the molecule uniquely stimulates placental calcium transport, thus allowing the fetus to maintain a 30% to 40% increased ionized calcium concentration gradient over the dam. This *fetal hypercalcemia* also stimulates fetal calcitonin release, which promotes bone formation (i.e., accretion). Fetal vitamin D, a fat-soluble vitamin, reflects maternal levels yet does not appear to be significant in fetal calcium metabolism.

Fetal Pancreas

Although fetal pancreatic islets are functional in the first trimester, insulin and glucagon secretion are relatively low. Neither appears to be critical for substrate metabolism, as glucose and amino acids are generally in plentiful supply from the mother. Fetal pancreatic α and β cells are reported to respond to their usual stimulators and suppressors in blunted fashion until birth, when responsiveness rapidly increases. Fetal insulin contributes to anabolism and to deposition of adipose tissue, and fetal glucagon may help to establish and maintain hepatic gluconeogenesis in ruminant animals, a metabolic process that is established early in fetal life. It should be noted, however, that if the mother is diabetic and therefore chronically hyperglycemic, the fetus could become the same. Fetal pancreatic β cells can become exhausted under sustained hyperglycemia, with the fetus born diabetic and unusually large.

Fetal Adrenal Gland

As previously discussed, the fetal adrenal cortex is identifiable early in the first trimester, with sex steroid biosynthesis occurring in the inner fetal zone (i.e., the zona reticularis). It differs anatomically and functionally from the adult gland in that the cortex increases to a mass that is considerably larger than its relative postnatal size. In most mammals, ACTH is thought to be somewhat less important for early fetal life, although later it is more important in stimulating glucocorticoid production. Catecholamine production in the inner adrenal medulla is critical during parturition and early postnatal development. During parturition, the newborn mounts an immediate "stress response," as shown by high circulating ACTH, cortisol, and epinephrine levels in umbilical cord blood (**Part E**). If endogenous ACTH and cortisol cannot be secreted at this time, death will ensue unless replacement therapy is provided.

20 Maternal Endocrine System

A

Gland	Hormone	Pattern of change during pregnancy
Adenohypophysis	GH	Unchanged
	LH, FSH	Low or basal levels
	ACTH	Unchanged until parturition
	TSH	Unchanged
	PRL	Rises to term in some mammals (e.g., primates)
Fetoplacental sex steroids	Estrone (E_1) and 17-β-estradiol (E_2)	Rise to term in varying amounts in most domestic animal species
	Estriol (E_3)	Rises to term in primates
	Equilin and equilenin	Rise to 240 days in mares, then decline slightly to term
	Testosterone	Rises to term, but free concentration falls
	DHEA	Declines to term
Placenta and CL	Progesterone	Variable in domestic animals, but rises to term in primates
	17-Hydroxyprogesterone	Levels in plasma correlate well with CL activity
Adrenal cortex	Glucocorticoids	Rise to term
	Mineralocorticoids	Rise to term
Thyroid	Total T_4 and T_3	Increase during first trimester, then plateau
	Free T_4 and T_3	Unchanged
Parathyroids	PTH	Rises to term
Pancreas	Insulin	Low in early pregnancy, but increases later
	Glucagon	Responsive to usual stimuli

Source: **Part A** modified from Greenspan FS, Strewler GJ. Basic and clinical endocrinology. 5th ed. Stamford, CT: Appleton & Lange, 1997:550–551.

Overview

- The maternal endocrine system exhibits important roles in the maintenance of pregnancy.

The fetus, like a successful parasite, manipulates the dam for its own gain, but normally avoids imposing excessive stress that would jeopardize this "host" and thus itself. Most endocrine function tests in the dam are significantly altered during pregnancy. Some changes are due to increased production of plasma-binding proteins by the liver, others to decreased circulating levels of albumin. Additionally, some endocrine changes are mediated by altered clearance rates owing to increased glomerular filtration, decreased hepatic excretion of metabolites, or metabolic clearance of steroid and protein hormones by the placenta. Although maternal endocrine adaptations to pregnancy (summarized in **Part A** and below) undoubtedly occur in all mammalian species, those in primates have been best detailed.

Maternal Anterior Pituitary

Maternal adenohypophyseal hormones generally have little influence on pregnancy after implantation. In some mammalian species, the pituitary gland enlarges somewhat during pregnancy, primarily due to hyperplasia of lactotrophs in response to high plasma estrogens. Prolactin, the product of lactotrophs, is the only maternal adenohypophyseal hormone to significantly increase during pregnancy, and established pregnancy can continue following hypophysectomy. In cases of pituitary hyperfunction, the fetus is generally unaffected unless hyperglycemia results.

Maternal Estrogens

As previously discussed, estrogen production by the placenta of most mammals depends on circulating precursors derived from the fetus. The estrogen 17β-estradiol (E_2) rises in varying amounts throughout gestation in the bitch, mare, cow, ewe, rat, sow, rabbit, goat, and primate (among others). Higher levels of estrone (E_1) are also noted in most domestic animal species. However, large elevations in maternal estriol (E_3) (e.g., by 1000-fold in humans) appear to be unique to primates. In the mare, rises in equilin and equilenin appear to parallel that of E_1. Immediately prior to parturition, estrogen levels generally rise while those for progesterone fall (a likely biochemical cue for the onset of labor).

Maternal Androgens

In addition to the placenta, the adrenal gland and ovaries also slightly increase the production of androgens during pregnancy. The most important determinant of androgen plasma concentration apparently is whether or not it binds to hepatic-derived sex hormone–binding globulin (SHBG). Levels of testosterone, which binds avidly, may increase into the normal male range by the end of the first trimester, yet free testosterone levels are actually lower than in the nonpregnant state. Dehydroepiandrosterone sulfate (DHEAS) does not bind to SHBG; therefore, plasma concentrations of this androgen reportedly decrease during pregnancy. Placental desulfation of DHEAS (see Chapter 14) and subsequent conversion of DHEA to E_1 and E_2 also appear to be important factors in its increased metabolic clearance.

Maternal Progestins

Progesterone synthesis relies on maternal cholesterol or the cholesterol precursor, acetate. Fetal death has no immediate influence on maternal plasma progesterone levels, thus indicating that the fetus is a negligible source of progesterone substrates. Maternal plasma progesterone concentrations rise in varying (species-dependent) amounts throughout pregnancy, then fall immediately before the onset of labor. Progesterone (meaning to *pro*long *gestation*) is necessary for the establishment and maintenance of pregnancy. Insufficient CL production of progesterone may contribute to implantation failure, and luteal phase deficiency is also implicated in some cases of infertility. Furthermore, progesterone is indispensable to a relatively quiescent state of the myometrium. Progesterone is also active as an immunosuppressive agent in some systems, inhibiting T-cell–mediated tissue rejection. Thus, high local concentrations of progesterone may contribute to immunologic tolerance by the uterus of invading embryonic trophoblast tissue. 17-Hydroxyprogesterone is considerably less active than progesterone, and because it originates from the CL, urinary levels indicate CL, not placental function (with the exception of ewes).

Maternal Adrenal Cortex

Plasma cortisol concentrations increase significantly by the third trimester in primates, yet mares may not exhibit similar increases. Most of the increase in primates is due to an increase in circulating *cortisol-binding globulin* (*CBG* or *transcortin,* which binds progesterone with equal affinity). Increased estrogen levels account for the increase in hepatic CBG synthesis, which in turn accounts for decreased catabolism of cortisol by the liver. The result is an increase in plasma cortisol half-life, while production of cortisol by the adrenal zona fasciculata is reduced. The net effect of these changes is an increase in plasma free cortisol that can be significant by late pregnancy and probably contributes to some of the insulin resistance experienced by the dam (though PL also causes insulin resistance). High progesterone levels may act as a glucocorticoid antagonist (because they compete for similar receptors), thus preventing excessive glucocorticoid effects.

Blood levels of aldosterone are markedly elevated during pregnancy, probably due to increased production by the adrenal zona glomerulosa (not to increased plasma protein binding or decreased clearance). Peak serum aldosterone levels are reached by mid-pregnancy and maintained until parturition. Renin substrate is increased by the influence of estrogen on hepatic synthesis, and both renin and angiotensin II levels are increased. In spite of these dramatic changes, normal pregnant animals show few signs of hyperaldosteronism. There is no tendency toward hypokalemia or hypernatremia, and blood pressure at mid-pregnancy, when changes in the renin–angiotensin system are maximal, tends to be lower than in the nonpregnant state.

Maternal Thyroid

The thyroid becomes palpably enlarged during the first trimester, with ^{131}I uptake by the gland increased. These changes are thought to be due in part to the increased renal clearance of iodide, which causes relative iodine deficiency. While total serum thyroxine (T_4) is elevated as a result of increased *thyroid-binding globulin (TBG)* synthesis by the liver, free T_4 and triiodothyronine (T_3) are normal. Although estrogen is known to stimulate thyroid-stimulating hormone (TSH) release, TSH is not elevated in pregnancy (perhaps due to negative feedback by T_4). Rhesus monkey chorionic gonadotropin (RhCG), which is similar in structure to TSH, is known to increase T_4 production, however.

Maternal Parathyroids

The Ca^{2+} demand imposed by fetal skeletal development is significantly increased by the third trimester. This is met by hyperplasia of the maternal parathyroids and elevated serum PTH. Total serum Ca^{2+} declines to a nadir late in the third trimester, largely due to the hypoalbuminemia of pregnancy. Serum ionized Ca^{2+}, however, is reportedly maintained at normal concentrations.

Maternal Pancreas

The size of pancreatic islets increases, and insulin-secreting β cells undergo hyperplasia. Basal levels of insulin are low or unchanged in early pregnancy but increase during the second trimester. Thereafter, pregnancy is diabetogenic, with resistance to peripheral metabolic effects of insulin apparent (perhaps due to glucocorticoids and PL). Increased insulin results from increased secretion rather than decreased metabolic clearance. The effects of pregnancy on the pancreas can be mimicked by appropriate treatment with estrogen, progesterone, PL, and glucocorticoids. Insulin is not transported across the placenta, but rather affects transportable metabolites. Pancreatic production of glucagon remains responsive to usual stimuli and is suppressed by glucose loading.

Excess carbohydrate during the first trimester is converted to fat, and fat is readily mobilized during the second half of pregnancy, particularly during periods of decreased caloric intake. Amino acid metabolism may also be altered during pregnancy at the expense of maternal needs. The normal effect of pregnancy, then, is to reduce glucose levels modestly, but to reserve glucose for fetal needs while maternal energy requirements are met increasingly by the peripheral metabolism of fatty acids. These changes in energy metabolism are beneficial to the fetus and generally innocuous to the mother (with an adequate diet). Even modest starvation, however, can cause ketosis.

21 Maternal Organ Systems

A

System and parameter	Pattern of change
Cardiovascular	
Heart rate	Gradually increases
Blood pressure	Gradually decreases until the end of pregnancy, then returns to prepregnancy values about the time of parturition
Stroke volume	Gradually increases
Cardiac output	Gradually increases
Peripheral venous distention	Progressively increases to term
Peripheral vascular resistance	Progressively decreases to term
Hematopoietic	
Blood volume	Progressively increases
Hematocrit	Decreases slightly
Fibrinogen	Increases
Electrolytes	Concentration unchanged (isotonicity)
Gastrointestinal	
Sphincter tone	Decreases
Gastric emptying	Decreases
Intestinal motility	Decreases
Respiratory	
Respiratory rate	Unchanged
Tidal volume	Increases
Expiratory reserve volume	Gradually decreases
Vital capacity	Unchanged
Respiratory minute volume	Increases
Renal	
Blood flow	Increases, then returns to normal before parturition
Glomerular filtration rate	Increases early, then plateaus
Urine formation	Increases slightly

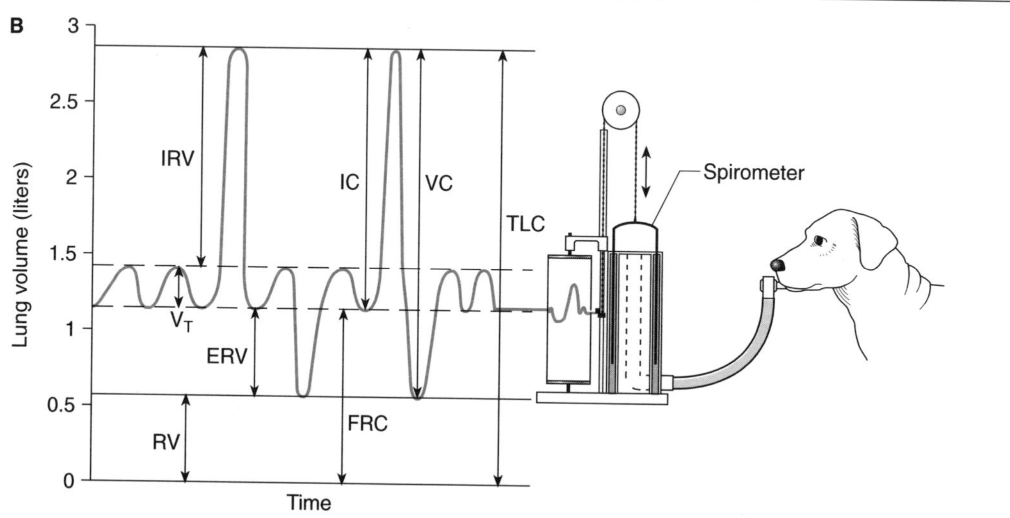

RV = residual volume (the amount of air remaining in the lungs after the most forceful expiration; V_T = tidal volume (the amount of air breathed in or out during one normal respiratory cycle); IRV = inspiratory reserve volume (the amount of air that may still be inspired after inhalation of the V_T); ERV = expiratory reserve volume (the amount of air that may still be expired after exhalation of the V_T); TLC = total lung capacity (the sum of all lung volumes); IC = inspiratory capacity (V_T plus IRV); FRC = functional residual capacity (the amount of air remaining in the lungs after a normal expiration); Respiratory minute volume (mL/min) = V_T (mL) × respiratory rate (breaths/min).

Source: Part A modified from Greenspan FS, Strewler GJ. Basic and clinical endocrinology. 5th ed. Stamford, CT: Appleton & Lange, 1997:555–556.

Overview

- Pregnancy affects the activity of virtually all maternal organ systems.
- The maternal blood pressure is normally low during pregnancy.
- Cardiac output is normally high throughout pregnancy.
- Blood volume and red blood cell mass normally increase, yet the hematocrit normally decreases during pregnancy.
- Intestinal motility decreases during pregnancy.
- Respiratory minute volume increases during pregnancy.
- Renal blood flow, GFR, and urine formation may increase during pregnancy.

Hormone production by the fetoplacental unit during pregnancy, as well as by the dam herself, results in physiologic adaptations of virtually every maternal organ system (**Part A**). These alterations are summarized in **Part A** and below.

Maternal Cardiovascular System

The first two trimesters of pregnancy are generally associated with low blood pressure (BP). In fact, a normal BP during this time may be associated with hypertension. Increased placental blood flow causes arteriovenous shunting of blood, which in turn causes peripheral vasodilation. Other contributors to low BP are increased endothelial synthesis of vascular relaxation factors in the placenta such as prostaglandins (PGE_2 and PGI_2) and nitric oxide (NO). The increased cardiac output during pregnancy is a result of cardiac afterload reduction (peripheral vasodilation). Because progesterone increases the ratio of β-adrenergic to α-adrenergic receptors in myometrial smooth muscle, it may similarly affect vascular smooth muscle, thereby lowering BP.

The rapid rise in arterial BP preceding parturition (preeclampsia or toxemia of pregnancy sometimes seen in bitches, mares, and primates) may be associated with loss of protein in urine due to an elevated glomerular filtration rate (GFR), or more probably to a rise in vasoconstricting placental thromboxanes (from circulating platelets). This rise in BP also has been associated with salt and water retention, weight gain, arterial compression by the fetus, and edema. The Ca^{2+} and Mg^{2+} drain by the fetus is also known to increase neuromuscular irritability, and it tends to elevate BP in the last trimester, when the majority of fetal growth occurs.

Maternal Hematopoietic System

Maternal blood volume (BV) shortly before term is above normal. The cause is mainly hormonal, as both aldosterone and estrogens increase renal fluid retention. Although there is an increase in red blood cell (RBC) mass (as PL increases erythropoietin production), hematocrit (Hct) decreases slightly because the degree of renal fluid retention is greater than that of erythropoiesis. Maternal estrogens also stimulate hepatic fibrinogen production. The electrolyte concentration of extracellular fluid (ECF) remains isotonic (i.e., unchanged) due to compensatory renal fluid retention.

Maternal GI Tract

Progesterone decreases not only uterine smooth muscle contraction, but also GI motility. This less desirable secondary effect can delay gastric emptying, cause generalized constipation, and decrease tension of the lower esophageal sphincter (LES). This latter effect of progesterone can result in gastroesophageal reflux.

Maternal Pulmonary System

Because the total oxygen requirement of the dam (and fetus) increases throughout pregnancy and a commensurate amount of carbon dioxide is produced, tidal volume and respiratory minute volume (**Part B**) steadily rise. Progesterone increases sensitivity of the medullary respiratory center to carbon dioxide, compounding the above effect and also effectively reducing alveolar (and arterial) P_{CO_2} significantly below that of nonpregnant animals. Because tidal volume increases and residual volume remains unchanged, expiratory reserve volume decreases. Physical compression of the fetus against the diaphragm can also have a tendency to limit total excursion of the diaphragm.

Maternal Renal System

Urine formation is slightly increased due to an increased load of excretory products from the fetus. Because electrolyte and water reabsorption is increased, the ECF volume is expanded. The increased BV leads to a progressive increase in the GFR until the second trimester, when it levels off throughout the remainder of pregnancy. Renal blood flow increases similarly, but for unexplained reasons returns toward normal during the final stage of pregnancy.

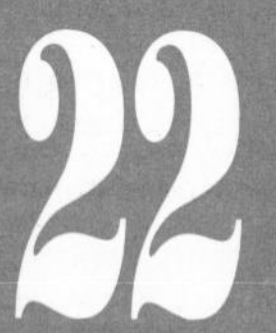

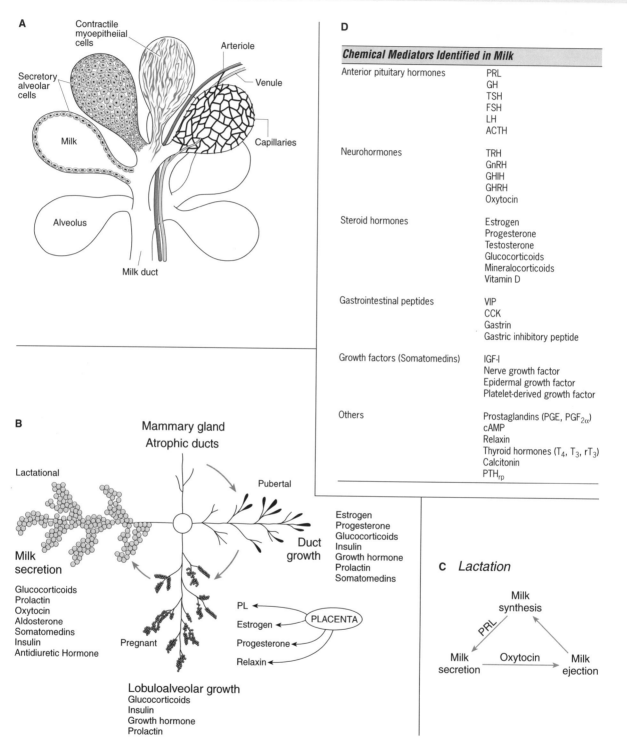

Mammary Glands and Prolactin: I

A

Contractile myoepitheiial cells
Arteriole
Secretory alveolar cells
Venule
Milk
Capillaries
Alveolus
Milk duct

D

Chemical Mediators Identified in Milk	
Anterior pituitary hormones	PRL GH TSH FSH LH ACTH
Neurohormones	TRH GnRH GHIH GHRH Oxytocin
Steroid hormones	Estrogen Progesterone Testosterone Glucocorticoids Mineralocorticoids Vitamin D
Gastrointestinal peptides	VIP CCK Gastrin Gastric inhibitory peptide
Growth factors (Somatomedins)	IGF-I Nerve growth factor Epidermal growth factor Platelet-derived growth factor
Others	Prostaglandins (PGE, $PGF_{2\alpha}$) cAMP Relaxin Thyroid hormones (T_4, T_3, rT_3) Calcitonin PTH_{rp}

B

Mammary gland
Atrophic ducts
Lactational
Pubertal
Milk secretion
Glucocorticoids
Prolactin
Oxytocin
Aldosterone
Somatomedins
Insulin
Antidiuretic Hormone
Duct growth
Estrogen
Progesterone
Glucocorticoids
Insulin
Growth hormone
Prolactin
Somatomedins
PL
Estrogen
Progesterone
Relaxin
PLACENTA
Pregnant
Lobuloalveolar growth
Glucocorticoids
Insulin
Growth hormone
Prolactin

C *Lactation*

Milk synthesis
PRL
Milk secretion
Oxytocin
Milk ejection

Source: Parts A and **B** modified from Cowie AT: Lactation. In Austin CR, Short RV [eds]: Hormonal control of reproduction. Reproduction in mammals, Vol 3, 2nd ed. Cambridge: Cambridge University Press, 1984:195–231.

Overview

- Mammary veins of lactating dairy cows are in effect varicose veins, thus sometimes giving rise to udder edema.
- Estrogen and progesterone are ineffective in stimulating mammogenesis in the absence of the pituitary.
- The placenta produces hormones that also stimulate mammogenesis.
- Lactogenesis is primarily controlled by PRL, PL, somatomedins, insulin, and corticosteroids.
- Milk ejection is controlled by a reflex mechanism.
- The first milk ejected by the mammary gland following pregnancy is called colostrum.

All mammals are uniquely dependent upon milk for nutrition during the neonatal period. Mammary glands have the capacity to synthesize a variety of essential nutritional compounds, including milk fat, proteins, and lactose, and to secure others from the blood stream.

The number and conformation of mammary glands, as well as the organization of ductular systems, varies somewhat between mammalian species. Pigs, for example, possess up to 18 separate mammary glands, each with 2 lobular sections that open to the exterior through independent canals. Primates, like pigs, have no gland sinus, and within the nipple there is a series of ducts that drain independent lobular systems. A similar arrangement can be found in cats, dogs, and rabbits. The udder of the cow has 4 mammary glands with independent ductular systems, so that milk formed in one gland cannot pass directly into adjacent glands. Posterior mammary glands of ruminants are generally larger, and hence produce more milk than anterior glands.

Mammary glands are essentially skin structures, and therefore they adopt the blood supply and lymphatic drainage of the skin in that region. As ruminant animals enter their first lactation, there is a significant increase in regional blood flow, placing severe stress upon regional veins. These veins distend and valvular incompetence sometimes develops. Mammary veins in lactating dairy cows are in effect varicose veins, reflecting the enormous strain imposed by lactation in a species manipulated by humans to produce milk greatly in excess of that required to fulfill the needs of its young. Lymph flow in the udders of lactating cows and sheep has been shown to be similar to the rate of milk secretion. Extensive edema of the udder sometimes seen in ruminant animals, can be attributed to the increased hydrostatic pressure within capillaries of the udder due largely to back pressure from veins, and an inability of distended lymphatic vessels to remove adequately the large amounts of interstitial fluid formed.

Growth and development of the mammary glands (*mammogenesis*), milk synthesis and secretion (*lactogenesis*), and *milk ejection* (letdown) are also regulated by hormones. Lactogenesis is primarily controlled by prolactin (PRL), whereas milk ejection is stimulated by oxytocin.

Mammogenesis

The internal structure of a functional mammary gland is highly vascularized, and it is organized into clusters of minute, sac-like structures known as *alveoli,* the glandular epithelium responsible for lactogenesis (**Part A**). Alveoli are continuous with ducts and their enlargements for storing milk. In addition, alveoli are surrounded by modified epithelial cells (*myoepithelial cells*) that contain muscle-like myofilaments. These cells can contract to cause ejection of milk from alveoli into the ductular system and out of the gland in the region of the nipple.

Androgens suppress mammary gland growth and are presumably responsible for their arrested development in the male fetus. Postnatal mammary development in females is conditioned by the degree of development achieved during each successive estrous cycle and involves hormones from the pituitary (ACTH, GH, and PRL), ovaries (estrogen and progesterone), pancreas (insulin), liver (somatomedins), and adrenal cortex (glucocorticoids). Estrogen is primarily responsible for ductular development, while progesterone stimulates lobuloalveolar development. However, in all mammals so far studied, estrogen and progesterone are ineffective in stimulating mammogenesis in the absence of the anterior pituitary hormones (ACTH, GH and PRL). During pregnancy, PL, relaxin, estrogen, and progesterone from the placenta continue stimulating expansion of alveoli, as do glucocorticoids, insulin, GH, and PRL. During lactation, continued milk secretion requires optimal physiologic levels of glucocorticoids, PRL, oxytocin, ADH, aldosterone, insulin, and somatomedins. **Part B** depicts mammary gland growth through the pubertal, pregnant, and lactation stages, and the hormones stimulating each.

Lactation

Lactation is generally separated into two separate phases. The first phase involves milk synthesis and secretion (lactogenesis), and the second phase involves milk ejection (**Part C**). If milk ejection is voluntarily halted, lactation ceases, milk is eventually reabsorbed, and functional alveoli are replaced by adipose tissue.

Although lactogenesis requires several hormones, it is primarily controlled by PRL, PL, growth factors (somatomedins), insulin, and corticosteroids. Lactogenesis involves alveolar cell synthesis of milk fat, protein, and lactose, and numerous vitamins and minerals are also secreted into the ductular lumen. Many hormones have been identified in milk, and their potential physiologic benefits to the neonate are being investigated (**Part D**).

Milk ejection is caused by a simple reflex mechanism controlled by oxytocin from the posterior pituitary (pars nervosa). Mechanical stimulation of the nipple (suckling) evokes release of oxytocin via a spinohypothalamic neuronal pathway (Chapter 24). Oxytocin then stimulates a contraction of myoepithelial cells that causes milk to be ejected from alveoli. Suckling young strip milk from the gland by expressing it between the tongue and hard palate. Prolactin is also released when milk is ejected, stimulating further milk synthesis.

The first milk ejected from the mammary gland following pregnancy is known as *colostrum* and has more protein and less carbohydrate than later milk. Colostrum contains antibodies (immunoglobulins) and other substances that protect the neonate against infection while its own immune system develops.

23 Mammary Glands and Prolactin: II

E

5-HT
END
(+)
(–)
Arcuate nucleus
DA
Hypothalamus
Hypothalamo-hypophyseal portal system
Adenohypophysis
(–)
(+)
DA (–)
GAP
GABA
VIP(+)
TRH
Estrogen
Lactotropes
PRL
(+)
Milk synthesis and secretion
Suckling reflex
Mammary gland

F

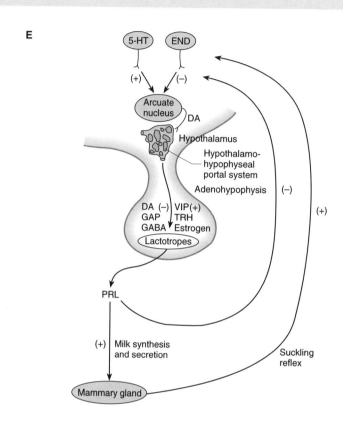

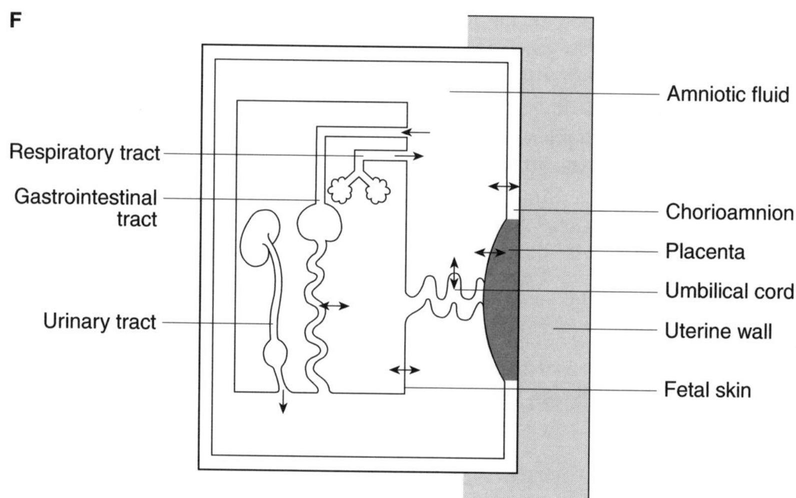

Source: Part F modified from Wallenburg HCS: The amniotic fluid. I. water and electrolyte homeostasis. J Perinat Med. 5: 193, 1977.

Overview

- PRL has at least 2 hypothalamic releasing hormones and 2 or 3 release-inhibiting hormones.
- Inhibitory control over PRL release from the anterior pituitary appears to be more important than stimulatory control.
- PRL may be the "mother-love" hormone, and has been detected in milk.
- Primary hypothyroidism may result in galactorrhea.
- Hyperprolactinemia in males may cause testicular atrophy.
- PRL may have an influence on amniotic fluid formation during pregnancy.

Control of Prolactin Secretion

Prolactin concentrations begin to increase progressively in the plasma of pregnant bitches, for example, about 35 days prior to parturition, peaking 1 to 2 days before whelping. They then decrease for about 36 hours before increasing to new peaks in response to each suckling experience.

Prolactin is the only pituitary hormone for which there is evidence of at least two releasing hormones, as well as two or three release-inhibiting hormones (**Part E**). Primary control over PRL release is inhibitory in mammals, with the pituitary releasing PRL when freed either surgically or chemically from hypothalamic control. This is in marked contrast to GH control, where both the presence of GHRH and the absence of somatostatin are necessary to elicit secretion.

Although there is some debate, most investigators believe that the physiologic mammalian PRL release–inhibiting hormone (PRIH) is the catecholamine neurotransmitter dopamine (DA), which is released into the hypothalamo-hypophyseal portal system from hypothalamic neurons in the arcuate nucleus. There is also some support for a peptide PRIH, namely the 56-amino-acid C-terminal fragment of the GnRH prohormone known as *GnRH-associated peptide (GAP)*. It remains to be demonstrated, however, that GAP is a physiologic regulator. Large amounts of γ-amino butyric acid (GABA) have also been shown to block PRL release by direct action on lactotropes. However, GABA also stimulates PRL release through actions on hypothalamic neurons. Because PRL itself increases GABA synthesis and release into the hypothalamo-hypophyseal portal system, GABA could be acting as part of PRL's major negative feedback loop. Serotonin (5-HT) also reduces PRL output by stimulating DA release from the arcuate nucleus.

The physiologic PRL-releasing hormone (PRH) was at first thought to be thyrotropin-releasing hormone (TRH). However, the neuropeptide known as *vasoactive intestinal polypeptide (VIP)* stimulates PRL release during suckling when TRH is ineffective. *Endogenous opiate peptides (END)* are also known to block the activity of DA-secreting neurons that normally prevent PRL release. Estrogen (in some mammals) tends to increase PRL secretion during the latter stages of pregnancy by increasing sensitivity of the lactotropes to hypothalamic PRHs. This effect may involve an estrogen-induced reduction in the sensitivity of lactotropes to DA by altering receptor levels and/or intracellular second messenger systems. Estrogen is also concentrated by certain GABA-secreting neurons that decrease their activity, thus increasing PRL release.

Prolactin and Galactorrhea

Secretion of lactescent (milky) fluid from the breasts of either males or females is called *galactorrhea*. It is generally caused by excessive PRL secretion and frequently occurs in primary hypothyroidism, characterized by decreased circulating levels of thyroid hormones, lack of their negative feedback, and therefore elevated circulating levels of TRH (and TSH). Prolactin release associated with primary hypothyroidism is thought to be evoked by high TRH levels (Chapter 51).

Prolactin, the "Mother Love Hormone", has been reported to promote maternal behavior and also nesting among the young.

Prolactin and Testicular Function

Circulating PRL concentrations in males are generally only slightly lower than those in nonlactating females. By itself, PRL apparently has little effect on the male reproductive apparatus. However, PRL receptors are present on the plasma membranes of testicular Leydig cells, where PRL is thought to potentiate the effect of interstitial cell–stimulating hormone (ICSH) on the steroidogenesis of testosterone. Prolactin may also increase the molecular population of androgen receptors on cells of the prostate and seminal vesicles.

Hyperprolactinemia in males is associated with a decrease in pituitary ICSH and FSH release, and with testicular atrophy. Although high circulating levels of PRL may exert inhibitory effects directly on the testes, inhibition of GnRH release is thought to be the major mechanism for reduced testosterone secretion, a hypogonadal state, decreased sperm production, and infertility.

Prolactin in Nonmammalian Vertebrates

Prolactin is also present in teleosts, amphibians, reptiles, and birds. In amphibians, PRL accelerates larval growth and blocks metamorphosis. It appears to be osmoregulatory in fishes and amphibians, where it is also, like PTH, a hypercalcemic factor. North American migratory birds exposed to a long day cycle release PRL, which induces premigratory fattening. As in mammals, TRH and VIP stimulate PRL release in birds.

Prolactin and Amniotic Fluid Formation

Amniotic fluid formation may be under hormonal control. It has been shown that PRL, which is present in amniotic fluid, can increase the permeability of the chorioamnion to water. Injection of PRL into the amniotic sac of rhesus monkeys in the third trimester of pregnancy significantly reduces the volume of amniotic fluid for 24 hours. Thus, prolactin's osmoregulatory role in amniotic fluid formation may be similar to its role in fish and amphibians.

Part F depicts the pathways involved in amniotic fluid formation. The placenta, umbilical cord, and chorioamnion exchange materials continuously; fetal skin exchange materials up to the time of keratinization; and the kidneys, respiratory tract, and gastrointestinal tract exchange materials phasically.

24 Oxytocin

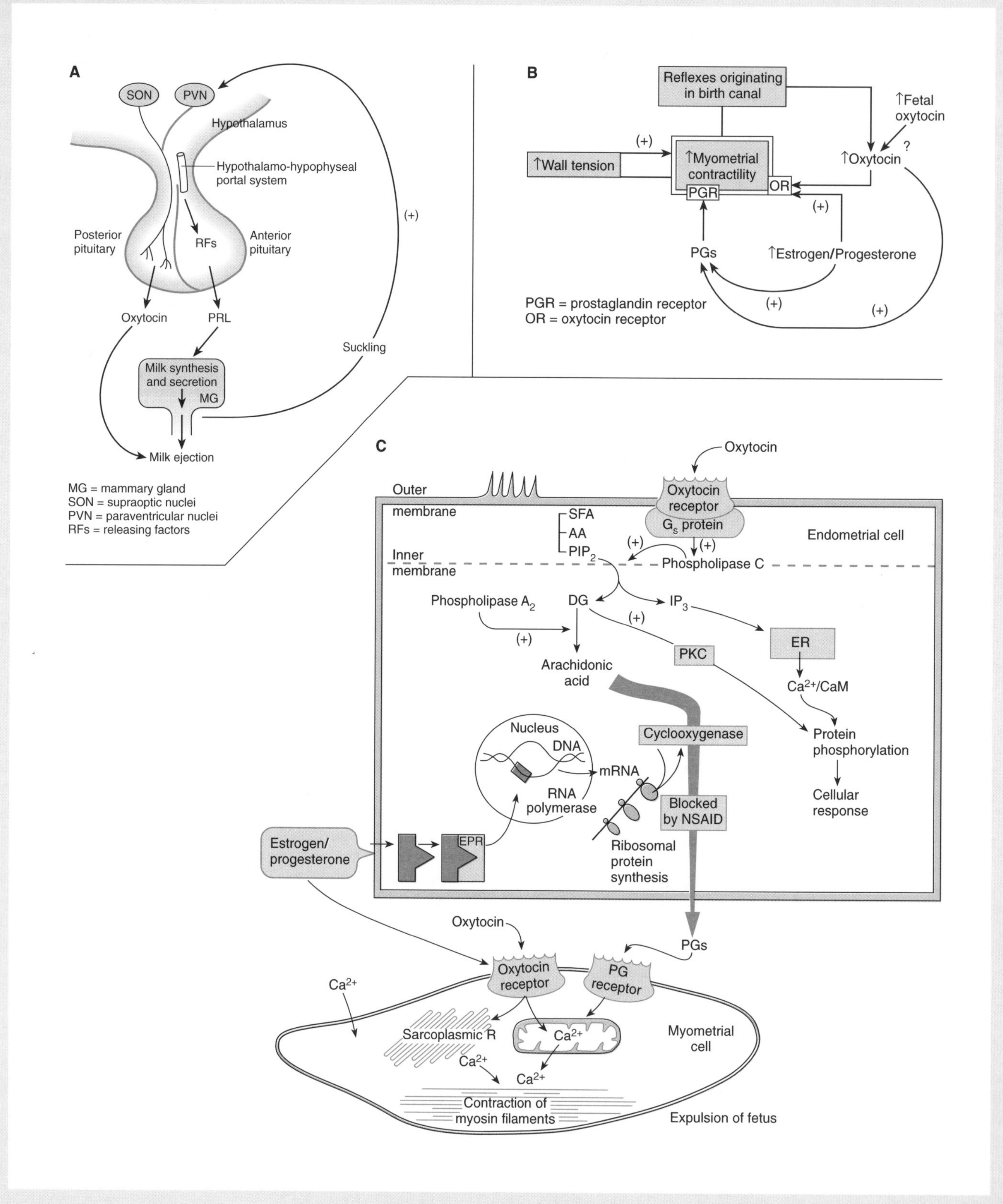

A
SON
PVN
Hypothalamus
Hypothalamo-hypophyseal portal system
Posterior pituitary
RFs
Anterior pituitary
(+)
Oxytocin
PRL
Suckling
Milk synthesis and secretion
MG
Milk ejection
MG = mammary gland
SON = supraoptic nuclei
PVN = paraventricular nuclei
RFs = releasing factors
B
Reflexes originating in birth canal
↑Fetal oxytocin
(+)
↑Wall tension
↑Myometrial contractility
PGR
OR
↑Oxytocin
?
(+)
PGs
↑Estrogen/Progesterone
PGR = prostaglandin receptor
OR = oxytocin receptor
(+)
(+)
C
Oxytocin
Outer membrane
Oxytocin receptor
G_s protein
SFA
AA
PIP_2
(+)
(+)
Endometrial cell
Inner membrane
Phospholipase C
Phospholipase A_2
DG
IP_3
(+)
(+)
ER
PKC
Arachidonic acid
Ca^{2+}/CaM
Nucleus
DNA
Cyclooxygenase
mRNA
Protein phosphorylation
RNA polymerase
Blocked by NSAID
Cellular response
Estrogen/ progesterone
EPR
Ribosomal protein synthesis
Oxytocin
PGs
Ca^{2+}
Oxytocin receptor
PG receptor
Sarcoplasmic R
Ca^{2+}
Myometrial cell
Ca^{2+}
Ca^{2+}
Contraction of myosin filaments
Expulsion of fetus

Overview

- Oxytocin plays important roles in both parturition and lactation.

Oxytocin is a nonapeptide (9 amino acids) synthesized in nuclei of the hypothalamus and stored in the posterior pituitary (see Chapter 25). Lesser amounts are also synthesized and secreted by the CL. In concert with estrogen and prostaglandin ($PGF_{2\alpha}$), CL-derived oxytocin may be involved with dissolution of the CL after an estrous cycle in which pregnancy did not occur.

Plasma levels of oxytocin are normally low in males and nongravid females. In pregnant females, however, concentrations increase substantially during parturition and following suckling during lactation. The two primary functions of pituitary-derived oxytocin appear to be: 1) contraction of myoepithelial cells that surround alveoli and ducts of mammary glands to eject milk; and 2) facilitation of uterine myometrial contraction during (and after) labor.

Oxytocin and Lactation

Exposure of mammary glands to estrogen during pregnancy causes development of myoepithelial cells that line ducts and alveoli, as well as development of oxytocin receptors on these cells so that they can respond to oxytocin following the suckling stimulus. As discussed in Chapter 18, PRL stimulates milk synthesis and secretion, while oxytocin causes contraction of myoepithelial cells for milk ejection (**Part A**). Oxytocin release is brought about through a neuroendocrine reflex, whereby suckling of the neonate sends neural impulses from the mammary gland to the hypothalamus, which then directs release of oxytocin from the posterior pituitary into the general circulation. Oxytocin may also have a stimulatory effect on PRL release (see Chapter 6); however, no distinct hormone-releasing role for this peptide has been established.

Lactation is generally considered a vegetative experience. Fright and stress are known to inhibit milk ejection through mobilization of catecholamines into the general circulation. Catecholamines, in turn, are thought to act at three levels to block milk ejection: 1) centrally by blocking oxytocin release; 2) peripherally by vasoconstricting arterioles, thus reducing the amount of oxytocin available to myoepithelial cells of mammary glands; and 3) directly as an antagonist to oxytocin on myoepithelial cells.

Oxytocin release may also be conditioned by a variety of visual, olfactory, and auditory stimuli (such as crying of the young or rattling of the milk bucket).

Oxytocin and Copulation

Genital stimulation involved in coitus releases oxytocin, which produces rhythmic contractions in the female reproductive tract as well as contraction of the vas deferens and epididymis in the male during ejaculation. The sensation of orgasm, which involves rhythmic contractions of reproductive smooth muscle in both males and females, may be induced by oxytocin. Whether the specialized contractions of the uterus and oviducts that propel sperm involve oxytocin has not been proven; however, it is possible that increased contraction of smooth muscle of the vas deferens and epididymis by oxytocin propels sperm toward the urethra.

Oxytocin and Parturition

The precise role of oxytocin in labor is enigmatic. Unquestionably, this peptide hormone causes myometrial contraction (providing the uterus is under estrogen dominance). Furthermore, its secretion can be reflexively increased by stretching the lower genital tract (**Part B**). However, maternal plasma oxytocin levels show no consistent rise immediately prior to or during early labor, although they do increase during the later stages. Fetal production is thought to contribute to this latter rise, and it has been suggested that the protracted labor seen in mothers carrying anencephalic fetuses (those lacking a brain) may be a consequence of the lack of fetal stimulus.

On the other hand, uterine oxytocin receptors do increase throughout gestation, and dramatically so at term (under the stimulatory effects of estrogen). While labor can proceed without oxytocin, its most important roles may be to: 1) work synergistically with estrogen in promoting endometrial prostaglandin synthesis, and 2) work synergistically with those prostaglandins in promoting maximal uterine contractions after delivery of the fetus, thereby minimizing blood loss.

A relatively low estrogen-to-progesterone ratio is important in maintaining uterine quiescence throughout pregnancy. An increase in this ratio precedes labor (due to increased fetal adrenal cortical activity and therefore estrogen precursor synthesis from pregnenolone) and is most likely a parturition-initiating event in most domestic animal species, because estrogen stimulates and progesterone inhibits endometrial prostaglandin and myometrial oxytocin receptor synthesis (**Part B** and **Part C**). Evidence also indicates that a placental progesterone-binding protein exists whose concentration may be increased by estrogen near term, causing an effective removal of free progesterone from the myometrium and thereby decreasing uterine quiescence. It has also been reported that unconjugated estrogen levels rise at term, thus increasing the amount of active estrogen available to enter target cells.

Estrogens and progesterone, respectively, act through receptor-mediated processes to stimulate and suppress the synthesis of mRNA essential for production of cyclooxygenase in the endometrium (**Part C**). The local decrease in the effectiveness of progesterone associated with continued action of estrogen also increases myometrial oxytocin receptor synthesis as well as prostaglandin (PG) levels in uterine fluid. In addition, PG production is increased by oxytocin, which also acts via receptor binding to the endometrium. Prostaglandins and oxytocin then act directly on uterine musculature to simulate contractions. Activation of contractile processes requires an increase in cytoplasmic Ca^{2+}, which is achieved by decreased binding of Ca^{2+} to subcellular membranes and by influx into the cell.

When oxytocin interacts with its plasma membrane receptors on endometrial cells, activation of membrane-bound phospholipase C (through G_s protein) catalyzes hydrolysis of the phosphatidylinositol 4,5-bisphosphate (PIP_2) moiety off membrane-bound phospholipid to produce diacylglycerol (DG) and inositol triphosphate (IP_3). Both DG and IP_3 act as intracellular messengers, DG as a membrane-associated activator of protein kinase C (PKC) and IP_3 as a water-soluble inducer of Ca^{2+} release from mitochondria and the endoplasmic reticulum (ER), thereby causing a transient rise in the Ca^{2+}/CaM concentration of the cytosol. These two effects initiate a cellular response (see Chapter 4). The DG is hydrolyzed further by phospholipase A_2 to form arachidonic acid (AA), a precursor to the prostaglandins, plus a monoglyceride (with a saturated fatty acid attached to the A_1 position). The monoglyceride is recycled into the membrane during the formation of another membrane-bound phospholipid. Cyclooxygenase inhibitors, such as nonsteroidal antiinflammatory drugs (NSAIDs) that reduce endometrial cell prostaglandin formation, can potentially abolish premature labor; however, they also close the ductus arteriosus, leading to fetal pulmonary hypertension.

Other Effects of Oxytocin

Oxytocin reduces blood pressure in birds, and severe water retention can occur in mammals who receive high doses of oxytocin to promote uterine contractions during labor. High doses of oxytocin also stimulate ADH receptors.

25 Antidiuretic Hormone and Diabetes Insipidus: I

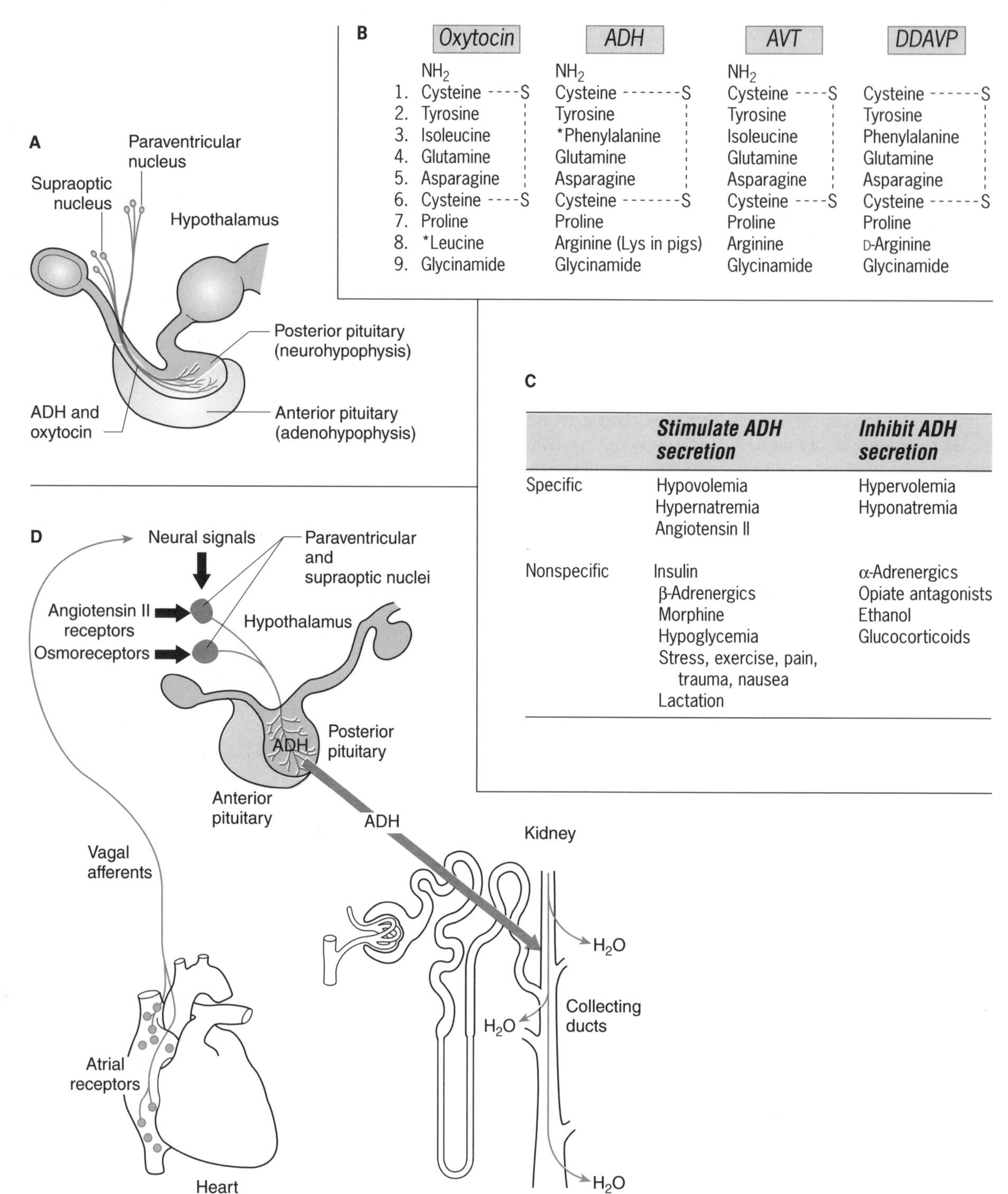

B

	Oxytocin	ADH	AVT	DDAVP
	NH_2	NH_2	NH_2	
1.	Cysteine ----S	Cysteine -------S	Cysteine ----S	Cysteine ------S
2.	Tyrosine	Tyrosine	Tyrosine	Tyrosine
3.	Isoleucine	*Phenylalanine	Isoleucine	Phenylalanine
4.	Glutamine	Glutamine	Glutamine	Glutamine
5.	Asparagine	Asparagine	Asparagine	Asparagine
6.	Cysteine ----S	Cysteine -------S	Cysteine ----S	Cysteine ------S
7.	Proline	Proline	Proline	Proline
8.	*Leucine	Arginine (Lys in pigs)	Arginine	D-Arginine
9.	Glycinamide	Glycinamide	Glycinamide	Glycinamide

C

	Stimulate ADH secretion	***Inhibit ADH secretion***
Specific	Hypovolemia Hypernatremia Angiotensin II	Hypervolemia Hyponatremia
Nonspecific	Insulin β-Adrenergics Morphine Hypoglycemia Stress, exercise, pain, trauma, nausea Lactation	α-Adrenergics Opiate antagonists Ethanol Glucocorticoids

Source: Part A modified from Chastain CB, Ganjam VK. Clinical endocrinology of companion animals. 1st ed. Philadelphia, PA: Lea & Febiger, 1986:47.

Overview

- Oxytocin and vasopressin (ADH) are neurohormones.
- Oxytocin and ADH are synthesized in the hypothalamus and secreted by the posterior pituitary.
- Arginine vasotocin (ACT) is secreted by the posterior pituitary of nonmammalian vertebrates.
- 1-Desamino-8-D-arginine (DDAVP) is a synthetic form of ADH used in the treatment of patients with diabetes insipidus.
- Secretion of ADH is regulated primarily by the osmolarity of plasma and changes in the blood volume and/or pressure.
- Lactation is a stimulus for ADH as well as oxytocin release.

Antidiuretic hormone (*ADH* or *arginine vasopressin, AVP*), a nonapeptide secreted by the posterior pituitary, inhibits diuresis and regulates urinary osmolarity by increasing permeability of the distal convoluted tubule and collecting ducts so that water is reabsorbed into the hypertonic interstitium. Without the effects of ADH, the urine produced is voluminous and hypotonic to plasma (hyposthenuric polyuria), a condition known as *diabetes insipidus* (DI).

Neuropeptides of the Posterior Pituitary

Although the posterior pituitary contains several neuropeptides that may possess important physiologic actions, the best characterized are oxytocin (see Chapter 24) and ADH. Both are neurohormones synthesized by paraventricular and supraoptic nuclei of the hypothalamus **Part A.** Each has a characteristic neurophysin associated with it as it passes down axons to be stored in granules of the neurohypophysis (posterior pituitary). Both the neuropeptide and its neurophysin are exocytosed into the general circulation following an action potential; however, they quickly dissociate in plasma. Neurophysins were originally thought to be binding polypeptides, but it now appears that they may be parts of their precursor.

In hippopotamuses and most pigs, arginine of the more typical mammalian AVP molecule is replaced by lysine to form *lysine vasopressin* (**Part B**). The posterior pituitary of some species of pigs and marsupials contains a mixture of arginine and lysine vasopressin. Each is a nonapeptide consisting of a six-member disulfide-containing ring. The structures of ADH and oxytocin differ by only two amino acids, and both are derived from a single precursor present in nonmammalian vertebrates, *arginine vasotocin (AVT)* (see **Part B**), that exhibits similar physiologic properties. The arginine in position 8 of ADH is critical to its pressor activity but not its diuretic action. Substitution of D-arginine in this position, along with removal of the terminal amino group of cysteine, produces a highly potent and long-acting antidiuretic peptide possessing virtually no pressor activity, namely 1-*desamino-8-D-arginine vasopressin (DDAVP)* (see **Part B**). This agent is the drug of choice in treating DI.

Factors Regulating ADH Secretion

Stimuli and inhibitors of ADH secretion are presented in **Part C.** Secretion of ADH is regulated mainly by the osmolarity of plasma and changes in blood volume and/or pressure. Hypothalamic nuclei that synthesize ADH (or some closely related nuclei) act as osmoreceptors, sensing modest changes in plasma osmolarity (namely the Na^+ concentration). An increase in plasma osmolarity of only 1% causes these osmoreceptors to shrink and to initiate nerve impulses that release ADH. Conversely, when plasma osmolarity is reduced, secretion is inhibited. Because ADH is rapidly degraded in plasma (plasma $t_{1/2}$ is approximately 5 to 10 minutes), circulating levels can be reduced to zero within minutes after secretion is inhibited. As a result, the ADH system can respond rapidly to fluctuations in plasma osmolarity.

A decrease in blood volume or pressure is sensed by low-pressure stretch receptors (i.e., baroreceptors) in the left atrium and high-pressure receptors in the aortic arch and carotid sinus. Signals from these receptors are relayed to ADH secretory neurons via afferent fibers in the vagus nerve. The sensitivity of this baroreceptor system is less than that of the osmoreceptors, and a 5% to 10% change in volume is required to alter ADH secretion.

Decreases in blood volume and/or pressure are also sensed by juxtaglomerular (JG) cells in the kidney that synthesize and secrete renin. As pressure declines, renin levels increase, which in turn elevates plasma levels of angiotensin II (see Chapters 39 and 40). Angiotensin II is a potent vasoconstrictor, as well as a stimulus for thirst and aldosterone and ADH release. **Part D** depicts the regulation of ADH secretion and its effect on water retention in the kidney.

26 Antidiuretic Hormone and Diabetes Insipidus: II

E Medullary Collecting Duct of the Kidney

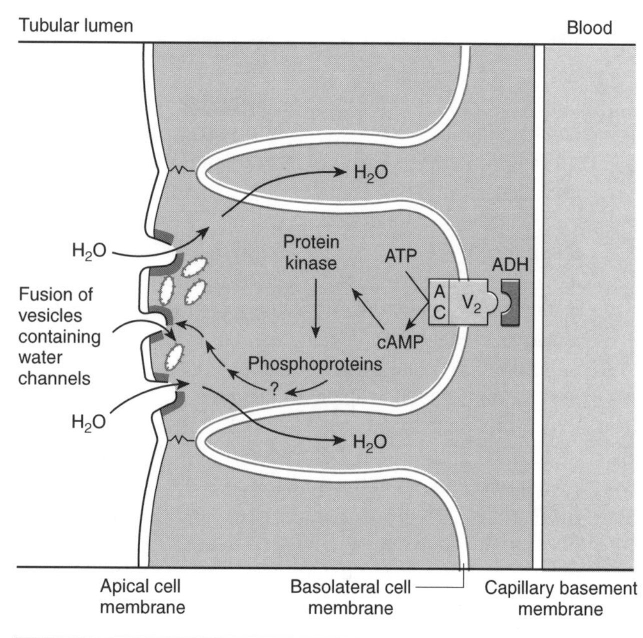

F

ADH Receptor	*Second Messenger*	*Function*
V_{1A}	↑IP_3, Ca^{2+}	Vasoconstriction, Hepatic glycogenolysis, CNS transmitter
V_{1B}	↑IP_3, Ca^{2+}	ACTH secretion
V_2	↑cAMP	Renal water retention

G

Causes of Diabetes Insipidus		
Central	CDI may result from any condition that damages the neurohypophyseal system (e.g., trauma, neoplasia, infections, vascular (aneurysms), cysts, autoimmune hypothalamitis. Permanent CDI usually requires an injury causing bilateral neuronal degeneration of supraoptic and paraventricular nuclei.	
Nephrogenic		
Primary (familial) NDI	Congenital defect involving impaired renal responsiveness to ADH	
Secondary (acquired) NDI	Pyometra:	*Escherichia coli*-associated pyometra can cause reversible renal tubular insensitivity to ADH.
	Hypercalcemia:	Damages renal tubular ADH receptors and inactivates adenyl cyclase.
	Hepatic insufficiency:	Decreased urea production decreases the renal medullary concentration gradient.
	Hyperadrenocorticism:	Cortisol interferes with ADH action.
	Hypoadrenocorticism:	Aldosterone deficiency, renal medullary solute washout, and loss of the medullary concentration gradient.
	Pyelonephritis:	Inflammation of the renal pelvis.
	Hypokalemia:	Collecting ducts are less responsive to ADH.
	Hyperthyroidism:	Mechanism unclear.

Source: Part E modified from Berne RM, Levy MN. Principles of physiology. 1st ed. St. Louis: Mosby, 1990:447.

Overview

- ADH is important in the minute-to-minute control of blood volume and pressure.
- ADH acts through cAMP in the collecting ducts of the kidney.
- ADH may act through the Ca^{2+}-calmodulin messenger system in other cell types.
- In large amounts ADH stimulates ACTH secretion, which in turn elevates circulating glucocorticoid levels.
- Patients with diabetes insipidus (DI) exhibit PU/PD.
- DI can be of central (CDI) or renal (i.e., nephrogenic, NDI) origin.
- DDAVP exhibits hemostatic as well as antidiuretic properties.

Primary Action of ADH

Blood pressure determines the glomerular filtration rate (GFR) in the kidneys. The filtrate normally lacks plasma proteins and cellular components of blood, and the initial concentrations of solutes like Na^+, glucose, and amino acids are identical to those in plasma. Numerous mechanisms operate to return solutes and most of the water back into blood; however, if something interferes with these reabsorption processes, a larger than normal amount of urine will be produced (i.e., diuresis). Should more reabsorption occur than normal, more fluid is reabsorbed and antidiuresis results. Regulation of water reabsorption in the kidney is essential in the maintenance of a normal blood volume and pressure.

As previously stated (see Chapter 25), an increase in the osmolarity of plasma or a decrease in blood pressure triggers release of ADH, which in turn causes increased water reabsorption in the kidneys and, thus, antidiuresis. Similarly, an increase in blood pressure and/or a decrease in the osmolarity of plasma represses ADH release, and causes diuresis with a corresponding drop in blood volume and pressure. Thus, ADH is important in the minute-to-minute control of blood volume and pressure because it is stored by the posterior pituitary, and can be released quickly upon demand. Another important action of ADH occurs in the brain, where it stimulates thirst (like angiotensin II). Consumption of water will also add fluid to the vascular system, and will thus increase blood pressure.

Antidiuretic hormone acts in the kidney to increase permeability of the collecting ducts to water.

A simplified model of this action is shown in **Part E.** ADH binds to a V_2 receptor on the basolateral membrane of renal target cells. Binding to this receptor, which is coupled to adenyl cyclase, increases intracellular levels of cAMP, which in turn activates one or more protein kinases. Phosphorylated proteins resulting from this next act to insert water channels (aquaporins) into the apical (i.e., luminal) membrane. Aquaporins are found not only in the collecting ducts of the kidney, but also in the brain, salivary and lacrimal glands, and respiratory tract.

There are at least three types of ADH receptors: V_{1A}, V_{1B}, and V_2. All are G protein–coupled (**Part F**).

Secondary Actions of ADH

The pressor actions of ADH include vasoconstriction of systemic, coronary, and pulmonary blood vessels, and dilation of cerebral and renal vessels. The dose of ADH that produces pressor activity is about 100 times the dose that provides its antidiuretic action; therefore, ADH is probably not a physiologic pressor agent in mammals. However, high doses of ADH can cause constriction of arteriolar smooth muscle and elevate the blood pressure. This may increase the glomerular filtration rate enough to override the antidiuretic action of ADH and, therefore, produce a net diuresis.

In large amounts, ADH also stimulates secretion of ACTH. An ADH response test using changes produced in serum cortisol levels has been recommended as an indicator of hypothalamic–pituitary function. An increase in serum cortisol after administration of ADH would indicate normal adenohypophyseal function. Conversely, high circulating levels of cortisol inhibit ADH release as well as its effects on the kidney (**Part C,** Chapters 35 and 37).

Diabetes Insipidus

Patients with diabetes insipidus (DI) produce rather large volumes of dilute, tasteless (i.e., insipid) urine, and therefore exhibit dire thirst.

Although several factors can cause polyuria/polydipsia (PU/PD) in domestic animals, DI is suspected when water consumption is greater than 100 mL/kg/day and urine production (without glucose) is greater than 50 mL/kg/day. The causes of DI can be of central (CDI) or renal origin (**Part G**). Central diabetes insipidus can result from destruction of ADH production sites in the hypothalamus (the supraoptic and paraventricular nuclei), loss of major axons that carry ADH to its storage sites in the posterior pituitary, or disruption of the ability to release stored ADH. Nephrogenic diabetes insipidus (NDI) can be caused by a number of etiologies that result in the inability of the kidneys to respond to ADH. Plasma ADH concentrations can be normal to elevated in NDI.

Many patients with DI are simply classified as being **idiopathic** (i.e., denoting that they possess a disease of unknown origin), and exhibit no other evidence of neuroendocrine dysfunction. Excessive water intake can also give rise to polyuria, and, therefore, is sometimes classified as a type of DI. Excessive drinking may be a behavioral problem (i.e., psychogenic polydipsia), or it may result from a malfunction in the thirst mechanism (dipsogenic DI).

Desmopressin (1-desamino-8-D-arginine vasopressin, DDAVP, **Part B**) is a synthetic analog of the naturally occurring ADH, and is the drug of choice for treating DI. Desmopressin not only has antidiuretic properties, but also hemostatic properties. It causes platelet aggregation and the release of hemostatic factors in dogs, and, therefore, is sometimes used in the treatment of bleeding disorders. The biological half-life of DDAVP is reported to be 4 to 8 times longer than the natural hormone, and is sometimes administered intranasally or instilled into the conjunctival sac. Although patients with idiopathic DI can sometimes be treated favorably, patients with nephrogenic DI and those with hypothalamic or pituitary tumors have a less favorable prognosis, particularly if neurologic signs are evident. Central DI due to head trauma has a variable prognosis, with some patients recovering satisfactorily.

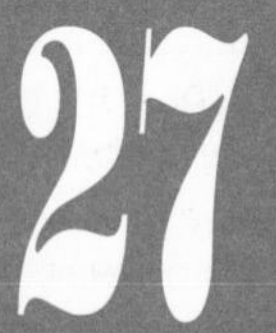

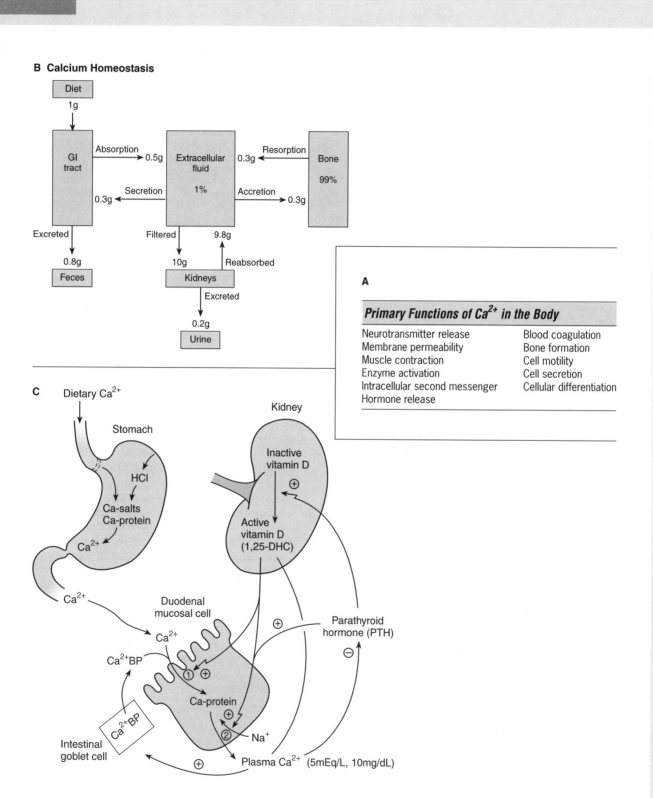

Calcium, Magnesium, and Phosphate: I

B Calcium Homeostasis

A

Primary Functions of Ca^{2+} in the Body	
Neurotransmitter release	Blood coagulation
Membrane permeability	Bone formation
Muscle contraction	Cell motility
Enzyme activation	Cell secretion
Intracellular second messenger	Cellular differentiation
Hormone release	

C

Overview

- Calcium (Ca^{2+}) is necessary for many body functions.
- The [Ca^{2+}] of extracellular fluid is normally about 1000 times greater than that in the cytoplasm of cells.
- Ca^{2+} is compartmentalized within cells.
- Only about 40% of the Ca^{2+} in the GI tract normally gets absorbed.
- About 40% of the calcium in plasma is complexed with protein and therefore does not get filtered by the kidneys.
- 1,25-DHC regulates Ca^{2+} absorption in the GI tract.
- PTH is a key Ca^{2+}-regulatory hormone.
- Acidosis can cause hypercalcemia, and therefore decreased neuromuscular excitability.

Serum calcium (Ca^{2+}), magnesium (Mg^{2+}), and phosphate (PO_4^{3-}) levels are closely regulated in all domestic animal species by the actions of vitamin D, PTH, and calcitonin on the GI tract, bone, and kidneys. The active form of vitamin D (1,25-dihydroxycholecalciferol, 1,25-DHC) and PTH tend to raise serum Ca^{2+} levels, which are counterbalanced by calcitonin. Other hormones such as glucocorticoids, estrogens, glucagon, and growth hormone play minor regulatory roles.

Calcium

The calcium concentration of extracellular fluid and that in the cytoplasm of cells must be regulated within narrow limits if normal body functions are to be maintained. Calcium ions serve many important roles in the body (**Part A**). They are important components of bones and teeth, they are responsible for excitation and contraction of muscle cells, as well as the induction of spontaneous excitations of cardiac pacemaker cells. Calcium ions are essential for exocytosis of secretion granules in neurons and glandular cells, and they serve as second messengers in many target cells. Certain key metabolic enzymes are activated by intracellular Ca^{2+}, and Ca^{2+} serves as a cofactor for several important blood-clotting proteins (factors VII, IX, and X).

Calcium is the fifth most abundant element in the body. Nearly 99% is found in the skeletal system, where calcium, together with phosphate, is essential for bone strength and serves as a storehouse to replenish serum deficits. However, less than 1% of skeletal Ca^{2+} is available normally for free exchange with extracellular fluid (ECF) (**Part B**).

The normal ECF concentration, which is carefully regulated at about 10 mg/dL (5 mEq/L), changes little over a lifetime despite major fluctuations in dietary Ca^{2+}, Ca^{2+} entering and leaving bone, renal Ca^{2+} excretion, and the additional demands of pregnancy or lactation. Intracellular Ca^{2+} is compartmentalized, yet the free cytoplasmic concentration (normally about 1000 times lower than the ECF concentration) can change dramatically as a result of release from intracellular stores and influx from the ECF.

An ordinary 75-kg adult mammal ingests about 1 g/day of calcium in food and liquid (as shown in **Part B**). Calcium also enters the gut in digestive secretions and as part of desquamated mucosal cells. Also, during active glucose absorption intercellular spaces between mucosal cells become swollen, and Ca^{2+} gets secreted into the lumen through tight junctions. Total Ca^{2+} entering the lumen by these means (less ingestion) amounts to about 0.3 g/day. Consequently, about 1.3 g/day is available for absorption. Approximately 0.5 g is absorbed (38% of that available), and 0.8 g is excreted in the stool. Although 0.5 g/day is absorbed, net absorption amounts to only 0.2 g/day.

Active absorption occurs primarily in the upper small intestine (i.e., duodenum) by a two-step mechanism (**Part C**). Calcium is not ionized at neutral pH. Instead, gastric HCl helps to solubilize calcium salts and free Ca^{2+} from dietary protein, thus permitting small intestinal absorption. Calcium is bound in the duodenum to a specific calcium-binding protein (Ca^{2+}BP) whose synthesis is stimulated by 1,25-DHC. Calcium-binding protein is synthesized and secreted into the intestinal lumen by mucus-secreting goblet cells. In the lumen it binds Ca^{2+}, and the complex is then absorbed through the luminal membrane into the epithelial cell. This step occurs by *facilitated diffusion* (step *1* in **Part C**), with the carrier molecule being responsive to 1,25-DHC. Calcium is sequestered within mucosal cells either by Ca^{2+}BP or by cell organelles, because it is important for the function of cells that the concentration of free Ca^{2+} in the cytoplasm be maintained at a low concentration (about 10^{-6}M). Calcium is then extruded into interstitial fluid by *active transport* (step *2* in **Part C**), where it then gains access to blood. Step *2* is positively affected by both PTH and 1,25-DHC. Continued removal of Ca^{2+} into blood sets up a concentration gradient for step *1* (which is saturable only at concentrations greater than those normally found in the lumen).

Serum Ca^{2+} exists in more than one form, yet about 50% is ionized. Ionized Ca^{2+} is the only form that influences secretion of PTH and can be used for the maintenance of neuromuscular excitability and blood coagulation. Approximately 10% to 15% of serum calcium is complexed with phosphate, citrate, or bicarbonate, while 40% is protein bound to albumin and, to a much lesser extent, α- and β-globulins. Complexed and protein-bound forms are circulating storage forms from which Ca^{2+} can be readily released.

Plasma proteins are more ionized when the ECF pH is high (alkalosis), providing more protein anion to bind with Ca^{2+}. Conversely, in acidosis plasma proteins become less ionized, thereby giving up their bound Ca^{2+}. Hypercalcemia, which can result from acidosis, also occurs with excessive resorption of bone or increased absorption from the GI tract. Hypercalcemia generally results in decreased neuromuscular excitability (as well as "bones, groans, and stones"), while hypocalcemia results in increased neuromuscular excitability (and tetany) (see Chapter 31).

28 Calcium, Magnesium, and Phosphate: II

D

Primary Functions of Mg^{2+} in the Body	
Enzyme activation (Cofactor for various kinases)	Regulation of protein synthesis. Complexes with ADP and ATP (holds ATP in position so that ATPase can attach)
Suppression of Ca^2 release from the sarcoplasmic reticulum	Structural component of bones and teeth

E Magnesium Homeostasis

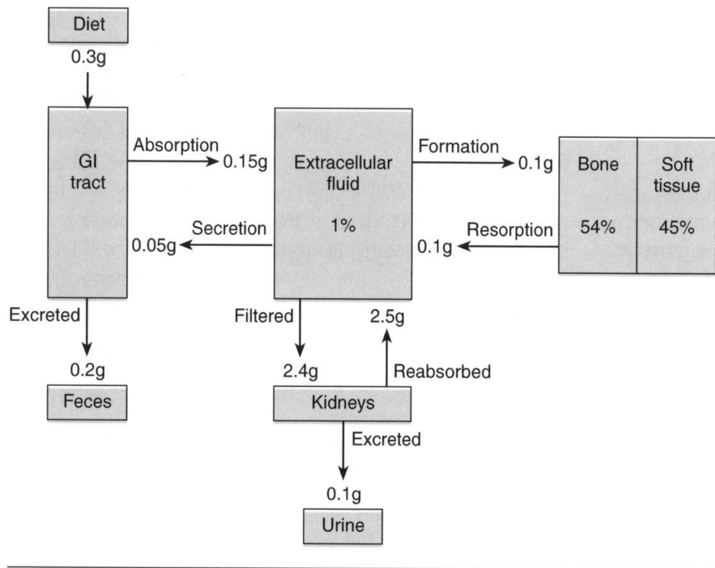

F

Primary Functions of PO_4^{3-} in the Body	
Major intracellular anion	Component of ADP and ATP
Component of all membranes (i.e., phospholipids)	Regulates enzyme action and protein function
Structural component of bones and teeth	Urinary buffer

G Phosphate Homeostasis

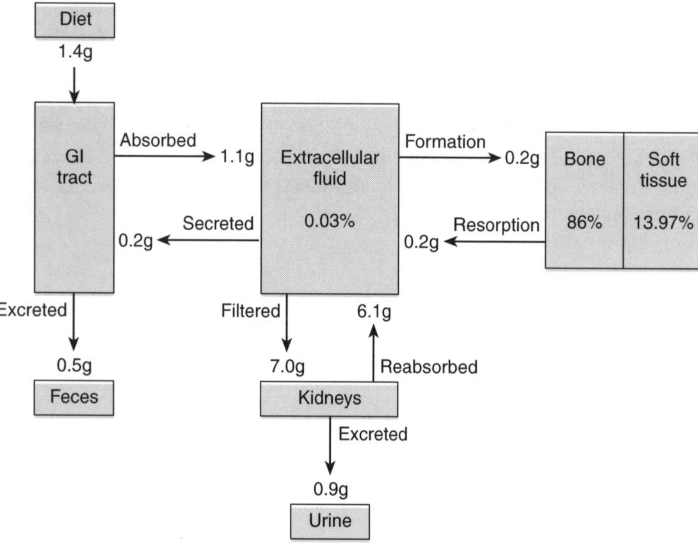

Overview

- Insulin stimulates translocation of Mg^{2+}, K^+, and PO_4^{3-} into cells.
- PO_4^{3-} is the most plentiful intracellular anion and Mg^{2+} is the second most plentiful intracellular cation.
- Ca^{2+} and Mg^{2+} are bound to serum protein but PO_4^{3-} is not.
- Mg^{2+} blocks Ca^{2+} channels.
- Urinary HPO_4^{2-} is an important buffer.
- Release of PO_4^{3-} from bone is stimulated by the same factors that release Ca^{2+}.
- Renal reabsorption of Ca^{2+}, Mg^{2+}, and PO_4^{3-} is hormone dependent.

Magnesium

Magnesium, the second most abundant intracellular cation in the body, has several roles including enzyme activation, regulation of protein synthesis, and suppression of Ca^{2+} release from the sarcoplasmic reticulum (**Part D**). About 54% of Mg^{2+} is in bone, 45% is in the intracellular fluid of soft tissue, and only 1% is in ECF (**Part E**). Effects of Mg^{2+} on central and peripheral nerves mimic those of Ca^{2+}; that is, Mg^{2+} enhances excitation when deficiencies exist and depresses it when excesses occur. The synthesis, release, and target cell effects of PTH also require Mg^{2+}, but excessive levels inhibit PTH secretion and possibly its action on target cells. Normal plasma Mg^{2+} concentrations are about 1.5 to 2.5 mEq/L. One-fourth of plasma Mg^{2+} is protein bound. Free plasma Mg^{2+} is freely filtered and extensively reabsorbed by the kidneys, a process that is increased by PTH. Serum Mg^{2+} concentrations decrease with acute PTH deficiency resulting from parathyroidectomy. Magnesium is by no means efficiently absorbed across the GI tract, and it is of variable bioavailability, depending on dietary composition. However, when dietary intake is restricted, intestinal absorption rises (although the hormones and factors responsible for this phenomenon remain unknown). It does not compete with Ca^{2+} for absorption, and *it is not actively absorbed across the GI tract.* Absorption generally depends on load. Magnesium, like Ca^{2+}, is wasted by the kidneys in acidosis, and an alkaline pH in the GI tract impairs absorption. Serious Mg^{2+} depletion can occur from intestinal malabsorption or diuretic overuse. In rare circumstances, dangerous ventricular arrhythmias have been observed.

Insulin stimulates the translocation of Mg^{2+}, K^+, PO_4^{3-}, and nucleosides into cells independent of its actions on glucose uptake (see Chapter 54). Therefore, insulin, secreted largely in response to a carbohydrate load, lowers serum Mg^{2+}, K^+, and PO_4^{3-}, and is considered to be an important regulator of K^+ balance [along with aldosterone and epinephrine (see Chapter 38)]. Insulin also assists in the reabsorption of K^+, Na^+, and PO_4^{3-} by the renal tubules. **Part E** shows the processes affecting magnesium homeostasis (based on the normal dietary intake of 0.3 g/day by a 75-kg mammal).

Phosphate

Calcium and PO_4^{3-} concentrations in the body are regulated in such a way that the product of the free plasma concentrations of each equals a constant $[([Ca^{2+}][PO_4^{3-}]) = k]$. This constant, however, will change according to different physiologic states or pathophysiologic conditions. For example, k is greater in growing, than in adult animals. This relationship implies that if there is an increase in the $[Ca^{2+}]$ of extracellular fluid, a corresponding decrease in the $[PO_4^{3-}]$ will occur. Likewise, an increase in the $[PO_4^{3-}]$ of extracellular fluid should cause a decrease in the $[Ca^{2+}]$. This generalization is useful for illustrating some of the relationships that exist between the regulatory mechanisms governing these two ions. Minute-to-minute adjustments in the concentrations of these two ions in extracellular fluid are accomplished primarily through a combination of bone destruction (resorption) or formation (accretion), an increase in the efficiency of absorption of these ions from the small intestine, and/or alterations in their renal excretion.

Phosphate is concentrated in cells, it is the most plentiful intracellular anion, and it is an important component of many organic molecules, including DNA, RNA, ATP, and intermediates of several metabolic pathways (**Part F**). Along with Ca^{2+}, it is a major constituent of bone [i.e., hydroxyapatite ($Ca_{10}[PO_4]_6[OH]_2$)]. In addition, urinary PO_4^{3-} is an important buffer (titratable acidity). Eighty-six percent of PO_4^{3-} is in bone, 13.97% is in intracellular fluid, and only 0.03% is in ECF (**Part G**). The plasma PO_4^{3-} concentration is normally about the same as the Mg^{2+} concentration: 2 mEq/L. Phosphate absorption in the intestinal tract occurs by both active and passive processes; it increases as dietary PO_4^{3-} rises, and is stimulated by 1,25-DHC (like Ca^{2+}). Unless otherwise needed for growth or lactation, the amount excreted in urine generally equals the net amount absorbed by the GI tract. Thus, the kidney plays a vital role in PO_4^{3-} homeostasis. Release of PO_4^{3-} is stimulated by the same factors that release Ca^{2+}, PTH and 1,25-DHC, and its entry into cells is stimulated by insulin. **Part G** shows the processes affecting phosphate homeostasis (based on the normal dietary intake of 1.4 g/day by a 75-kg mammal).

Unlike Ca^{2+} and Mg^{2+}, serum PO_4^{3-} is not protein bound, so it readily passes through glomeruli in the kidney. Usually, 85% to 90% of PO_4^{3-} in the glomerular filtrate is reabsorbed in the proximal convoluted tubule. This renal reabsorption process is inhibited by expansion of the ECF volume, hypercalcemia, and the hormones PTH, calcitonin, and cortisol (all are phosphaturic). Elevated serum PO_4^{3-} tends to enhance the secretion of PTH indirectly by binding with Ca^{2+}, thereby suppressing the free ionized Ca^{2+} level.

29 Parathormone, Calcitonin, and Vitamin D: I

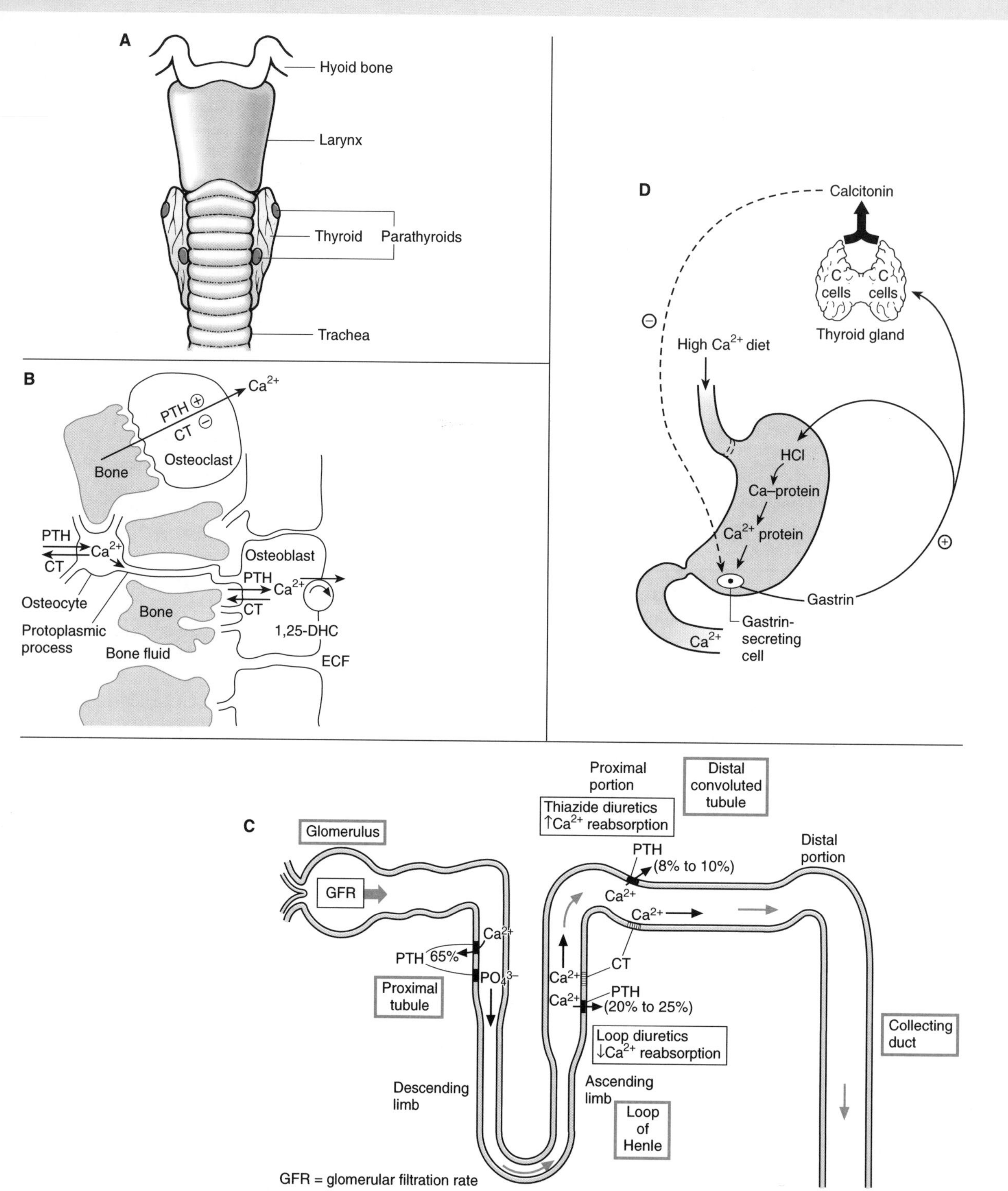

Source: Part A modified from Chastain CB, Ganjam VK. Clinical endocrinology of companion animals, 1st ed. Philadelphia, PA: Lea & Febiger, 1986:180. **Part B** modified from Ganong WF. Review of medical physiology. 10th ed. Los Altos, CA: Lange Medical Publications, 1981:310.

Overview

- PTH, CT, and vitamin D help to maintain Ca^{2+}, Mg^{2+}, and PO_4^{3-} homeostasis.
- PTH and vitamin D act to elevate the plasma ionized Ca^{2+} concentration, while CT acts to lower it.
- PTH, like CT, is phosphaturic.
- PTH_{rp} exhibits all the actions of PTH on bone and kidney.
- CT may help to protect the mother from excessive bone loss during pregnancy.

Parathormone (PTH), a protein hormone of 84 amino acid residues, is the only known secretion of the parathyroid glands. The biologic activity of PTH resides in the first 34 amino acids, and it interacts with calcitonin and vitamin D to maintain calcium (Ca^{2+}), phosphate (PO_4^{3-}), and magnesium (Mg^{2+}) homeostasis.

Parathyroid Glands and PTH

The parathyroid glands are found in all air-breathing vertebrates, and appear first in amphibians coincident with their transition to terrestrial life. Investigators have suggested that the appearance of parathyroid glands may have arisen from a need to protect against the development of hypocalcemia, as well as the necessity to maintain skeletal integrity. Terrestrial animals, compared to their aquatic cousins, live in a relatively low calcium, high phosphate environment.

The parathyroids may be embedded within the thyroid glands (as in mice, dogs, cats, and humans) or lie separately near the thyroids (as in goats and rabbits) (**Part A**). Consequently, thyroidectomy may result in a lowered plasma Ca^{2+} concentration because of simultaneous removal of parathyroid tissue.

The parathyroids have two types of cells: *chief cells* (or "principal" cells) and *oxyphil cells.* Chief cells have a clear cytoplasm and are the PTH-secreting cells. They are also part of the amine precursor uptake and decarboxylation (APUD) series of cells (see Chapter 63). Oxyphils, which represent only 1% of total parathyroid tissue, are apparently inactive. The number of oxyphils is reported to increase with age, however, and oxyphils are generally more rare in some species than in others (e.g., horses have comparatively more oxyphils than dogs and cats).

Serum ionized Ca^{2+} (not protein-bound calcium) **has the greatest influence on PTH release.** Although Mg^{2+} is only one-half to one-third as potent as Ca^{2+} on PTH secretion, it appears that a basal level of Mg^{2+} is needed for optimal release, as wide fluctuations in the serum Mg^{2+} concentration ($>\uparrow\downarrow Mg^{2+}$) inhibit PTH release. Also, chief cells are known to contain β-adrenergic and glucocorticoid receptors, indicating that "physiologic stress" may also increase PTH release.

Parathormone is degraded by its target cells. Metabolic degradation by the kidney, for example, involves specific proteases on the surface of renal tubular epithelial cells, as well as lysosomal enzymes within those cells. The circulating half-life of PTH in mammals is generally less than 20 minutes.

The primary function of PTH is to elevate the serum ionized Ca^{2+} concentration by stimulating bone resorption (dissolution), renal Ca^{2+} reabsorption (and PO_4^{3-} excretion), and renal vitamin D activation. Because Ca^{2+} is partially bound to PO_4^{3-} in the circulation, the phosphaturic effect of PTH has a tendency to elevate the serum free ionized Ca^{2+} concentration.

Actions of PTH on bone involve activation of adenyl cyclase, with consequent increased formation of cAMP. This action may first involve prostaglandin formation. The hormone increases activity of osteoclasts, osteocysts, and osteoblasts in moving Ca^{2+} into the ECF (**Part B**). On a long-term basis, PTH promotes formation of more osteoclasts while inhibiting osteoblast formation. Local release of lysosomal enzymes from osteoclasts and end products of glycolysis create an environment that favors dissolution of bone. Osteoclasts appear to phagocytize bone, digesting it in their cytoplasm. This is why bone around an active osteoclast has a ruffled or "chewed-out" edge. Osteocytes, which communicate anatomically with osteoblasts through protoplasmic processes, ramify throughout bone. As PTH stimulates the osteocyte, Ca^{2+} moves through these protoplasmic processes into osteoblasts, where it is next pumped into ECF (with the help of 1,25-DHC).

Parathormone promotes renal reabsorption of Ca^{2+} in the proximal nephron, the ascending thick limb of the loop of Henle (LOH), and the proximal portion of the distal convoluted tubule (DCT) (**Part C**). It also decreases reabsorption of PO_4^{3-}, primarily in the proximal nephron (where the bulk of PO_4^{3-} reabsorption occurs). Loop diuretics, which inhibit Na^+ reabsorption in the ascending thick limb of the LOH, also decrease Ca^{2+} reabsorption, whereas thiazide diuretics, which act similarly on the proximal portion of the DCT, enhance Ca^{2+} reabsorption. Consequently thiazide diuretics are sometimes used to treat patients with Ca^{2+}-containing renal stones. The primary actions of PTH can be summarized as follows:

- Increase bone resorption
  - Increase osteoclast formation and activity
  - Move Ca^{2+} from osteocytes to osteoblasts
  - Move Ca^{2+} from osteoblasts to ECF
- Increase renal vitamin D activation
  - Increase 1α-hydroxylase activity
- Increase renal Ca^{2+} reabsorption
- Decrease renal PO_4^{3-} reabsorption

Parathormone-Related Protein

Parathormone-related protein (or peptide; PTH_{rp}) was originally identified as a product of nonparathyroid tumors of squamous cell origin that resulted in severe, if not fatal, hypercalcemia. This molecule is now known to be expressed by at least some normal tissues as well, including skin keratinocytes, lactating mammary epithelium, and probably fetal parathyroid glands. The structure of PTH_{rp} is similar to PTH (with few amino acid substitutions), and PTH_{rp} exhibits all the actions of PTH on bone and kidney. In addition, a completely different segment of PTH_{rp}, that between amino acids 75 and 84, uniquely stimulates placental Ca^{2+} transport. The PTH_{rp} in mammary tissue may aid in the uptake of Ca^{2+} into milk, and that present in milk may aid Ca^{2+} absorption in the neonatal GI tract.

Calcitonin

In nonmammalian vertebrates, the source of calcitonin (CT; a 32-amino-acid peptide with a five-minute biologic half-life) is the ultimobranchial bodies, a pair of glands derived embryologically from the neural crest. These bodies have become incorporated primarily into the thyroid gland of mammals, where ultimobranchial tissue is found as *parafollicular cells,* also known as C ("clear") cells. Total thyroidectomy does not, however, reduce circulating CT levels to zero, indicating that this hormone also originates from other tissues (e.g., pituitary, thymus, lung, gut, liver, bladder, etc.). Like chief cells of the parathyroids, mammalian C cells exhibit APUD characteristics.

The exact physiologic role of CT is unknown. There is general agreement, however, that **PTH has a far greater impact on Ca^{2+} homeostasis than does CT,** and although some patients with medullary carcinoma of the thyroid have been reported to have high circulating titers of CT and watery diarrhea, most have no abnormalities in Ca^{2+} homeostasis. Similarly, a syndrome due to CT deficiency has not been described.

This hormone may be more active in young animals and may play a role in skeletal development. It has been suggested that CT protects against postprandial hypercalcemia, and it may protect the bones of the mother from excess Ca^{2+} loss during pregnancy. Bone formation in the infant and lactation can be major drains on Ca^{2+} stores, and plasma concentrations of 1,25-DHC and CT are both elevated during pregnancy. Besides hypercalcemia, estrogens also enhance CT release, as does the gut hormone gastrin **Part D.** It appears that a high-Ca^{2+} diet releases gastrin, which in turn acts as an anticipatory hormone causing CT release. Gastrin also increases gastric HCl secretion, which releases dietary Ca^{2+} bound to protein (a prerequisite for absorption). Calcitonin in turn feeds back negatively on gastrin.

30 Parathormone, Calcitonin, and Vitamin D: II

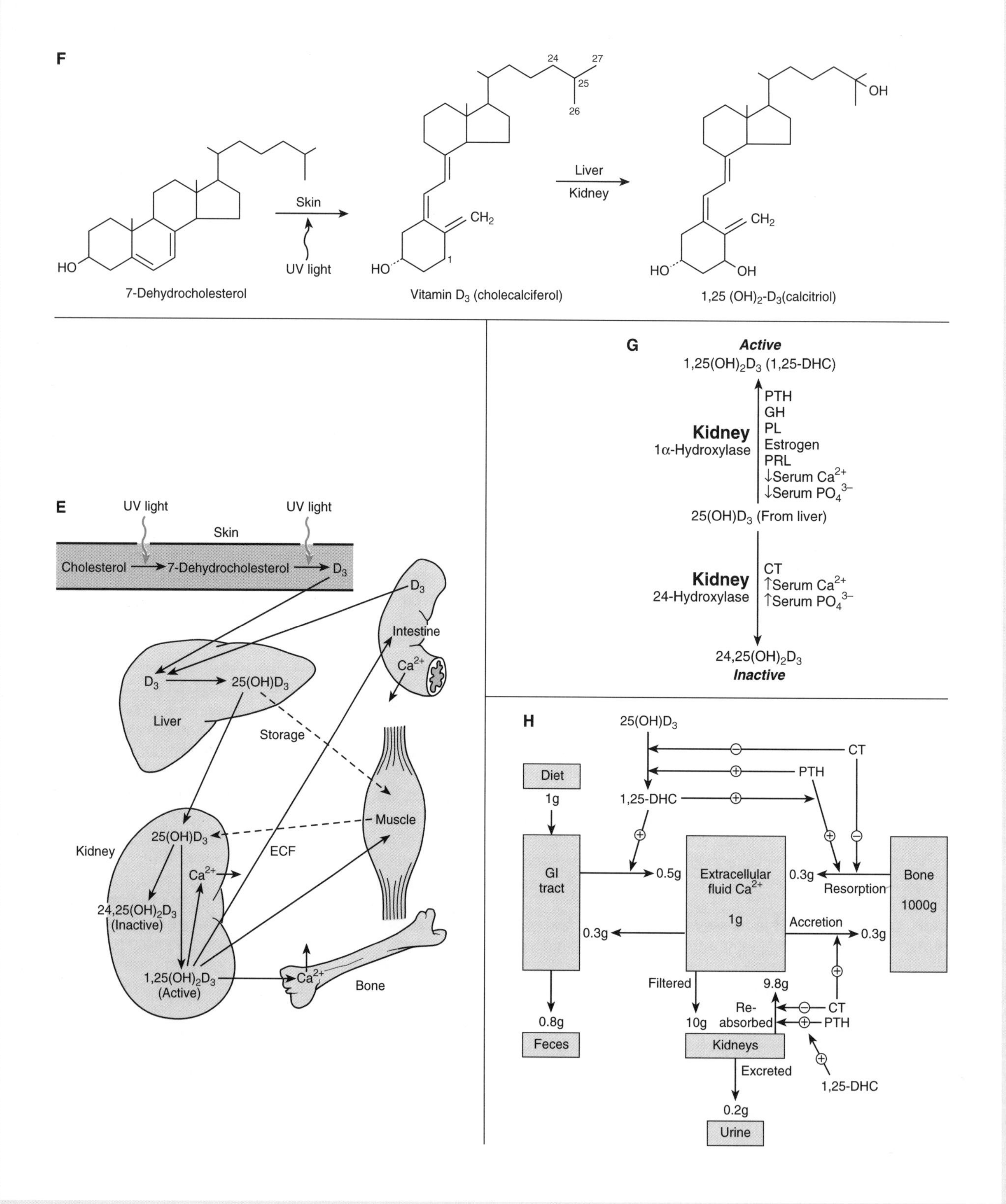

Overview

- UV light helps to promote vitamin D synthesis.
- The active form of vitamin D requires hydroxylation reactions that occur in the liver and kidneys.
- Vitamin D may also be deactivated by the kidneys.
- Several hormones promote the renal activation of vitamin D.
- The placenta may also be a source of vitamin D.
- In general, vitamin D assists PTH in carrying out its physiologic actions.
- Vitamin D increases the efficiency of Ca^{2+} absorption from the small intestine.
- Parathyroid glands are present in mammals, birds and herptiles, but absent in fishes.

Calcitonin apparently prevents bone resorption by interfering with PTH activation of adenyl cyclase by prostaglandins (see above). It also reduces Ca^{2+} reabsorption in the ascending thick limb and early distal part of the nephron (**Part C**), thus increasing urinary Ca^{2+} excretion.

The physiological actions of calcitonin can be summarized as follows:

- Primary
    - Protect the skeleton
        - Antiosteoclastic
- Secondary
    - Osteoblastic effect on bone
    - Decrease renal reabsorption of Ca^{2+} and PO_4^{3-}
    - Renal inactivation of vitamin D

Vitamin D

The actions of PTH on bone; kidneys, and the intestine are enhanced by the active form of the steroid vitamin D, namely 1,25-DHC (**Part E**). Although several molecular forms of vitamin D exist, the most metabolically important forms are D_3 and 1,25-DHC.

Various Forms of Vitamin D

	Generic Name
D_2	Ergocalciferol
Reduced D_2 (DHT)	Dihydrotachysterol
D_3	Cholecalciferol
$25(OH)D_3$	Calcifediol
$1,25(OH)_2D_3$ (1,25-DHC)	Calcitriol (1,25-Dihydroxycholecalciferol)

The first steps in 1,25-DHC formation involve ultraviolet (UV) light–stimulated conversion of cholesterol to 7-dehydrocholesterol in the skin, and then to cholecalciferol (vitamin D_3) (**Parts E** and **F**). This fat-soluble vitamin can also be obtained via the diet, but sunlight-activated D_3 formation is probably the largest source for domestic animals. Although UV light is filtered out by hair coat, pigmented layers of the skin, and window glass, it is thought that the nose of hairy mammals may be a particularly important location for D_3 formation.

The next step in 1,25-DHC formation is transport of D_3 to the liver, which is facilitated by a binding protein in plasma with a high affinity for cholecalciferol. Vitamin D_3 is converted by the liver (in a nonregulated fashion) to 25-hydroxycholecalciferol, and then by the kidney (in a regulated fashion) to $1,25(OH)D_3$ (i.e., calcitriol or 1,25-DHC) (**Parts E** and **F**). Hypocalcemia, PTH, and hormones associated with growth, pregnancy, and lactation stimulate activity of renal 1α-hydroxylase, whereas hypercalcemia, hyperphosphatemia, and CT inactivate 25 $(OH)D_3$ by causing hydroxylation in the 24 position rather than in the 1 position (**Part G**).

During pregnancy, the placenta may also synthesize 1,25-DHC (Chapter 17), which could augment intestinal Ca^{2+} uptake in the dam. Vitamin D deficiency leads to rickets in the young and osteomalacia in adults.

Major physiologic actions of **1,25-DHC** are as follows:

- Increase Ca^{2+} and PO_4^{3-} intestinal absorption
- Increase Renal Ca^{2+} and PO_4^{3-} reabsorption
- Increase bone resorption

In general 1,25-DHC assists PTH in carrying out its physiologic actions (with the exception that PTH decreases while 1,25-DHC enhances renal PO_4^{3-} retention). Therefore, this lipid-soluble steroid, which can be absorbed from the intestinal tract, is used to treat patients with PTH deficiency. Since PTH is a protein, if given orally it is destroyed in the GI tract.

The stimulatory and inhibitory interactions of **PTH, CT** and **1,25-DHC** on the GI tract, kidney, and bone in Ca^{2+} homeostasis is shown diagramatically in **Part H.** Those actions, along with other hormones affecting Ca^{2+} homeostasis, can be summarized as follows:

Hormone	**Action**
PTH	Stimulates bone resorption, renal Ca^{++} retention and vitamin D activation
CT	Primary antiosteoclastic effect; secondary osteoblastic effect
1,25-DHC	Facilitate intestinal Ca^{++} absorption and the action of PTH on bone and kidney
Estrogens	Inhibit action of PTH on bone; stimulate TCT secretion and renal vitamin D activation
GH	Stimulate bone and cartilage growth
IGFs	Mediators of GH action on cartilage and bone
Cortisol	High levels stimulate PTH release yet inhibit the action of 1,25-DHC on the intestine, and the action of PTH on the kidneys

Nonmammalian Vertebrates

Although fish lack parathyroid glands, Ca^{2+} regulation appears to be accomplished by a hypercalcemic pituitary factor (PRL or hypercalcin) and by a hypocalcemic factor (hypocalcin) from the corpuscles of Stannius embedded in the kidneys. Scales are important Ca^{2+} stores. The hypercalcemic factor appears to be important to freshwater fish, and the hypocalcemic factor to saltwater fish. Salmon CT, which is used clinically, is a more potent hypocalcemic factor in mammals than is mammalian CT.

Parathyroid glands are present in birds and herptiles, with the effects of PTH and parathyroidectomy similar to those observed in mammals.

31 Disorders of Calcium Homeostasis

A

Hypercalcemia		*Hypocalcemia*
Decreased neuromuscular excitability		Increased neuromuscular excitability
		Muscle cramps and pain
Bones:	dissolution of bone, pain, and fractures	Irritability
		Impaired mentation
		Seizures
Groans:	constipation, anorexia, dyspepsia	Prolonged Q-T intervals (ECG)
		Congestive heart failure
Stones:	nephrocalcinosis, kidney stones, PU/PD, metabolic acidosis	Laryngospasm
		Bronchospasm
		Tetany
Moans:	fatigue, myalgia, muscle weakness, joint pain	Cataracts
		Coagulopathies
		Eclampsia
Overtones:	depression, memory loss, confusion, lethargy, and coma	Milk fever

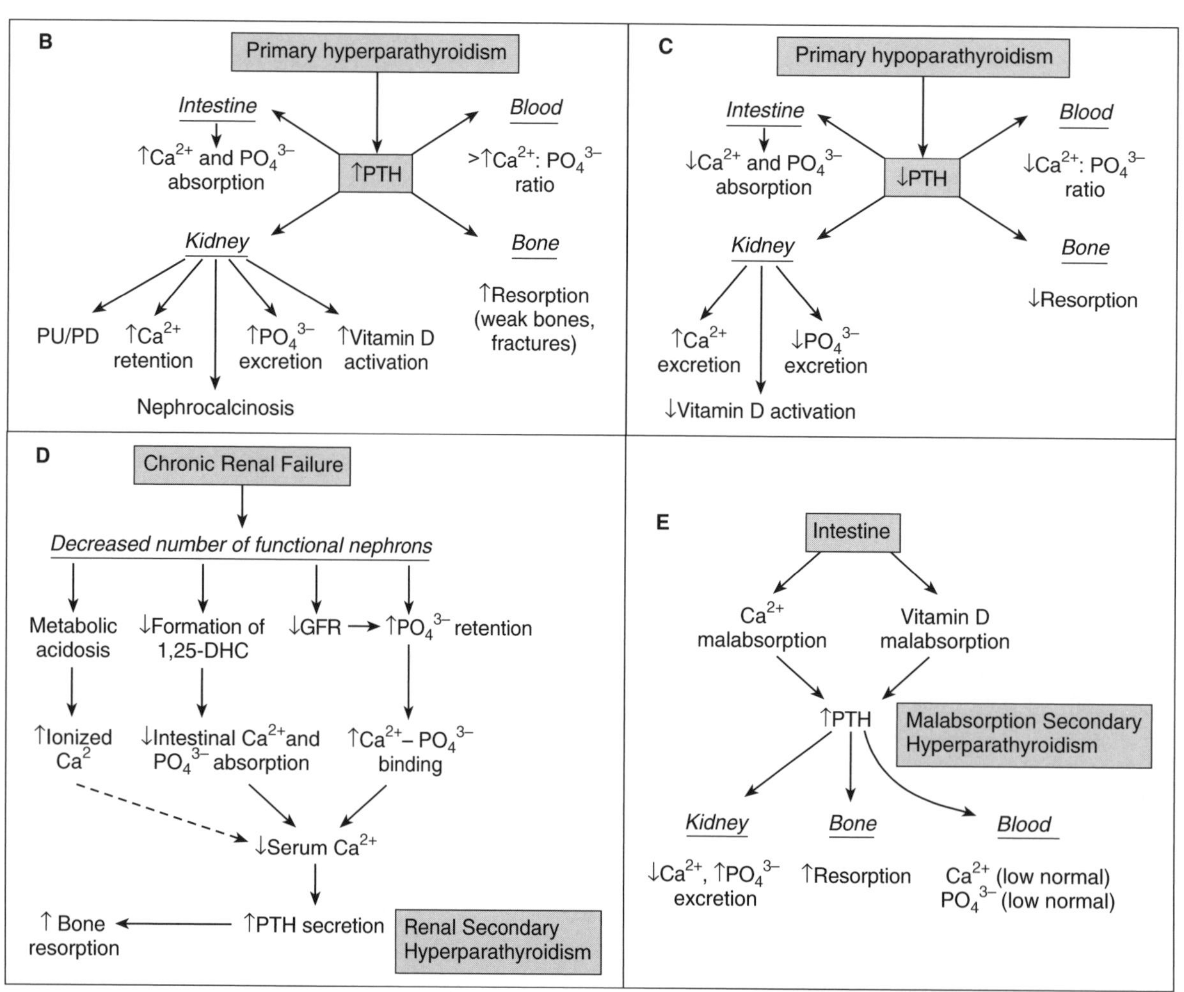

When intricate control mechanisms maintaining the normal plasma free ionized Ca^{2+} concentration fail, the result is either hyper- or hypocalcemia. Hyperparathyroidism indicates overproduction of PTH; however, this is not always associated with *hypercalcemia*. The term *primary hyperparathyroidism* is used to describe excess parathyroid tissue secreting PTH that has not been suppressed by a high plasma Ca^{2+} concentration. *Secondary hyperparathyroidism* (of various causes) refers to parathyroid hyperplasia and high circulating PTH levels that are an appropriate response to prolonged *hypocalcemia*. *Pseudohyperparathyroidism* is used to describe any hypercalcemia resulting from malignancy (not caused by bone metastasis).

Hypercalcemia

Primary Hyperparathyroidism

Clinical signs of primary hyperparathyroidism are produced by hypercalcemia, bone resorption, and calcium nephropathy ("bones, groans, stones, moans, and overtones") resulting from excessive PTH secretion (**Part A**). Most cases are associated with polyuria/polydipsia (PU/PD) from hypercalcemic nephropathy. Except for rare carcinomas, parathyroid tumors are not generally palpable.

Symptoms include hypercalcemia, hypercalciuria, hypophosphatemia, hyperphosphaturia, and reduced creatinine clearance. Whether hypercalcemia is the **cause** or **consequence** of renal disease must be carefully determined. Because PTH decreases renal reabsorption of PO_4^{3-}, the plasma Ca^{2+}-to-PO_4^{3-} ratio significantly increases. **Part B** shows the pathogenesis of primary hyperparathyroidism.

Pseudohyperparathyroidism

Hypercalcemia resulting from malignancy is most frequently associated with squamous cell carcinoma and lymphosarcoma in dogs and cats, probably due to these tumors producing high levels of PTH_{rp} or a lymphokine (osteoclast-activating factor). The second most reported cause of hypercalcemia in dogs is apocrine gland adenocarcinomas of the anal sacs. Symptoms are similar to primary hyperparathyroidism; however, PTH levels are low (because normal parathyroids are being suppressed by high titers of Ca^{2+}). As hypercalcemia of malignancy can be a near terminal event in some patients, treatment should be based on relieving the biochemical effects of PTH_{rp} and lowering serum Ca^{2+} levels.

Vitamin D Toxicosis

Hypercalcemia and hyperphosphatemia are anticipated signs in animals with vitamin D toxicity. Increased bone resorption and increased intestinal absorption of Ca^{2+} and PO_4^{3-}, are the causes. Cholecalciferol rodenticide toxicosis in dogs and cats reportedly causes weakness, lethargy, and anorexia within two days of exposure. Diffuse gastric and intestinal hemorrhage may follow. Excessive administration of vitamin D to hypoparathyroid cats that have been surgically treated for hyperthyroidism is an additional concern. Some house plants also contain vitamin D (e.g., *Cestrum diurnum, Solanum malacoxylon,* and *Trisetum flavescens*), and consumption can also cause vitamin D toxicosis.

Other Causes of Hypercalcemia

These include hydrochlorothiazide diuretics (increase renal Ca^{2+} reabsorption), lithium (causes excessive PTH secretion), vitamin A toxicity (causes excessive osteoclast activation), excessive Ca^{2+} ingestion, acute or chronic renal failure, and hibernation or prolonged immobilization (osteoporosis).

Hypocalcemia

Primary Hypoparathyroidism

Although some animals exhibit naturally occurring hypoparathyroidism, a more common cause of PTH deficiency is surgical damage or removal of parathyroid tissue during thyroid surgery. Severe hypomagnesemia also causes hypocalcemia because optimal amounts of Mg^{2+} are required for PTH synthesis and secretion. Parathyroid hypofunction leads to declining Ca^{2+} and increasing PO_4^{3-} levels in plasma. Urinary Ca^{2+} excretion rises acutely, then declines with plasma concentrations. Urinary PO_4^{3-} excretion also diminishes. All of these alterations are explained by loss of PTH effects on: 1) bone resorption, 2) renal retention of Ca^{2+} and excretion of PO_4^{3-}, and 3) intestinal absorption of both Ca^{2+} and PO_4^{3-} (**Part C**). Other pathophysiologic effects of hypocalcemia are listed in **Part A.**

Detection of antibodies against parathyroid tissue in human patients has led to speculation that some forms of primary hypoparathyroidism in animals may be caused by autoimmune processes.

Pseudohypoparathyroidism

Pseudohypoparathyroidism is a rare disorder characterized by target tissue resistance to PTH. Although it has been described in humans, reports of domestic animals with this specific disease are lacking. Symptoms in humans are hypocalcemia, increased serum concentrations of PTH (a form of secondary hyperparathyroidism), and a variety of skeletal development defects. Renal tubular resistance to PTH causes hypercalciuria and diminished phosphaturia.

Renal Secondary Hyperparathyroidism

Patients with this syndrome generally exhibit modest hypocalcemia and a more pronounced hyperphosphatemia. Like primary hyperparathyroidism, renal secondary hyperparathyroidism is characterized by excessive PTH secretion leading to excessive bone resorption (**Part D**). The driving force for PTH secretion is a low (normal) plasma Ca^{2+} concentration. Chronic renal insufficiency can result from several different causes, but when it progresses to the point where the number of functional nephrons is significantly reduced, hyperphosphatemia and azotemia develop. Although serum PO_4^{3-} has no direct regulatory influence on PTH secretion, it may, when elevated, contribute to parathyroid stimulation by virtue of its ability to bind Ca^{2+}, and thus lower the plasma free ionized Ca^{2+} concentration. Intestinal Ca^{2+} and PO_4^{3-} absorption may also be impaired by a defect in renal vitamin D hydroxylation. However, renal disease also causes metabolic acidosis, and this has a tendency to offset reductions in the free ionized Ca^{2+} concentration.

Malabsorption Secondary Hyperparathyroidism

Decreased intestinal absorption of dietary Ca^{2+} and increased fecal excretion lead to this syndrome. The degree of Ca^{2+} malabsorption is generally proportional to the extent of small bowel disease. An additional factor is inadequate absorption of vitamin D. As in pancreatitis or liver disease, clinical signs in malabsorption/maldigestion are generally gastrointestinal. Consequences of Ca^{2+} and vitamin D malabsorption are secondary hyperparathyroidism leading to bone loss, modest hypocalcemia, hypophosphatemia, hypocalciuria, and hyperphosphaturia (**Part E**).

Nutritional Secondary Hyperparathyroidism

Animals fed all-meat diets with low Ca^{2+}-to-PO_4^{3-} ratios can develop a secondary hyperparathyroidism that leads to skeletal abnormalities. Although serum Ca^{2+} and PO_4^{3-} concentrations may remain within normal range, these animals generally exhibit hypocalciuria and hyperphosphaturia.

Other Causes of Hypocalcemia

These include long-term anticonvulsant therapy (phenobarbital and phenytoin), ethylene glycol toxicity (acute renal failure with severe hyperphosphatemia), PO_4^{3-}-containing enemas (hyperphosphatemia), transfusion with citrated or ethylenediaminetetraacetic acid (EDTA)-containing blood (calcium chelators or laboratory error because EDTA was used), and osteoblastic metastases.

32 Mineral Imbalances

A Pathophysiologic effects associated with hyper- and hyponatremia

Hypernatremia	
↑**ECF volume** *(Hypertension;* ***e.g., NaCl engorgement)***	↓**ECF volume** *(e.g., diabetes insipidus,* ***excessive free water loss)***
Increased cardiac output	Concentrated serum electrolytes
Increased renal blood flow	Concentration alkalosis
Decreased aldosterone and ADH	Increased Aldosterone and ADH
Cellular dehydration	Cellular dehydration
Increased neuromuscular irritability	

Hyponatremia	
↓**ECF volume** *(Hypotension; e.g., diarrhea, sweating and* ***diabetes mellitus)***	↑**ECF volume** ***(e.g., water intoxication)***
Decreased cardiac output	Dilute serum electrolytes
Decreased renal blood flow	Dilutional acidosis
Increased aldosterone	Decreased aldosterone and ADH
Increased intracellular fluid volume (hypotonic hypovolemia with cellular hydration)	

B Pathophysiologic effects associated with hyper- and hypokalemia

Hyperkalemia	*Hypokalemia*
Increased neuromuscular excitability	Decreased neuromuscular excitability
Cardiac toxicity (arrhythmia,weak contractions, and bradycardia)*	Tachycardia*

*Note: The effect of either hyper- or hypokalemia on cardiac rhythm is complex, and virtually any arrhythmia may be seen. Various brady-arrhythmias, including impaired AV conduction and complete AV block, may occur with hyperkalemia. Hyperkalemia may also produce sinus bradycardia, sinus arrest, slow idioventricular rhythm, and asystole. In other circumstances, tachycardias may result, including sinus tachycardia, ventricular extrasystole, ventricular tachycardia, and ventricular fibrillation. The rate of K^+ elevation appears to influence the type of arrhythmia produced. For example, a slow elevation in K^+ produces widespread block and depressed automaticity, while more rapid infusions produce ventricular ectopic rhythms and, terminally, ventricular fibrillation. Obviously, care must be taken in the administration of K^+-containing fluids to patients.

C Pathophysiologic effects associated with hyper- and hypophosphatemia

Hyperphosphatemia	*Hypophosphatemia*
Increased neuromuscular excitability	Decreased neuromuscular excitability
Hypocalcemia (↑Ca^{2+} binding)	Aciduria
	Rickets and osteomalacia

D

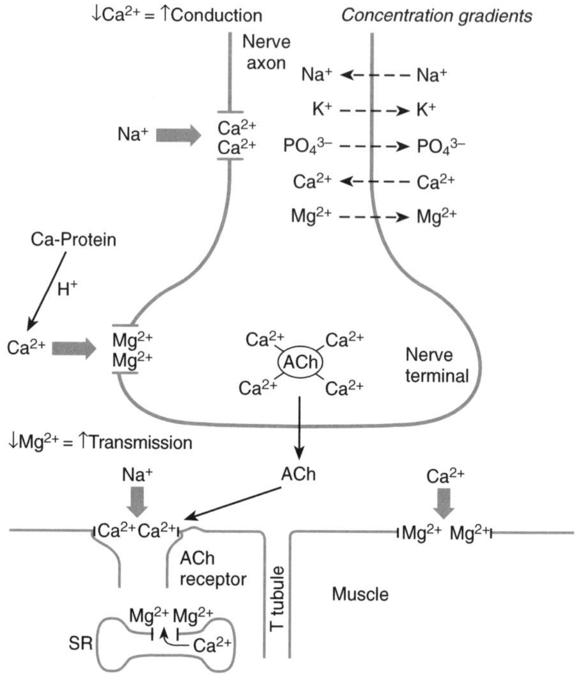

Intracellular Mg^{2+} also dampens release of Ca^{2+} from the sarcoplasmic reticulum (SR). Severe hypocalcemia, as occurs with milk fever, will decrease transmission of action potentials (because Ca^{2+} entry into nerve terminals is required for exocytosis of neurotransmitters).

E Pathophysiologic effects associated with hyper- and hypomagnesemia

Hypermagnesemia	*Hypomagnesemia*
Decreased neuromuscular excitability	Increased neuromuscular excitability
Depressed respiration	Cardiac arrhythmia
Depressed deep tendon reflexes	Generalized tremors
Depressed sinoatrial node and cardiac conducting system	Grass tetany (or wheat pasture poisoning) in ruminants
Decreased vascular smooth muscle contraction, decreased blood pressure	

Overview

- Neuromuscular irritability (NI) is directly proportional to the plasma concentrations of Na^+, K^+, and PO_4^{3-}, and inversely proportional to the plasma concentrations of Ca^{2+}, H^+, and Mg^{2+}.
- The most potent influence on plasma osmolarity is Na^+ (and its accompanying anions [Cl^- and HCO_3^-]).
- Rapid correction of acidemia can sometimes dangerously decrease serum K^+ levels.
- Hypotonic dehydration may be associated with cellular hydration.
- Hypomagnesemia is associated with grass tetany in ruminant animals.
- Hyperphosphatemia is more common in domestic animals than hypophosphatemia.
- "Milk fever" is associated with severe hypocalcemia.

All organ systems are dependent on normal plasma concentrations of calcium (Ca^{2+}), phosphate (PO_4^{3-}), sodium (Na^+), potassium (K^+), and magnesium (Mg^{2+}). These concentrations in turn largely depend on dietary intake, acid/base balance, and renal, gastrointestinal, and endocrine function. The physiologic processes most affected by these minerals are neuromuscular function and blood volume/pressure homeostasis.

The effects of PTH and CT on Ca^{2+} and PO_4^{3-} balance were discussed in previous chapters, and the effects of aldosterone on Na^+ and K^+ balance are discussed in Chapters 38–40. Other important interactions between these minerals will be the subject of this chapter.

The effects of changes in the extracellular fluid (ECF) concentrations of these minerals (and H^+) on *neuromuscular irritability (NI)* can be depicted in the following expression:

$$\mathbf{NI \propto (Na^+ \times K^+ \times PO_4^{3-})/(Ca^{2+} \times H^+ \times Mg^{2+})}$$

Plasma K^+ and Ca^{2+} concentrations are inversely correlated with pH (i.e., acidosis tends to displace K^+ from cells and liberate ionized Ca^{2+} from plasma protein binding sites, while alkalosis has the opposite effects). Because respiratory changes develop more rapidly than renal changes, the free ionized plasma Ca^{2+} concentration is more commonly influenced by respiratory alterations in pH. Hypocalcemia, for example, sometimes becomes symptomatic by reducing serum ionized Ca^{2+} levels through hyperventilation (as caused by heat or pain). Also, rapid correction of acidemia can sometimes dangerously decrease serum K^+ by encouraging reentry of K^+ into cells (by reducing the H^+ concentration within cells).

The most potent influence on blood volume and pressure is Na^+, along with its accompanying anions, Cl^- and HCO_3^-. Together these ions account for about 93% of ECF tonicity. The Na^+ concentration generally affects ECF volume in two ways: 1) it helps maintain ECF volume when more water than electrolyte is lost (largely by pulling water out of intracellular fluid sites), and 2) it helps deplete ECF volume when more Na^+ than water is lost (by allowing water to move into intracellular fluid sites) (**Part A**). When isotonic fluids are lost (e.g., by hemorrhage), Na^+ has no direct affect on ECF volume; however, through the renin–angiotensin system (Chapters 39 and 40), aldosterone-mediated Na^{2+} retention contributes to restoration of plasma volume (at the expense of K^+ depletion). Increasing the ECF Na^+ concentration increases its concentration gradient into excitable tissue, which tends to be depolarizing. For this reason, Na^+ appears in the numerator of the NI equation.

When the extracellular K^+ concentration rises, its diffusion gradient out of cells decreases; therefore, it has less of a hyperpolarizing effect (and more of a depolarizing effect on excitable tissue). The depolarizing nature of hyperkalemia can also be depicted by the Nernst equation: $E_{K^+} = 61.5\log([K^+_E]/[K^+_I])$.

If normal K^+ concentrations for extracellular fluid ($[K^+_E]$) and intracellular fluid ($[K^+_I]$) are given as 5.5 and 150 mEq/L, respectively, then the equilibrium potential for K^+ (E_{K^+}) is -90 mV. When $[K^+_E]$ increases to 6.5 mEq/L, for example, E_{K^+} becomes -84 mV (i.e., a depolarizing effect).

Modest increases in extracellular K^+ have a tendency to depolarize pacemaker cells of the heart and, thus, decrease intracellular negativity. This, in turn, decreases Na^+ and Ca^{2+} conductance into pacemaker cells, which effectively decreases the rate of rise of the prepotential (phase 4) and decreases the amplitude of phase 0. This decreased Na^+ and Ca^{2+} conductance prolongs the pacemaker action potential and slows heart rate. Larger increases in extracellular K^+, however, may have the opposite effects (**Part B**).

Because phosphate is concentrated within cells and is a part of membrane-bound phospholipids, ATP, and other important compounds within cells, hypophosphatemia is associated with a decrease in NI. Conversely, hyperphosphatemia, which is more common in domestic animals, increases NI, partially because PO_4^{3-} binds Ca^{2+} and creates a secondary hypocalcemia (**Part C**).

As seen in **Part D,** Ca^{2+} has a tendency to align itself in Na^+ neuronal channels. Thus, when the Ca^{2+} concentration rises Na^+ has a more difficult time entering neurons (i.e., paresis), and when it falls nerve depolarization increases (hypocalcemic tetany). Potassium administration, because it is depolarizing, would obviously aggravate symptoms of hypocalcemic tetany.

However, when severe decreases in the plasma Ca^{2+} concentration occur, as in milk fever of dairy cows, transmission of action potentials can be compromised, with reduced acetylcholine (ACh) release at neuromuscular junctions (i.e., paresis). Most animals that experience milk fever, however, first experience a short period of enhanced excitability before becoming "downer cows."

The Mg^{2+} ion has a tendency to block Ca^{2+} channels (similar to the way Ca^{2+} blocks Na^+ channels; see **Part D**). Hypermagnesemia will therefore decrease Ca^{2+} entry into nerve terminals (i.e., cause decreased transmission and paresis) as well as Ca^{2+} movement into the cytoplasm of cardiac and smooth muscle cells (from both inside and outside the cell) (**Part E**). Although Mg^{2+} administration would aggravate hypocalcemic paresis in dairy cows, it helps to alleviate symptoms of hypocalcemic tetany in other animals (because the release of ACh is inversely related to the ECF Mg^{2+} concentration).

33 ACTH and Glucocorticoids: I

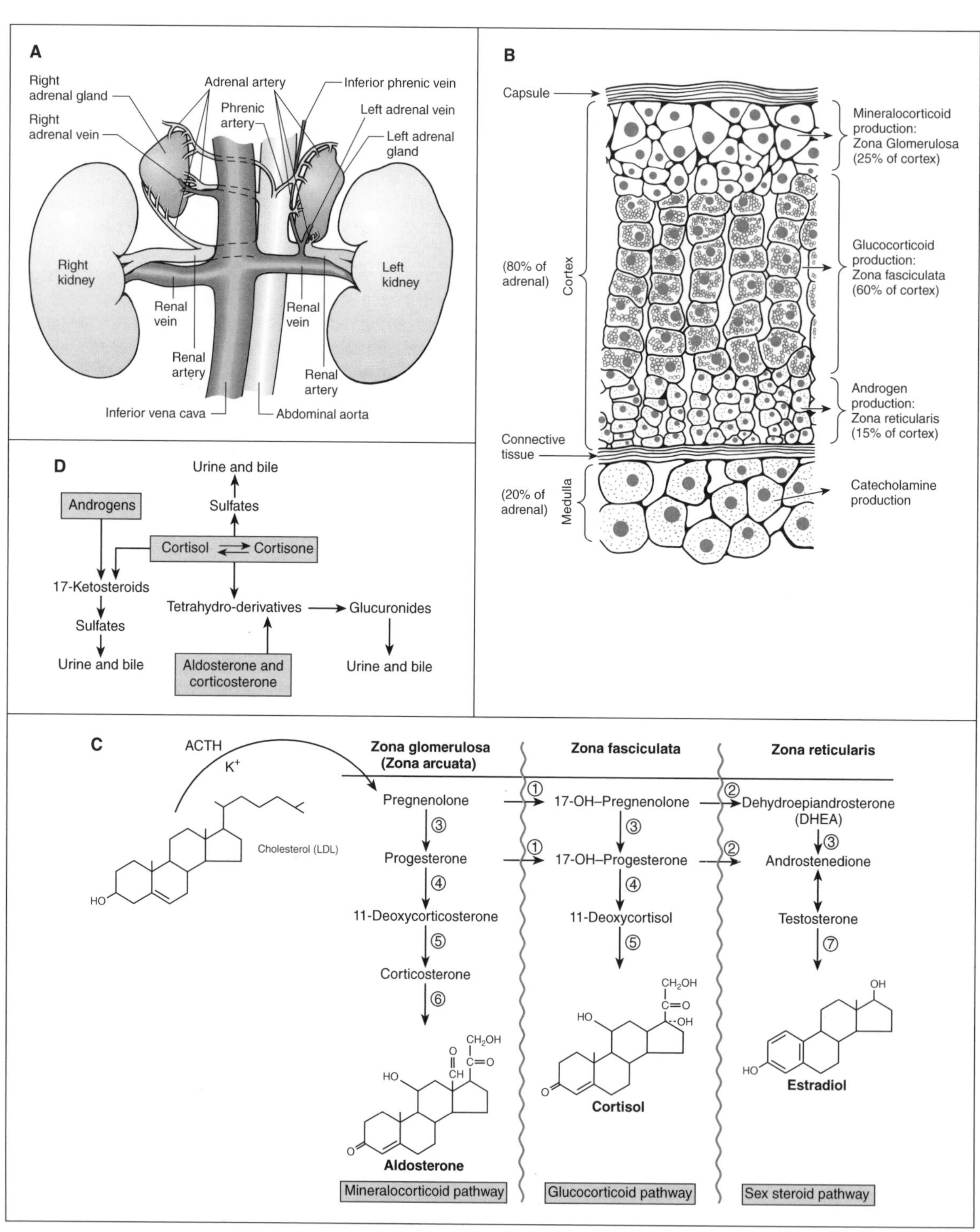

A
Right adrenal gland
Right adrenal vein
Adrenal artery
Phrenic artery
Inferior phrenic vein
Left adrenal vein
Left adrenal gland
Right kidney
Left kidney
Renal vein
Renal vein
Renal artery
Renal artery
Inferior vena cava
Abdominal aorta
B
Capsule
Mineralocorticoid production: Zona Glomerulosa (25% of cortex)
(80% of adrenal)
Cortex
Glucocorticoid production: Zona fasciculata (60% of cortex)
Androgen production: Zona reticularis (15% of cortex)
Connective tissue
(20% of adrenal)
Medulla
Catecholamine production
D
Urine and bile
Sulfates
Androgens
Cortisol
Cortisone
17-Ketosteroids
Sulfates
Urine and bile
Tetrahydro-derivatives
Glucuronides
Aldosterone and corticosterone
Urine and bile
C
ACTH
K+
Cholesterol (LDL)
HO
Zona glomerulosa (Zona arcuata)
Zona fasciculata
Zona reticularis
Pregnenolone
① 17-OH–Pregnenolone
② Dehydroepiandrosterone (DHEA)
③
Progesterone
① 17-OH–Progesterone
② Androstenedione
④
11-Deoxycorticosterone
11-Deoxycortisol
Testosterone
⑤
⑦
Corticosterone
⑥
CH2OH
C=O
OH
Aldosterone
Cortisol
Estradiol
Mineralocorticoid pathway
Glucocorticoid pathway
Sex steroid pathway

Overview

- Adrenal steroids are produced in the outer adrenal cortex.
- Pheochromocytes, which secrete catecholamines, are located in the inner adrenal medulla.
- The cortex normally accounts for about 80% of adrenal tissue.
- The zona reticularis and zona fasciculata of the adrenal cortex can be regenerated from cells originating in the zona glomerulosa.
- The adrenal cortex is capable of synthesizing all steroid hormones (except vitamin D).
- Adrenal steroids are generally inactivated by the liver.

The adrenal glands of birds and mammals are small oval structures located bilaterally at the anterior aspects of the kidneys (**Part A**). Each gland consists of two primary endocrine segments: an outer adrenal cortex that secretes steroid hormones, and a smaller inner medulla that secretes the catecholamines, epinephrine [comes from the Greek words *epi* (the top) and *nephros* (the kidney)], and norepinephrine. In birds, medullary tissue is mixed with cortical tissue. In mammals, however, the dark red medulla is distinct from the pale yellow cortex. Medullary tissue is composed of a spongework of chromaffin cells (or *pheochromocytes*). In addition, small groups of nerve cells (paraganglia) are scattered throughout the medulla, which can be regarded as a specialized ganglion of the sympathetic nervous system (because secretory cells are richly innervated by cholinergic preganglionic fibers from lower thoracic segments of the spinal cord).

The cortex, which normally accounts for about 80% of adrenal tissue, consists of cells with well-marked nuclei aligned in three distinct functional zones (**Part B**). The outermost zone in most mammals is called the *zona glomerulosa* (because cells form clusters resembling glomeruli in the kidney). In dogs and cats, the arc-like configuration of this zone causes it to sometimes be referred to as the *zona arcuata*. The second zone inward from the capsule is called the *zona fasciculata*, and the innermost zone the *zona reticularis* (sometimes referred to as the cortical graveyard).

The adrenal medulla does not regenerate following injury, but when the inner two zones of the cortex are removed, they are regenerated from glomerulosa cells. Following hypophysectomy (i.e., loss of ACTH), the zona fasciculata and zona reticularis atrophy, whereas the zona glomerulosa remains almost unchanged because nonpituitary factors (e.g., angiotensin II and K^+) maintain aldosterone synthesis. Conversely, injections of ACTH cause hypertrophy of the inner two zones but do not affect the size of the zona glomerulosa.

Biosynthesis of Adrenal Steroids

Cholesterol is the starting material from which all steroid hormones are synthesized, and at the adrenals it is largely derived from low-density lipoprotein (LDL). Adrenal cortical cells can also synthesize cholesterol from its primary precursor (acetate). Although pregnenolone is used to synthesize all corticosteroids, it is not used for glucocorticoid biosynthesis in the zona fasciculata if 17α-hydroxylase activation (process *1* in **Part C**), which normally requires the presence of ACTH, has not occurred. However, activation of 3β-de[illegible]drogenase (process *3*), 21β-hydroxylase (process *4*), 11β-hydrox[illegible]cess *5*), and 18-OH-dehydrogenase (process *6*) by angio[illegible] levels of serum K^+ will result in aldosterone biosynthe[illegible] *mineralocorticoid pathway*. Hydroxylation of either pregnen[illegible] progesterone in the 17 position is also required prior to [illegible] and estrogen formation in the zona reticularis. Androgen formation (process *2*) requires side chain cleavage of the 21-carbon 17-hydroxy derivatives of pregnenolone and progesterone to 19-carbon derivatives. Further conversion to estrogen requires activation of the aromatase enzyme that converts testosterone to estrogen (process *7*).

The *mineralocorticoids* (namely aldosterone, corticosterone, and 11-deoxycorticosterone) are steroids that have very little direct effect on general metabolism but do affect ionic equilibrium by controlling renal Na^+ and K^+ excretion. In contrast, the *glucocorticoids* (namely cortisol and its derivative, cortisone) have pronounced effects on carbohydrate, protein, and lipid metabolism. Although cortisone is an active glucocorticoid, it is not secreted in appreciable quantities by the adrenals.

The *progestogens* (or progestins, namely pregnenolone and progesterone) function mainly as precursors to all of the other corticosteroids, including the androgens and estrogen. Biosynthetic pathways for the adrenal sex hormones (androgens, i.e., DHEA, androstenedione, and testosterone; and estrogen, i.e., estradiol) are probably more important in fetal than in adult life. Secretion of these hormones is controlled by ACTH (not pituitary gonadotropins), and there appears to be no sex difference in secretion (i.e., it is low and normally the same in both adult males and adult females).

Catabolism of Adrenal Steroids

Adrenal steroids are catabolized and inactivated principally by the liver and kidneys (**Part D**). Tetrahydroglucuronides of aldosterone, cortisol, cortisone, and corticosterone are freely soluble in water; about 15% of these metabolites appear in feces, with the remainder appearing in urine.

A smaller portion of cortisol (but not corticosterone) is converted in the liver to 17-ketosteroid derivatives of cortisol and cortisone that are conjugated to sulfate and excreted in urine and bile (see **Part D**). Most androgens secreted by the adrenal cortex and testes have a keto group in the 17 position; therefore, they are also found in urine. The daily urinary 17-ketosteroid excretion in males is normally greater than that in females.

The rate of hepatic inactivation of steroid hormones, including the sex steroids, is decreased in liver disease, and therefore their concentrations in blood remain elevated over time. During surgery and other stresses, glucocorticoid levels in plasma sometimes rise higher than they do with maximal ACTH stimulation (in the absence of stress).

34 ACTH and Glucocorticoids: II

E

Steroid	*Glucocorticoid activity*	*Mineralo-corticoid activity*	*Approximate normal plasma concentration (μg/dL)*
Naturally occurring			
Cortisol	1.0	1.0	10
Cortisone	0.8	0.8	—
Corticosterone	0.5	15	1
Deoxycorticosterone	0.01	100	0.07
Aldosterone	0.3	3000	0.009
Synthetic			
Prednisone	4	<0.1	—
6α-Methylprednisone (Medrol)	5	<0.1	—
9α-Fluoro-16α-OH-prednisolone (triamcinolone)	5	<0.1	—
9α-Fluoro-16α-Methylprednisolone (dexamethasone)	30	<0.1	—
9α-Fluorocortisol	10	500	—

All potencies are relative to the glucocorticoid and mineralocorticoid activity of cortisol (liver glycogen deposition and renal Na^+/K^+ balance, respectively), which have been assigned the arbitrary value of 1.0. (Data from various sources.)

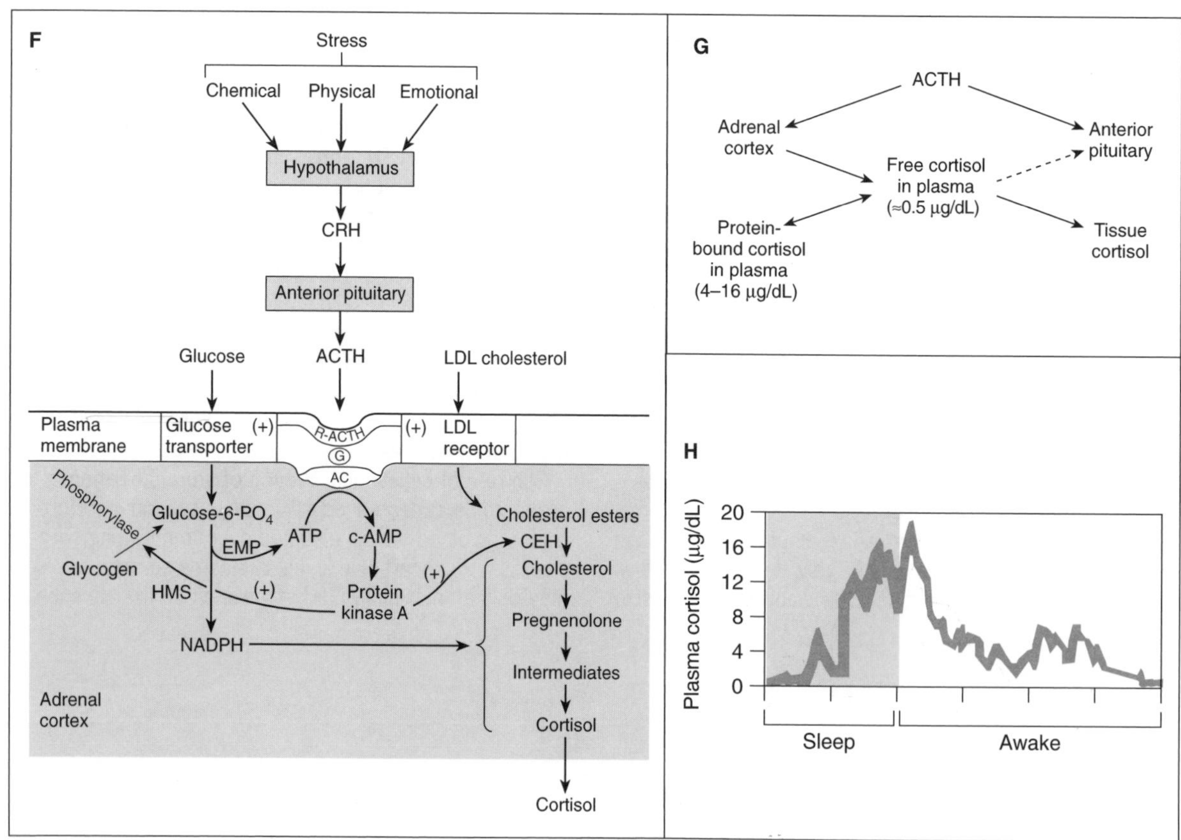

Source: Part G modified from Ganong WF: Review of medical physiology. 17th ed. Stamford, CT: Appleton & Lange, 1995: 337. **Part H** redrawn from Weitzman ED, et al: J Clin Endocrinol Metab 33:14, 1971. The Endocrine Society.

Overview

- Normal plasma concentrations of glucocorticoids are over 1000 times greater than those for the mineralocorticoids, but their potencies on aldosterone receptors are small.
- ACTH (from the anterior pituitary) regulates glucocorticoid synthesis and secretion.
- Cortisol is bound in plasma to a protein, transcortin, which is produced by the liver.
- Cortisol secretion from the adrenal cortex normally increases during sleep.
- NADPH, derived from the HMS of adrenal cortical cells, is required for steroid biosynthesis.
- Synthetic corticosteroids are highly effective because of their long biologic half-lives.

Adrenal Steroid Potency

Relative potencies of naturally occurring and synthetic corticosteroids are shown in **Part E.** Corticosterone and deoxycorticosterone have more mineralocorticoid activity than cortisol, and cortisone (which is produced in target cells from cortisol) is a slightly weaker glucocorticoid than cortisol. Note that normal plasma concentrations for cortisol are approximately 1100 times greater than those for aldosterone, and that cortisol has a potency 3000 times lower than aldosterone on mineralocorticoid receptors. Although a plasma concentration for cortisone is not given, cortisol is in equilibrium with cortisone in its target tissues through the activity of 11β-dehydrogenase, therefore rendering exogenous cortisone an effective source of glucocorticoid activity.

The activity of the corticosteroids can be changed by altering their structure. Of the synthetic corticosteroids, prednisone and prednisolone possess primary glucocorticoid activity, and 9α-fluorocortisol has primary mineralocorticoid activity. These synthetic corticosteroids are highly effective because they have long biologic half-lives.

ACTH Secretion

The primary regulator of adrenal cortical activity is the anterior pituitary hormone, ACTH. It controls growth of the inner two zones of the cortex, maintains structural and functional integrity of all cells in the cortex, and stimulates secretory activity, particularly of cortisol.

Many adverse conditions cause secretion of *ACTH-releasing hormone (CRH)* from the hypothalamus (which in turn causes ACTH release from the anterior pituitary). Such conditions include chemical, physical, and emotional stress (e.g., overcrowding, extreme external cold or heat, severe exercise, traumatic shock, toxins, hemorrhage, infections, starvation, hypoglycemia, etc.) (**Part F**). The mechanism of action of ACTH on adrenal cortical cells in the inner two zones is as follows: When ACTH binds to its receptor (*R-ACTH*), adenyl cyclase (*AC*) is activated through a guanosine-binding protein (*G*). In addition, binding of ACTH to its receptor favors transport of glucose into cortical cells (as well as cholesterol from LDL). Glucose is oxidized via the Embden-Meyerhof pathway (*EMP*). This yields ATP, as well as NADPH via the hexose monophosphate shunt (*HMS*). Through activation of AC, ATP is converted to cAMP, which in turn activates protein kinase A. Protein kinase A activates a phosphorylase needed for glycogenolysis, and also phosphorylates cholesterol ester hydrolase (*CEH*), thus increasing its activity. Consequently, more free cholesterol is formed and converted to pregnenolone and then to intermediates of cortisol biosynthesis. Note that NADPH derived from the HMS is required for steroid biosynthesis.

Unlike other glandular cells, steroid-producing cells do not store hormones, but rather synthesize them on demand. Stimulation by ACTH increases cortisol secretion within 1 to 2 minutes, with peak rates occurring in about 15 minutes.

Cortisol Transport

Cortisol is bound in plasma to an α-globulin called *transcortin* (or *corticosteroid-binding globulin, CBG*), and to a lesser extent to albumin. The plasma half-life for cortisol is about 60 to 90 minutes. Bound cortisol is inactive, yet it serves as a circulating reservoir of the hormone. At normal plasma concentrations of cortisol and transcortin, there is very little free cortisol available to tissues (**Part G**). When binding sites on CBG become saturated (cortisol concentrations >20 μg/dL), however, free and tissue cortisol levels rise. Transcortin is synthesized in the liver, and its production is increased by estrogen (e.g., during pregnancy) and decreased by liver disease (e.g., cirrhosis). Some patients with nephrosis (loss of CBG in urine) have low total plasma cortisol, yet exhibit few symptoms of glucocorticoid deficiency because free cortisol levels change minimally.

Cortisol Circadian Rhythmicity

Plasma concentrations of cortisol vary within a normal range in mammals of about 4 to 16 μg/dL and show circadian rhythmicity, with normal concentrations rising during the sleeping hours (**Part H**). Because of this circadian rhythmicity, the time of blood sampling should be taken into account when interpreting clinical concentrations of plasma cortisol.

35 ACTH and Glucocorticoids: III

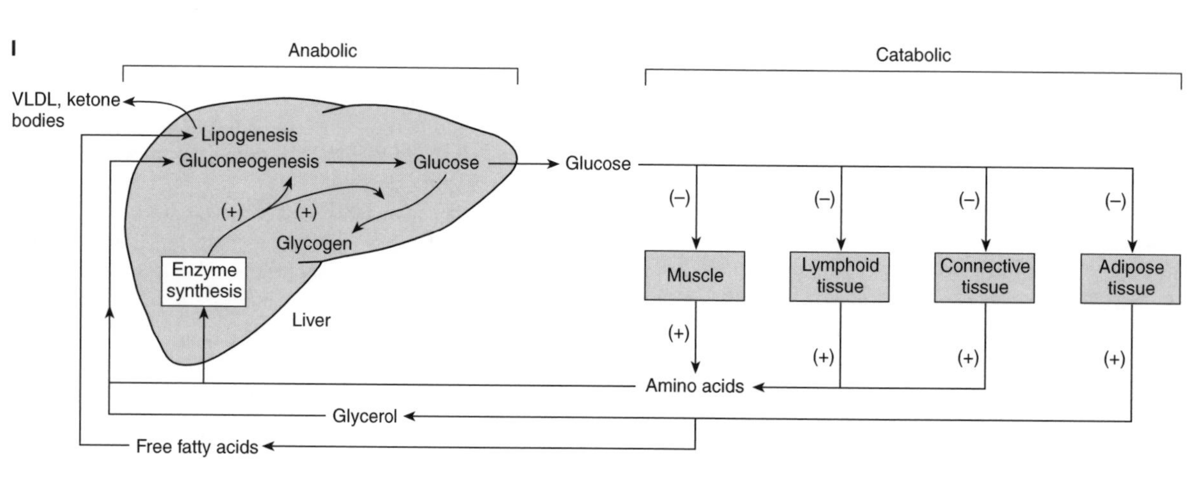

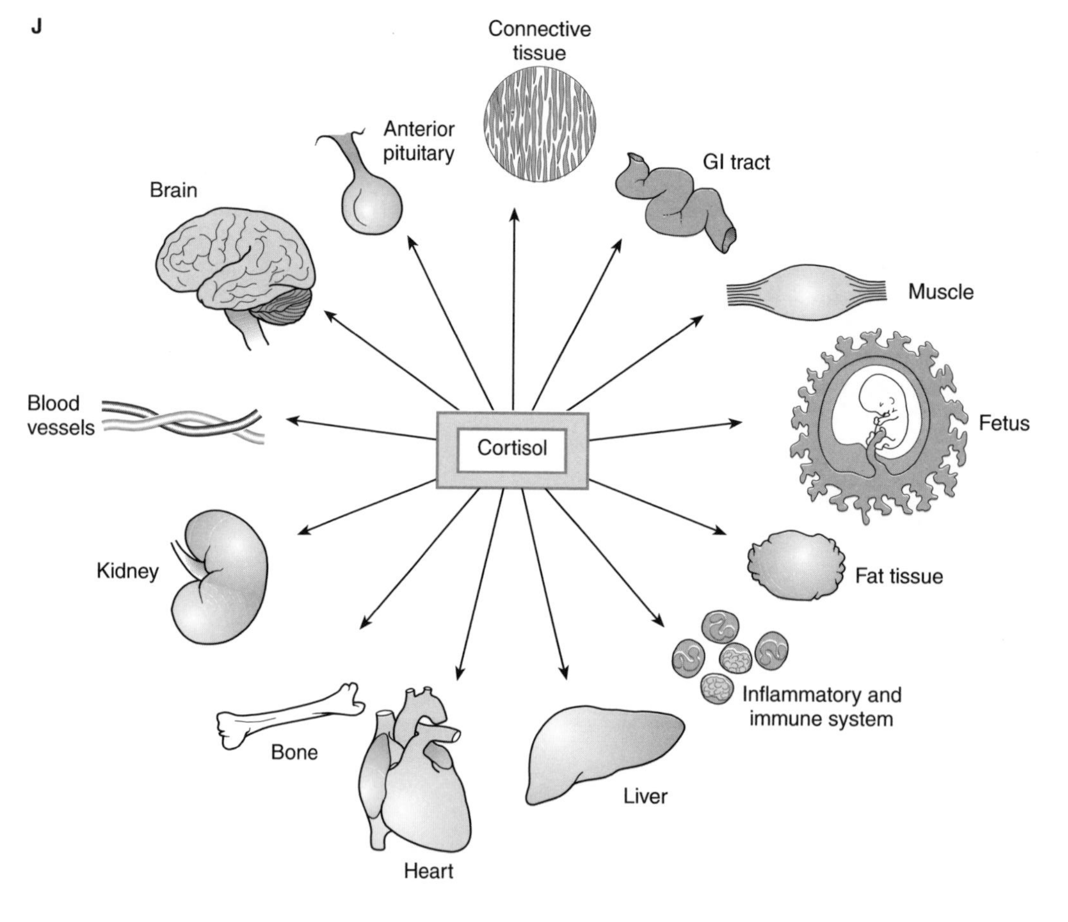

Overview

- In general, the effects of glucocorticoids on intermediary metabolism are opposite to those of insulin.
- Cortisol acts permissively to mobilize fuel in times of need (e.g., starvation).
- Cortisol increases β-adrenergic receptor synthesis (like thyroxine and progesterone).
- Cortisol has a hyperlipidemic action.
- Cortisol helps to maintain the blood glucose concentration between meals.
- Glucocorticoids are contraindicated in osteoporosis.

The glucocorticoids exert profound influences on intermediary metabolism. Primary effects on carbohydrate metabolism are increased hepatic gluconeogenesis and glycogenesis and decreased glucose utilization in extrahepatic insulin-sensitive tissues (**Part I**). Free fatty acid mobilization from adipocytes also occurs, with conversion of the fatty acids in the liver to triglycerides and ketone bodies. Protein synthesis is reduced, and there is a generalized breakdown of muscle protein into amino acids for hepatic gluconeogenesis. In general, the actions of glucocorticoids on carbohydrate, fat, and protein metabolism are opposite to those of insulin.

In large amounts, glucocorticoids inhibit several steps associated with the inflammatory and immune responses evoked by, for example, tissue trauma, chemical irritants, infection, or foreign proteins. Therefore, they are frequently used therapeutically.

In this chapter, both the physiologic and the supraphysiologic (i.e., pharmacologic) actions of glucocorticoids (summarized in **Parts J** and **K**) will be discussed.

Starvation

Cortisol acts permissively to facilitate fuel mobilization in times of need. The nocturnal surge of cortisol discussed in Chapter 25 supports the enhanced gluconeogenesis and lipolysis necessary for overnight metabolic stability and, if food continues to be unavailable, for longer periods of time. The rate of amino acid mobilization from muscle is noticeably increased during starvation. Therefore, when liver glycogen stores have been depleted (by exercise, for example), deficient gluconeogenesis from amino acids may lead to death from hypoglycemia if glucocorticoid secretion is also deficient. Cortisol also antagonizes the actions of insulin on glucose metabolism, thereby inhibiting insulin-stimulated glucose uptake into muscle, lymphoid, connective, and adipose tissue (which leaves more glucose in blood to go to insulin-insensitive tissue such as nerves) (**Part I**). Cortisol also increases appetite, probably by inducing neuropeptide-Y synthesis in the hypothalamus. In short, cortisol is an important diabetogenic, anti-insulin hormone during starvation. Its primary hyperglycemic and lipolytic actions and secondary proteolytic and ketogenic actions are usually exhibited only when its secretion is greatly stimulated by metabolic stress. Cortisol then potentiates and extends the duration of hyperglycemia evoked by glucagon, epinephrine, and growth hormone and accentuates loss of body protein.

Effects on Muscle

At low concentrations, cortisol has an inotropic effect on muscle that may be exerted via an increase in acetylcholine synthesis at the neuromuscular junction. Cortisol also increases β-adrenergic receptor synthesis (like thyroxine and progesterone). Cortisol excess, however, causes insulin insensitivity (decreased glucose uptake), muscle proteolysis, and consequently reduced muscle mass and strength (particularly of slow oxidative type I muscle fibers).

Effects on Fat Tissue

Cortisol enhances the synthesis of *adipolytic triglyceride lipase* (i.e., hormone-sensitive lipase), thereby enhancing the actions of other lipolytic hormones, and decreases glucose uptake into adipocytes, thereby reducing triglyceride deposition (because glucose is required for adipocyte glycerol formation). However, when food intake is increased, glucocorticoid excess induces fat redistribution to centripetal areas, with deposits occurring in the face ("moonface") and suprascapular regions ("buffalo hump"). Excessive fat distribution can also lead to a pendulous abdomen.

Hyperlipidemic Action

As previously stated, cortisol increases lipolysis by epinephrine, ACTH, and GH during starvation by decreasing glucose entry into adipocytes and increasing hormone-sensitive lipase synthesis. Free fatty acids enter the circulation and are removed into liver cells, where they are repackaged into triglyceride and exocytosed into the circulation as very-low-density lipoprotein (VLDL), thereby creating a hypertriglyceridemia. Cortisol also decreases sensitivity of the anterior pituitary to TRH, thereby reducing TSH output. The relative hypothyroid state that follows can cause hypercholesterolemia, as T_4 is required to maintain LDL receptor synthesis in liver cells.

Effects on the Liver

Cortisol enhances the gluconeogenic effects of glucagon, GH, and epinephrine enough to restore depleted glycogen levels. It also promotes the resynthesis of triglyceride and facilitates VLDL formation and exocytosis. When free fatty acids are in excess, cortisol also increases the hepatic production of ketone bodies (see **Part I**). By increasing hepatic angiotensinogen production, cortisol excess can lead to hypertension.

Effects on Bone

Cortisol reduces Ca^{2+} availability to bone by: 1) opposing the action of vitamin D in the intestine, 2) decreasing Ca^{2+} and PO_4^{3-} reabsorption in the nephron, and 3) increasing the rate of bone resorption. Cortisol also reduces the synthesis of type I collagen, a fundamental component of bone matrix. Consequently, a major consequence of cortisol excess is a reduction in bone mass (i.e., osteoporosis).

36 ACTH and Glucocorticoids: IV

K

Effector	Response
Blood	Hypertriglyceridemia* Hypercholesterolemia* Hyperglycemia* ↑Erythrocytes, leukocytes, platelets, neutrophils* ↓Lymphocytes, eosinophils, basophils* ↓Antibodies
Bone	↑Resorption + ↓Accretion = ↓Bone mass* ↓Type I collagen*
Connective Tissue	↓Collagen synthesis* ↓Fibroblast activity*
CNS	↑Appetite ↑Sensory acuity ↓REM sleep* Insomnia* Mood swings* ↓Seizure threshold* ↓CRH secretion
Fat Tissue	↑Hormone-sensitive lipase synthesis ↑Lipolysis ↓Glucose uptake Fat redistribution (facial, suprascapular, abdominal)
Fetus	Maturation of: CNS Retina GI tract Lungs ↑Surfactant synthesis
GI Tract	Stomach (ulcerogenic)*: ↑HCl secretion ↓HOC_3^- secretion ↓Prostaglandin production Duodenum: ↓Ca^{2+} absorption

*Actions occurring when plasma titers of cortisol are substantially elevated (e.g., during therapeutic application, Cushing's-like syndrome or disease, or severe chemical, physical, or emotional stress).

Effector	Response
Immune System	↓Immune response ↓Macrophage interleukin-1 release ↓T-cell interleukin-2 and -6 release ↓Tumor necrosis factor α ↓T-cell proliferation ↓B-cell proliferation ↓Antibody production
Inflammatory System	↓Inflammatory Response* ↓Phospholipase A_2 ↓Arachidonic acid ↓Leukotrienes ↓Neutrophil function ↓Bacterial killing ↓Cyclooxygenase ↓Prostaglandins ↓Thromboxanes Vasodilation ↓Platelet-activating factor ↓Nitric oxide
Kidneys	↑Excretion of H_2O load Maintain GFR (↓Cortisol → ↓Urine volume) Blunt ADH release and renal effects* PU/PD* ↓Ca^{2+} and PO_4^{3-} reabsorption* Glutamine → NH_4^+ + glucose
Liver	↑Gluconeogenesis ↑Glycogenesis ↑Lipogenesis ↑Ketogenesis ↑Angiotensinogen
Muscle	Inotropic ↑β-Adrenergic receptor synthesis ↑Proteolysis* ↓Glucose uptake (insulin insensitivity)*
Pituitary	↓ACTH secretion (acute) and synthesis (chronic) ↓TSH → ↓T_4 → ↓LDL receptors → ↑Cholesterol ↓GH ↓ADH
Vasculature	Assist in maintaining normal blood volume and pressure

Overview

- Cortisol excess causes capillary fragility.
- Cortisol assists in maintaining normal blood pressure and volume.
- Cortisol aids in the excretion of a water load.
- Cortisol excess can precipitate gastric and/or duodenal ulceration.
- Cortisol aids fetal development.
- Glucocorticoids are used to treat lymphomas and lymphocyte leukemia.
- Glucocorticoids, in pharmacological amounts, have antiinflammatory and immunosuppressive properties.

Effects on Connective Tissue

Cortisol excess inhibits collagen synthesis and fibroblast activity, producing thinning of skin and the walls of capillaries (which can result in capillary fragility, rupture, and intracutaneous hemorrhage).

Effects on the Vascular System

Cortisol helps to maintain normal blood pressure and volume by: 1) sustaining myocardial performance, 2) permitting normal responsiveness of arterioles to the constrictive actions of catecholamines and angiotensin II, 3) decreasing production of vasodilator prostaglandins from the vascular endothelium, and 4) decreasing permeability of the vascular endothelium.

Effects on the Kidneys

Cortisol aids in the excretion of a water load by: 1) helping to maintain the glomerular filtration rate, 2) suppressing ADH release, and 3) decreasing ADH effects on collecting tubules. With cortisol excess, PU/PD is evident. Cortisol is also required for generation of NH_4^+ from glutamine, and aids in the renal gluconeogenic conversion of glutamine hydrocarbons to glucose. As mentioned above, cortisol reduces renal Ca^{2+} and PO_4^{3-} reabsorption.

Effects on the GI Tract

Although cortisol facilitates maturation of the fetal GI tract, glucocorticoid excess in adult animals increases parietal cell HCl secretion and decreases epithelial neck cell HCO_3^- and prostaglandin production in the stomach, thereby reducing the gastric mucosal barrier and favoring peptic ulcer formation. Cortisol also blunts the action of 1,25-DHC on the duodenum, thereby reducing Ca^{2+} absorption.

Effects on the CNS and Pituitary

Cortisol increases appetite, decreases rapid eye movement (REM) sleep, and modulates excitability, mood, and behavior. In excess, cortisol can cause insomnia, elevate or depress moods, decrease memory, and lower the threshold for seizure activity. Cortisol excess also decreases the ability to detect a salty taste and dampens acuity to sensory stimuli. Glucocorticoid therapy can depress CRH and ACTH output, thereby making it more difficult for the pituitary to rebound once therapy has been discontinued. High levels of cortisol also suppress ADH, TSH, and GH release from the pituitary.

Effects on the Fetus

Cortisol facilitates maturation of the fetal CNS, retina, skin, GI tract, and lungs. Immediately prior to parturition, cortisol (and epinephrine) increases surfactant synthesis in type II alveolar epithelial cells.

Effects on Formed Elements of Blood

Cortisol increases the number of circulating erythrocytes by stimulating their production and decreasing their destruction, and increases the number of circulating leukocytes, platelets, and neutrophils by increasing their release from bone marrow and decreasing their removal from the circulation (i.e., inhibiting diapedesis). Cortisol decreases the number of circulating lymphocytes, eosinophils, and basophils four to six hours following a dose by redistributing them away from the periphery rather than by increasing their destruction. Because cortisol decreases the mass of lymphoid tissue by directly inhibiting mitosis, it can be used therapeutically to treat lymphomas and lymphocyte leukemia. Involution of lymph nodes, the thymus, and the spleen leads to decreased antibody production, which may aid in the reduction of an immune response by an organ transplant recipient; however, antibiotics would be necessary adjunct therapy in order to counteract possible infections.

Effects on Inflammatory and Immune Responses

Although cortisol is required for survival of stressed, traumatized, or infected animals, many defense mechanisms engaged in the response to these insults appear to be inhibited by high titers of glucocorticoids. This apparent paradox can be explained by the following: Basal or modestly elevated levels of cortisol may be beneficial during the initial metabolic, inflammatory, and immune responses; however, when local inflammatory reactions become more intense and spread to adjacent uninjured sites, higher titers of glucocorticoids may be required to limit inflammatory and immune responses so that they do not destroy normal tissues.

High levels of cortisol inhibit phospholipase A_2 and cyclooxygenase, thereby reducing eicosanoid biosynthesis (i.e., prostaglandins, thromboxanes, and leukotrienes) from arachidonic acid. Cortisol also inhibits synthesis of nitric oxide and platelet-activating factor, thereby impairing the vascular component of inflammation. Inhibition of leukotriene synthesis impairs neutrophil phagocytosis and the bactericidal abilities of the organism. Further inhibition of antigen presentation and macrophage lymphokine release (i.e., interleukin-1) impairs proliferation and further cytokine release from T cells. Ultimately, B-cell function is reduced, antibody production declines, and both cellular and humoral immunity are affected.

Although the antiinflammatory and immunosuppressive effects of glucocorticoids may be useful in treating various disease states, when these hormones are administered therapeutically over long periods of time, they may: 1) increase susceptibility to bacterial, fungal, and viral infections and allow their dissemination; 2) delay wound healing; 3) exacerbate the symptoms of diabetes mellitus, osteoporosis, and psychiatric disorders; and 4) seriously retard anterior pituitary release of ACTH and adrenal release of cortisol once discontinued. Therefore, **judicious care must be exercised in their use.**

37 Cushing's-Like Syndrome and Disease

A

Signs and Symptoms of Cushing's-Like Syndrome	
Physical	**CBC**
Cutaneous hyperpigmentation	Mature leukocytosis
Short stature and immature hair coat in young animals	Neutrophilia
PU/PD	Lymphopenia
Polyphagia	Eosinopenia
Abdominal enlargement	Erythrocytosis (mild)
Thin skin (bilateral alopecia)	
Bruising	**Plasma Profile**
Exercise intolerance (muscle weakness and wasting)	↑Alkaline phosphatase, ↑alanine aminotransferase (ALT)
Increased respiratory rate	↑Cholesterol
Lethargy and obesity	Hypertriglyceridemia (↑VLDL)
Heat intolerance	Hyperglycemia, ↑insulin
Skin infections	↓Blood urea nitrogen (BUN)
Hypothyroidism	↓T_4, T_3, TSH, GH, FSH, LH
Calcinosis cutis	
Exophthalmos	**Urinalysis**
Anestrus, clitoral hypertrophy	↓Specific gravity
Testicular atrophy	Urinary tract infection
Osteoporosis	Glucosuria
Hepatomegaly	Urinary calculi (calcium phosphate or calcium oxalate)
Hypertension, congestive heart failure	↑Cortisol: creatinine ratio

B

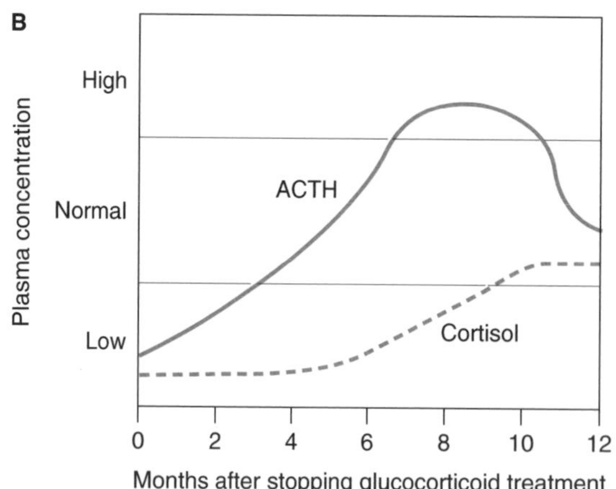

Source: **Part B** modified from Ganong WF. Review of medical physiology. 18th ed. Stamford, CT: Appleton & Lange, 1997: 352.

Overview

- Most animals with PDH have a pituitary tumor.
- Not all animals with PDH exhibit hyperpigmentation due to excessive ACTH secretion.
- Cushing's-like syndrome is associated with muscle weakness and wasting, as well as numerous other clinical signs.
- Mitotane (o,p'-DDD) is used to treat adrenocortical tumors.
- Excessive long-term administration of glucocorticoids can cause iatrogenic Cushing's-like syndrome, inhibit adrenocortical synthesis and secretion of cortisol, hypothalamic release of CRH, and pituitary release of ACTH for extended periods of time.

In 1932, Harvey Cushing published his observations that basophilic tumors of the pituitary were associated with secondary adrenocortical hyperplasia. The collective condition including tumors of the pituitary with associated hyperadrenocorticism was thus called *Cushing's disease* in humans, and *Cushing's-like disease* in animals. The term *Cushing's syndrome* was originally used to denote primary hypersecreting tumors of adrenal cortices (in order to differentiate them from ACTH-secreting tumors of the pituitary). However, today Cushing's syndrome (or Cushing's-like syndrome) is used as a general term to denote the clinical and pathophysiologic manifestations resulting from chronic exposure to excessive amounts of glucocorticoids. Therefore, Cushing's syndrome can have several origins (e.g., pituitary-dependent hyperadrenocorticism, PDH; ectopic ACTH-secreting tumors; primary hyperadrenocorticism; or chronic excesses of exogenously administered ACTH or glucocorticoids). The term Cushing's disease is still applied to those cases of Cushing's syndrome resulting from PDH, which accounts for the majority of cases in domestic animals.

Cushing's-Like Disease

Pituitary-dependent hyperadrenocorticism in animals is caused by chronic excessive ACTH secretion, which results in excess cortisol secretion and, eventually, adrenocortical hyperplasia. Although ectopic ACTH-secreting tumors have been described in humans, they have not yet been reported in animals.

Pituitary-dependent hyperadrenocorticism is characterized by a lack of glucocorticoid feedback inhibition on ACTH secretion and loss of hypothalamic control. Normal stimuli such as physical stress or hypoglycemia fail to cause additional ACTH secretion. Possible causes include pituitary hyperplasia, pituitary adenoma, pituitary carcinoma, and CNS dysfunction resulting in excessive stimulation of pituitary corticotrophs by CRH. Most animals with PDH have a pituitary tumor.

Because ACTH shares a common amino acid sequence with α-MSH (see Chapters 7 and 8), patients with PDH would be expected to exhibit hyperpigmentation. Although hyperpigmentation may be evident, not all animals with PDH exhibit this sign. Also, hyperpigmentation has been described in animals with either pituitary or adrenal causes for Cushing's-like syndrome.

Primary Hyperadrenocorticism

Functional adrenocortical tumors (adenomas or carcinomas) causing signs and symptoms of Cushing's-like syndrome can usually be identified by ultrasonography. These tumors function independent of ACTH control, and both CRH and ACTH blood levels are usually low or undetectable. If the tumor is unilateral, cortical atrophy of the uninvolved adrenal will also be evident. Histologically, the zona reticularis will be severely reduced; however, the zona glomerulosa may be near normal. Mitotane (o,p'-DDD, Ortho para'DDD, Lysodren) is used in the treatment of adrenocortical tumors. Although closely related to the insecticides DDD and DDT, mitotane is the prototype of a drug with selective antitumor activity against adrenocortical carcinoma; however, it is also toxic to normal adrenal cortical cells. As most adrenal tumors are handled surgically, this drug is used almost exclusively for adrenal hyperplasia.

Iatrogenic Cushing's-Like Syndrome

Chronic exposure to excessive amounts of exogenous glucocorticoids may also result in the development of the classic signs and symptoms of Cushing's-like syndrome (**Part A**). Reports of chronic exposure to excessive amounts of injectable, oral, topical, or ophthalmic glucocorticoids indicate the importance of this source of the syndrome. **Due to sustained negative feedback effects of long-term exposure to glucocorticoids, the pituitary and adrenal glands may take weeks to months to recover before they can secrete normal amounts of ACTH and cortisol (Part B).**

Excess glucocorticoids can also inhibit normal pituitary and hypothalamic function, resulting in secondary hypothyroidism (decreased TSH), testicular atrophy and anestrus (decreased gonadotropins), and short stature among young animals (decreased GH).

38 Mineralocorticoids

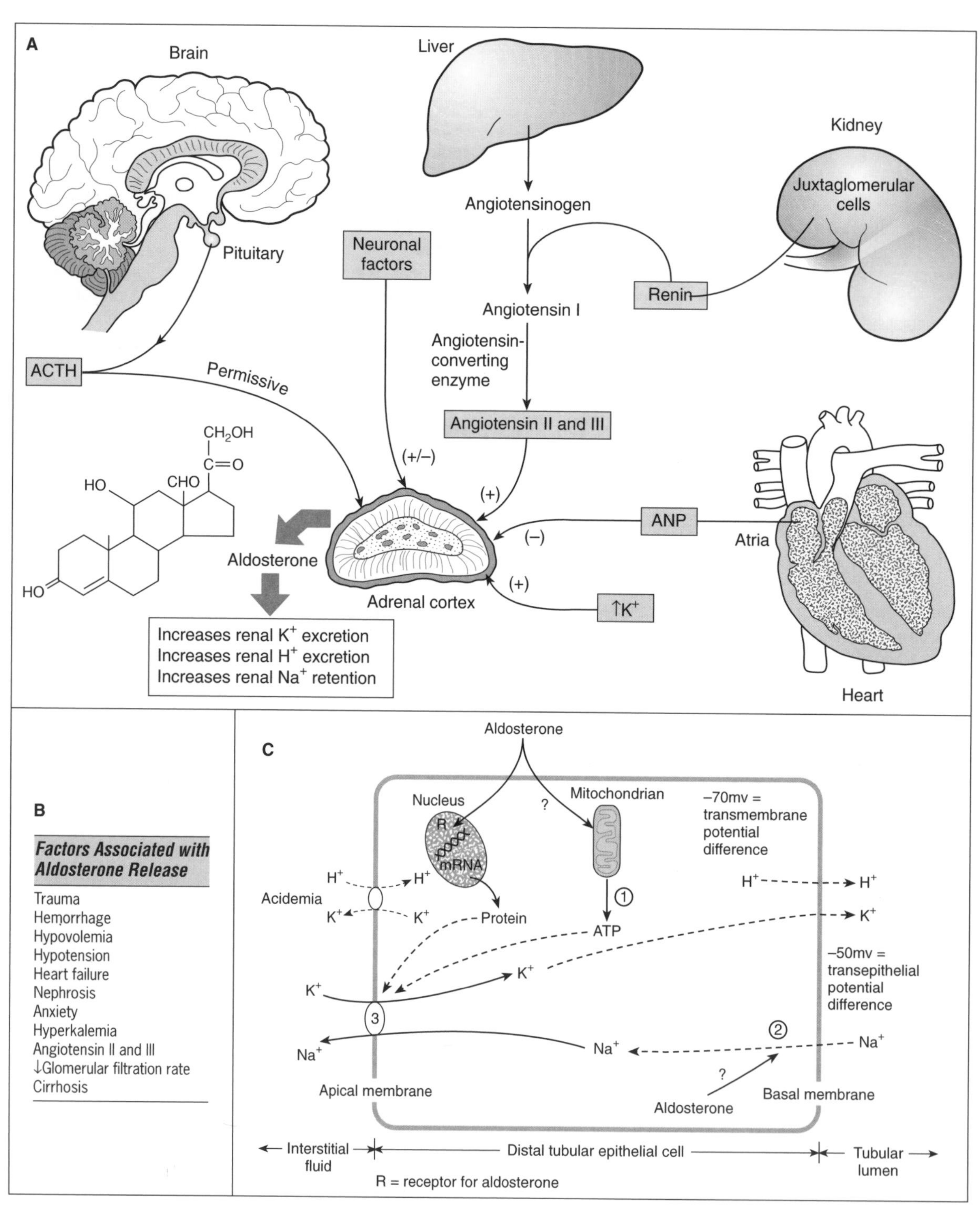
A
Brain
Pituitary
ACTH
Permissive
Liver
Angiotensinogen
Kidney
Juxtaglomerular cells
Renin
Angiotensin I
Angiotensin-converting enzyme
Angiotensin II and III
Neuronal factors
(+/–)
(+)
ANP
(–)
Atria
Heart
↑K+
(+)
CH2OH
C=O
HO
CHO
HO
Aldosterone
Adrenal cortex
Increases renal K+ excretion
Increases renal H+ excretion
Increases renal Na+ retention
B
Factors Associated with Aldosterone Release
Trauma
Hemorrhage
Hypovolemia
Hypotension
Heart failure
Nephrosis
Anxiety
Hyperkalemia
Angiotensin II and III
↓Glomerular filtration rate
Cirrhosis
C
Aldosterone
Nucleus
R
mRNA
?
Mitochondrian
–70mv = transmembrane potential difference
Acidemia
H+
H+
K+
K+
Protein
1
ATP
H+
H+
K+
K+
–50mv = transepithelial potential difference
K+
3
Na+
Na+
2
Na+
?
Aldosterone
Apical membrane
Basal membrane
Interstitial fluid
Distal tubular epithelial cell
Tubular lumen
R = receptor for aldosterone

Overview

- The adrenal cortex secretes aldosterone due largely to the presence of two non-pituitary factors, K^+ and angiotensin II.
- Aldosterone primarily causes the distal tubules of the kidney to save Na^+ and to secrete K^+ and H^+ into the filtrate.

The zona glomerulosa of the adrenal cortex secretes *aldosterone,* its major mineralocorticoid, independent of direct pituitary control. *Corticosterone* and *11-deoxycorticosterone* are additional mineralocorticoids secreted by the adrenal cortex; however, they possess less than 3% of the activity of aldosterone (see Chapter 34).

Although ACTH appears to play a permissive role in maintaining biosynthetic stability and responsiveness of the zona glomerulosa to other controlling factors (e.g., increased serum K^+ and the angiotensins; **Part A**), it does not directly stimulate aldosterone release. The major target sites for aldosterone are the distal convoluted tubules and cortical collecting ducts of the kidney, where it facilitates Na^+ reabsorption as well as K^+ and H^+ secretion.

Factors Stimulating Aldosterone Release

A 1% increase in the plasma K^+ concentration (<0.1 mEq/L) is a potent stimulus for aldosterone release from the zona glomerulosa. Aldosterone secretion is also increased in the hyponatremic, volume-depleted patient (**Part B**). This is largely due to the presence of angiotensin II and III, which are formed in blood after a drop in blood pressure or volume (see Chapter 39). The angiotensins and K^+ stimulate conversion of cholesterol to pregnenolone, and corticosterone to aldosterone, in the zona glomerulosa (see Chapter 33). They do not, however, increase secretion of 11-deoxycorticosterone. Although ACTH increases cAMP levels in adrenocortical cells, the angiotensins increase diacylglycerol levels and the activity of protein kinase C. Also, K^+ apparently depolarizes cells of the zona glomerulosa, opening voltage-gated Ca^{2+} channels and thus increasing intracellular Ca^{2+} levels (see Chapters 3 and 4).

Chronically elevated blood volume or pressure stretches atria of the heart, causing release of *atrial natriuretic peptide (ANP),* which in turn inhibits aldosterone release from the adrenal cortex (**Part A**) and stimulates renal Na^+ excretion. This peptide also inhibits ADH release from the posterior pituitary and renin release from juxtaglomerular cells in the kidney (see Chapters 39 and 40).

The adrenal cortex is also well supplied with neurons that secrete a variety of products. Serotonin, norepinephrine, acetylcholine, vasoactive intestinal polypeptide, vasopressin, and prostaglandins are all found in the adrenal cortex, and all can stimulate aldosterone release. Somatostatin may also be produced locally and is known to inhibit angiotensin II–induced aldosterone release. Although neuronal regulation of aldosterone release may occur, it is not considered a primary physiologic control mechanism.

In normal animals, plasma aldosterone secretion increases during the active portion of the day. Aldosterone is secreted at a rate 100 times slower than cortisol and 50% to 60% of aldosterone is bound in plasma to albumin. Its biologic half-life is about 20 minutes.

Mineralocorticoid Target Sites

Aldosterone and other mineralocorticoids increase Na^+ reabsorption and K^+ and H^+ secretion predominantly in the distal nephron and cortical collecting ducts. To a lesser extent, Na^+/K^+ ATPase activity is also increased in sweat and salivary glands, the gastric mucosa, and the large intestine. Aldosterone has also been shown to stimulate K^+ uptake by muscle, liver, adipose and nerve tissue.

Aldosterone and Renal Na^+ Reabsorption

The primary effect of aldosterone on Na^+ transport in the distal nephron is to increase its movement from the tubular lumen to the interstitium, and then to the bloodstream. Because H_2O is passively reabsorbed with Na^+, there is little increase in the plasma Na^+ concentration, and ECF volume expands in an isotonic fashion. Although only 3% of total Na^+ reabsorption is regulated by aldosterone, deficiency of this hormone produces a significantly negative Na^+ balance, while excess produces hypertension.

Aldosterone, like other steroid hormones, binds to nuclear receptors and enhances DNA-dependent mRNA synthesis in its target cells (**Part C**). The mRNA, in turn, stimulates protein synthesis at the ribosomal level.

The functions of aldosterone-induced protein synthesis remain unsettled; however, three hypotheses have evolved (see numbered processes in **Part C**):

1. *Metabolic hypothesis:* Aldosterone increases mitochondrial oxidation of substrates (perhaps free fatty acids) in its target cells, thus providing reduced nicotinamide adenine dinucleotide (NADH) for ATP production.
2. *Permease hypothesis:* Aldosterone increases (passive) permeability of basal membranes to Na^+.
3. *Na^+ pump hypothesis:* Aldosterone increases synthesis of Na^+/K^+ ATPase, and when these pump molecules are inserted into apical membranes, Na^+ extrusion is increased.

Although all three hypotheses may be correct, the third appears to be the most widely accepted.

Aldosterone fails to exert any effect on Na^+ reabsorption for 10 to 30 minutes or more when injected directly into the renal artery, and for 1 to 2 hours when secreted endogenously. This latent period represents the time needed to increase protein synthesis within its target cells.

Aldosterone and Renal K^+ Secretion

As most filtered K^+ is reabsorbed in the proximal nephron, urinary K^+ excretion largely reflects the quantity secreted from epithelial cells of the distal tubules and cortical collecting ducts.

Aldosterone-stimulated Na^+ reabsorption leaves the relatively impermeable chloride anion behind in the tubular filtrate, thus increasing the *transepithelial potential difference.* This relatively high negativity of the tubular filtrate (about −50 mV; **Part C**) allows K^+ to diffuse down its concentration gradient into the tubular lumen. As aldosterone also increases Na^+/K^+ ATPase activity in apical membranes, more K^+ is available for secretion. Chronic high levels of aldosterone will thus result in hypokalemia.

Aldosterone and Renal H^+ Secretion

Aldosterone also enhances distal tubular secretion of H^+ as the transepithelial potential difference increases. Aldosterone excess causes hypokalemia, which eventually leads to an increase in the intracellular H^+ concentration of distal tubular epithelial cells (relative to K^+). This favors distal tubular secretion of H^+, thus leading to the development of metabolic alkalosis. In contrast, aldosterone deficiency produces hyperkalemia and metabolic acidosis. If acidemia is the primary originating event, there is cellular exchange of K^+ for H^+ (**Part C**), leading to increased aldosterone-stimulated renal H^+ secretion and hyperkalemia.

Hypothyroidism

Aldosterone-stimulated renal Na^+/K^+ ATPase activity is dependent on adequate titers of the thyroid hormones (T_3 and T_4). With thyroid deficiency, the aldosterone Na^+ conservation mechanism is impaired and renal Na^+ excretion is enhanced (see Chapter 51). This leads primarily to osmotic dilution of body fluids (i.e., hyponatremia), because the ADH mechanism for renal H_2O retention remains intact to maintain the ECF volume.

39 Renin–Angiotensin System: I

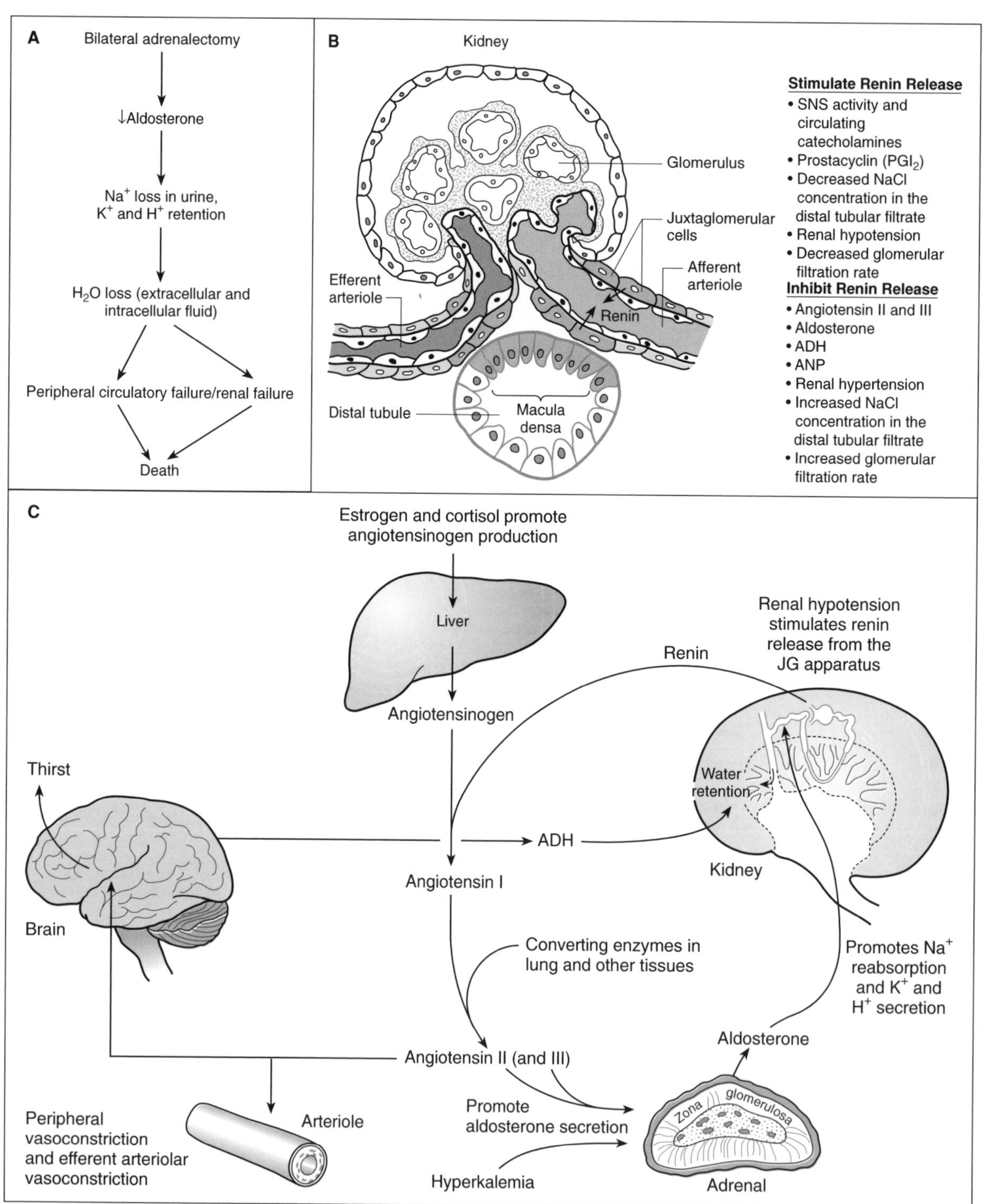

Source: Part B modified from Ham AW. Histology. 7th ed. Philadelphia: JB Lippincott, 1974:753, and Ganong WF: The renin-angiotensin system and the central nervous system. Fed Proc 1977;36:1771.

Overview

- The renin-angiotensin-aldosterone system aids in the long-term control of blood pressure and volume.
- JG cells located in afferent arterioles of the kidney secrete renin.
- Angiotensinogen is a circulating plasma protein produced by the liver.
- Angiotensin converting enzyme (ACE) is located primarily in capillaries of the lungs.
- Angiotensin II is a potent vasoconstrictor; it stimulates catecholamine, ADH, and aldosterone release and promotes thirst.
- A decrease in the GFR is indirectly sensed by specialized cells in the distal renal tubules (the macula densa). These cells in turn promote renin release from adjacent JG cells.

Although hypophysectomy is not life-threatening, bilateral adrenalectomy is fatal (**Part A**). The life-maintaining principles supplied by the adrenal cortices are cortisol, a glucocorticoid, and perhaps more importantly the renal Na^+-retaining mineralocorticoid, aldosterone, which is produced by cells of the zona glomerulosa (see Chapter 38). Aldosterone deficiency, whether it occurs in an experimental animal or in a patient, results in hyperkalemia, metabolic acidosis, hyponatremia, peripheral circulatory failure, renal failure, and inexorably, death.

An important factor controlling aldosterone secretion is the renin–angiotensin system, a multifactorial physiologic control system for maintaining blood pressure and volume. A major component of the renin–angiotensin system is the *juxtaglomerular (JG) apparatus* of the kidney. The JG apparatus is a combination of specialized vascular and tubular cells located near the glomerulus, where afferent and efferent arterioles come into close contact with the distal tubule (**Part B**). The JG cells are specialized myoepithelial cells of the afferent arteriole that synthesize, store, and secrete into blood a proteolytic enzyme called *renin. Macula densa cells* are specialized distal renal tubular epithelial cells that sense the NaCl concentration of the filtrate and can signal the JG cells to secrete renin.

Part C depicts the processes involved in the renin–angiotensin system. Circulating renin splits the end off a liver-derived plasma protein called *angiotensinogen* (or renin substrate), thus generating the decapeptide *angiotensin I.* Within a few seconds, two additional amino acids are split off angiotensin I to form *angiotensin II.* This conversion occurs mainly in pulmonary capillary endothelial cells through the activity of dipeptidyl carboxypeptidase, otherwise known as *angiotensin-converting enzyme (ACE).* This enzyme is found to a lesser degree in blood plasma and renal tissue. Angiotensin II persists in blood for approximately 1 minute, but it is rapidly inactivated by a number of different blood and tissue enzymes collectively called *angiotensinase.* While active in blood, angiotensin II stimulates aldosterone synthesis and release from the adrenal cortex, among other actions.

The Angiotensins

Angiotensin II is one of the most potent known vasoconstrictors. It promotes norepinephrine release from sympathetic nerve endings, as well as epinephrine and norepinephrine release from the adrenal medulla. It also vasoconstricts peripheral arterioles, efferent arterioles of the kidney, and to a lesser extent, veins. Primary stimuli for angiotensin generation are a decrease in blood volume and/or pressure (e.g., hemorrhage) and a decrease in the glomerular filtration rate (GFR).

Arteriolar constriction increases peripheral resistance, thereby raising arterial pressure back toward normal. Also, mild constriction of veins increases mean circulatory filling pressure, sometimes by as much as 20%, which promotes an increased tendency for venous return of blood to the heart, helping it to pump against the extra pressure load.

Other effects of angiotensin are primarily related to more long-term body fluid volume restoration: 1) it has a direct effect on proximal tubules of the kidneys to enhance NaCl reabsorption; 2) it stimulates aldosterone secretion; 3) it stimulates thirst; and 4) it promotes ADH secretion.

A metabolic product of angiotensin II, des-Asp-angiotensin II or *angiotensin III,* is as potent as angiotensin II in releasing aldosterone but is a less effective pressor agent. It is probably most important in rats, where it accounts for almost 60% of angiotensin activity. In humans and dogs, only about 10% of angiotensin activity is attributable to angiotensin III.

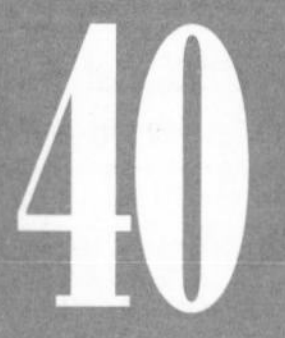

Renin – Angiotensin System: II

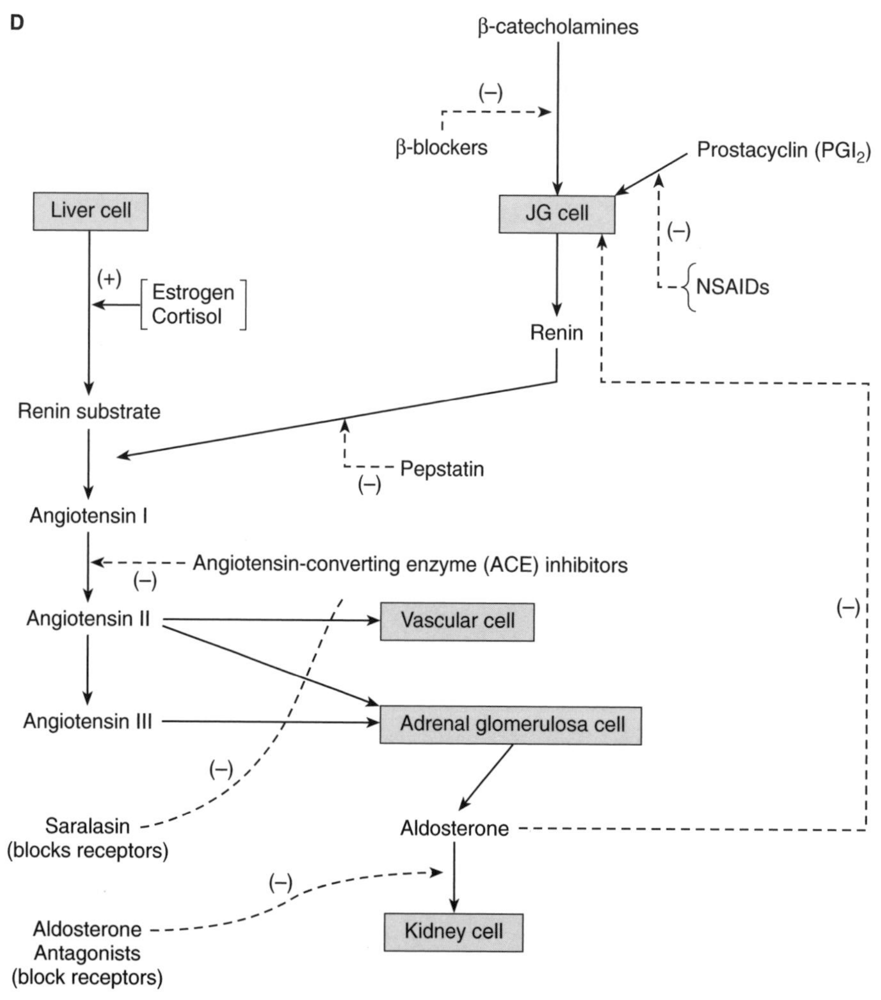

Overview

- Nonsteroidal antiinflammatory drugs (NSAIDs) and those that block β-adrenergic receptors reduce renin release.
- Estrogens and glucocorticoids enhance hepatic angiotensinogen release.
- Hypertensive patients with adrenal tumors may have low-renin hypertension and therefore may not respond to ACE inhibitors, NSAIDs, or β-adrenergic blocking agents.
- There may be a separate renin-angiotensin system within the brain for the control of cerebral blood pressure.
- The afferent arteriole, which releases renin, is a modified stretch receptor.

Factors Regulating Renin Secretion

Renin secretion is regulated by several variables (see **Part B**). The sympathetic nervous system (SNS) plays a role in stimulating renin release via renal sympathetic nerves and circulating catecholamines. Adrenergic effects on JG cells are exerted via β_1-adrenergic receptors (and intracellular cAMP) and are thus enhanced by *isoproterenol,* a β-agonist, and attenuated by *propranolol,* a β-blocker (**Part D**). Although renal innervation is not a requisite for renin release, the SNS can modulate the secretion of renin and thus have an indirect effect on aldosterone release.

Locally produced prostaglandins (mainly prostacyclin, PGI_2) stimulate renin release, apparently by a direct action on JG cells.

Intrarenal arteriolar pressure is monitored by *stretch receptors* (i.e., high pressure baroreceptors) in the JG body (i.e., afferent arterioles). When blood pressure falls, renin is released. In addition, a drop in GFR due to pressure and volume depletion reduces the filtered load and increases time for NaCl reabsorption in the proximal nephron. These combined events reduce delivery of NaCl to cells of the macula densa, which in turn sense the reduced NaCl concentration of the filtrate and signal adjacent JG cells to secrete renin into the circulation.

Negative feedback on renin release is exerted by angiotensin II and III, aldosterone, ADH, ANP, volume repletion, and restoration of the GFR. Evidence indicates that atrial stretching, volume expansion, and high-Na^+ states elicit elaboration of ANP into the circulation. At the renal level, ANP reduces renin release and causes renal vasodilation, natriuresis, and diuresis. It also inhibits aldosterone release from the adrenal cortex.

Renin Substrate

Angiotensinogen, also called renin substrate, is an α_2-globulin synthesized in the liver. It is the prohormone of the angiotensins and appears in higher concentrations in plasma as a result of hepatic glucocorticoid or estrogen stimulation. Although the amount of available renin substrate is not rate-limiting under ordinary circumstances, an increase in its concentration may lead to the production of inappropriately high amounts of angiotensin and thus aldosterone. Increases in plasma renin substrate concentrations during pregnancy inevitably lead to increases in angiotensin and aldosterone production. In spite of these dramatic changes, however, normal pregnancy elicits few signs of hyperaldosteronism. There is no tendency toward hypokalemia or hypernatremia, and blood pressure at mid-pregnancy, when changes in the renin–angiotensin system are maximal, tends to be lower than in the nonpregnant state. It has been postulated that edema of late pregnancy is due to these changes, but hyperaldosteronism of nonpregnancy leads to hypertension, not edema. Estrogen therapy and pharmacologic amounts of glucocorticoids also elevate renin substrate levels. In severe liver disease or adrenocortical insufficiency, plasma renin substrate levels may be low.

Renin-Angiotensin System Pharmacology

When the design of a complex physiologic regulatory system becomes apparent, it is sometimes possible to modify that system at several points with drugs. The renin–angiotensin system is a good example (**Part D**).

Pharmacologic intervention into this system is usually beneficial. In some instances, however, the system may be adversely affected by drugs that are being administered for purposes unrelated to blood volume and pressure regulation.

Because the JG cell is stimulated by catecholamine β-agonists, its secretion can be reduced by β-blocking agents such as propranolol. These β-blockers are sometimes used to treat high-renin hypertension. Additionally, aspirin, indomethacin, and other nonsteroidal anti-inflammatory drugs (NSAIDs) reduce cyclooxygenase activity and, therefore, inhibit local prostacyclin release.

Renin's action on angiotensinogen can be blocked by pepstatin, and although angiotensin I is biologically inactive, the effects of excessive production of renin can be additionally neutralized through administration of ACE inhibitors, which reduce angiotensin II and III synthesis by the converting enzyme. Saralasin is another drug that binds to stereospecific plasma membrane receptors for angiotensin II and III, thus preventing them from illiciting biologic responses.

Drugs that inhibit renin secretion and reduce production of the angiotensins or prevent their actions can also be useful diagnostic agents in characterizing the contribution of the renin–angiotensin system to the hypertension of individual patients. For example, hypertensive patients with aldosterone-secreting tumors would be expected to exhibit low-renin hypertension; therefore β-blockers, NSAIDs, ACE inhibitors, and saralasin would have minimal effects in normalizing blood pressure and volume in these patients. However, the spirolactones, which are structural analogues of aldosterone, compete with aldosterone for its receptors and thus reduce its effects in the kidney. These are effective therapeutic agents for treating low-renin hypertension as well as edematous states.

Independent Renin-Angiotensin Systems

Renin, angiotensinogen, ACE, and angiotensin II have all been found in the brain, pituitary, gonads, and adrenal cortex. This has led some investigators to speculate that the complete renin–angiotensin system may exist independently within each of these structures. The significance of these observations, however, remains to be elucidated.

41 Addison's-Like Disease

A

Causes of Addison's-Like Disease

Primary Hypoadrenocorticism	Secondary Hypoadrenocorticism
Idiopathic	Naturally occurring
Autoimmune-mediated destruction of the Adrenal Cortex*	↓CRH or ↓ACTH (hypothalamic or pituitary failure);
Spontaneous	from inflammation, tumors, trauma, or congenital defects
Infections	Iatrogenic
Hemorrhage	Prolonged glucocorticoid administration*
Neoplasms	
Trauma	
Amyloidosis	
Iatrogenic (adrenal suppressive therapeutic agents)	
Cytotoxic (e.g., from Mitotane* (o,p'DDD)	
Ketoconazole (blocks ACTH actions)	
Megestrol acetate (a synthetic progestin in cats)	

o,p'DDD = Mitotane (Ortho para'DDD); ACTH = Adrenocorticotropic Hormone; CRH = ACTH Releasing Hormone
*Most common causes

B

Signs and Symptoms of Addison's-Like Disease

Physical	Blood	Urine
Anorexia; thin and weak	CBC (normocytic, normochromic anemia)	↓Specific gravity
Ectomorphy	↓–↑ Hematocrit	
Vomiting, diarrhea (bloody), and dehydration	↓(Mild) erythrocytes, leukocytes, platelets, and neutrophils	
PU/PD	↑(Mild) lymphocytes, eosinophils, and basophils	
Weak pulses and bradycardia	Hyponatremia	
Painful abdomen	Hyperkalemia	
Hypotension	↓Na^+/K^+ ratio	
	Hypochloremia	
	Hypercalcemia	
	Hypoglycemia	
	↑BUN	
	↑ACTH, ↓Cortisol, ↓Aldosterone	
	↑Creatinine	
	Acidemia	

Overview

- Iatrogenic secondary hypoadrenocorticism is the most common cause of adrenal insufficiency (i.e., Addison's-like disease) in domestic animals.
- Hypoglycemia, hypercalcemia, hyponatremia, hypochloremia, metabolic acidosis, and hyperkalemia are common signs in patients with Addison's-like disease.
- Animals with Addison's-like disease sometimes exhibit other endocrinopathies.
- Animals with Addison's-like disease have difficulty dealing with physiologically stressful situations (e.g., trauma, surgery, starvation).
- Cutaneous hyperpigmentation may be seen in patients with primary hypoadrenocorticism.

Thomas Addison described the signs and symptoms of human adrenocortical insufficiency in 1855. Naturally occurring adrenocortical insufficiency in animals, however, was not reported until the 1950s. Hypoadrenocorticism is referred to today as *Addison's disease* in humans, and either Addison's disease or *Addison's-like disease* in animals. It appears to be more frequent in young to middle-aged females.

Causes of Hypoadrenocorticism

The causes of Addison's-like disease are listed in **Part A.** *Idiopathic primary hypoadrenocorticism* is usually bilateral and apparently has an immune-mediated basis in animals as in humans. Animals with this disease may sometimes exhibit additional endocrinopathies (e.g., hypothyroidism, diabetes mellitus, or hypogonadism). *Iatrogenic primary hypoadrenocorticism* may follow administration of the adrenocorticolytic drug mitotane (o,p′-DDD, Ortho para′DDD, Lysodren) for the treatment of Cushing's-like syndrome (see Chapter 37).

Iatrogenic secondary hypoadrenocorticism is the most common cause of adrenal insufficiency and occurs following prolonged administration of glucocorticoids. Exogenous glucocorticoids (i.e., oral, injectable, or topical) inhibit ACTH release and can cause adrenal atrophy. **Depending on the amount and length of glucocorticoid administration, a return to normal pituitary–adrenal function can take weeks to months following steroid withdrawal** (see Chapter 37).

Signs and Symptoms of Hypoadrenocorticism

The signs and symptoms of this disease are first reflected in a glucocorticoid deficiency, and later in both a glucocorticoid and a mineralocorticoid deficiency (see Chapters 33 and 34 and **Part B**). However, more than 90% of the adrenal cortex is reportedly destroyed before clinical signs and symptoms become obvious. As animals encounter stressful situations (e.g., starvation, trauma, surgery, or kennel boarding), they have more difficulty recovering.

As physical signs of this disease can mimic those of others, a definitive diagnosis usually requires a judicious physical exam combined with a CBC, serum chemistry profile, and urinalysis. An additional assessment of adrenal reserve capacity through an ACTH stimulation test may also be needed.

In severe cases, *ectomorphy,* in which tissues derived from ectoderm predominate, may be evident. There may be a preponderance of linearity and fragility, a large surface area with thin muscles and subcutaneous tissue, and slightly developed digestive viscera (as contrasted with endomorphy and mesomorphy).

Although changes in the CBC are generally secondary to glucocorticoid deficiency (see Chapters 35 and 36), dehydration due to mineralocorticoid deficiency can complicate interpretation of the hemogram until patients become rehydrated. An unchanged hemogram in an ill, stressed patient, however, would be abnormal.

Hyponatremia, hypochloremia, hyperkalemia, and a Na^+/K^+ ratio less than 20:1 are not uncommon in patients with hypoadrenocorticism, and the hyperkalemia may require therapy to prevent cardiac arrhythmia (see Chapter 32). Although other causes of a low Na^+/K^+ ratio exist (e.g., renal failure or severe GI disorders), hypoadrenocorticism is indicated when the low ratio is associated with other signs and symptoms listed in **Part B.** Because hypoaldosteronism also impairs distal renal tubular H^+ secretion, a metabolic acidosis may also develop. Hypotension and decreased tissue perfusion will exacerbate the acidemia.

Hypercalcemia associated with hypoadrenocorticism most likely develops because of a decrease in urinary Ca^{2+} excretion. Glucocorticoids normally suppress renal Ca^{2+} reabsorption, and in their absence excessive reabsorption is thought to occur.

Glucocorticoids are required to maintain the plasma glucose concentration between meals by stimulating hepatic gluconeogenesis and decreasing insulin sensitivity in peripheral tissues. Therefore, their absence due to hypoadrenocorticism may result in hypoglycemia. It should be noted, however, that not all animals with hypoadrenocorticism exhibit hypoglycemia.

Blood urea nitrogen (BUN) and creatinine concentrations may also increase due largely to dehydration and ECF volume contraction. The hyponatremia that develops in this disease due to hypoaldosteronism will eventually lead to renal medullary solute washout, diuresis, and a decreased urine specific gravity.

Cutaneous hyperpigmentation would also be expected in patients with primary hypoadrenocorticism, because deficient adrenal cortices remove inhibitory feedback control on the hypothalamus and anterior pituitary. The resulting high titer of ACTH, and potentially α-MSH, would stimulate dermal melanophores, because both hormones contain the polypeptide chain that is responsible for melanosome dispersion (see Chapter 8). For unknown reasons, however, some animals reportedly fail to exhibit this melanophore response in spite of high titers of ACTH.

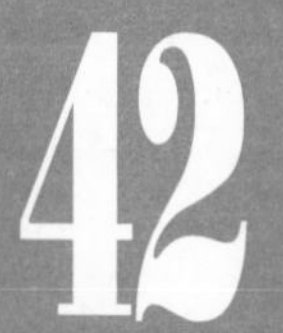

42 Erythropoietin

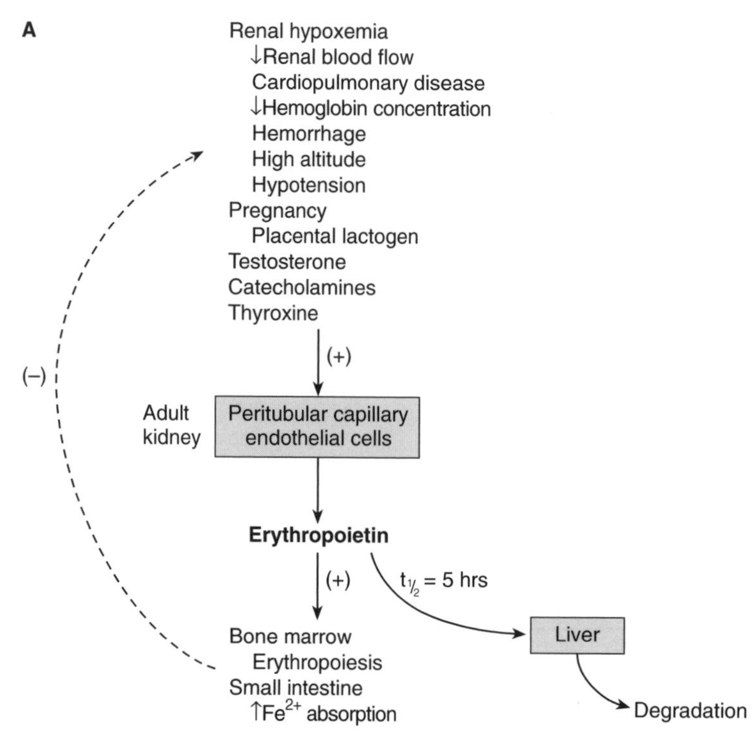
A
Renal hypoxemia
↓Renal blood flow
Cardiopulmonary disease
↓Hemoglobin concentration
Hemorrhage
High altitude
Hypotension
Pregnancy
Placental lactogen
Testosterone
Catecholamines
Thyroxine
(+)
(–)
Adult kidney
Peritubular capillary endothelial cells
Erythropoietin
(+)
$t_{1/2}$ = 5 hrs
Liver
Degradation
Bone marrow
Erythropoiesis
Small intestine
↑Fe^{2+} absorption

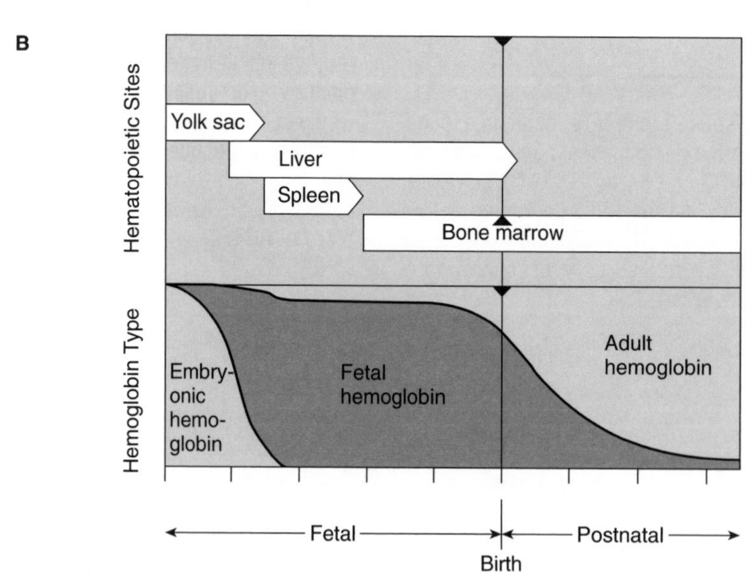
B
Hematopoietic Sites
Yolk sac
Liver
Spleen
Bone marrow
Hemoglobin Type
Embryonic hemoglobin
Fetal hemoglobin
Adult hemoglobin
Fetal
Postnatal
Birth

Overview

- Erythropoietin (EPO) is produced by the fetal liver and the adult kidney.
- Erythropoiesis occurs in the fetal liver and in the adult bone marrow.
- EPO stimulates erythropoiesis in bone marrow and Fe^{2+} uptake by the small intestine.
- The Po_2 of blood perfusing the kidneys primarily controls EPO output.
- Recombinant human erythropoietin alfa (rHuEPO alfa) has been used to treat anemic animals.

The glycoprotein hormone *erythropoietin (EPO)* is produced by peritubular capillary endothelial cells of the adult kidney in response largely to renal hypoxemia. Erythropoietin, containing 166 amino acid residues, stimulates erythropoiesis in bone marrow and Fe^{2+} uptake by the small intestine (**Part A**). Iron is an essential component of the heme fraction of hemoglobin.

As the kidneys maintain a rather constant blood flow (compared with other tissues and organs of the body), it seems appropriate that nature selected them as major sites for EPO production in adult mammals.

Fetal Versus Adult Hemoglobin

In many mammalian species, the fetus has a different hemoglobin from that of the adult. Also, fetal hemoglobin (HbF) does not bind erythrocytic 2,3-diphosphoglycerate (2,3-DPG) with as great an affinity as does adult hemoglobin (HbA), thus giving HbF a greater oxygen-binding affinity. Theoretically, this helps to enhance the oxygen diffusion gradient from maternal to fetal blood. Fetal and adult hemoglobins can be distinguished from one another by their mobility when subjected to electrophoresis and by amino acid analysis, ultraviolet absorption spectra, oxygen dissociation curves, and other tests.

Erythropoiesis (and thus Hb production) occurs in the embryonic yolk sac, then subsequently in the fetal liver and spleen. Bone marrow does not normally establish full erythropoietic potential until the second half of pregnancy, when changeover to the adult type of hemoglobin begins. This changeover continues on into neonatal life, when HbA quickly becomes predominant (**Part B**). In sheep, HbF has been detected up to 35 days of age, but this is thought to be a residue from that made before birth. Fetal hemoglobin in calves has been reported to account for 41% to 100% of total hemoglobin at birth, yet diminishes rapidly as it is replaced with HbA at 2 to 3 months of age. By the end of the first year, HbF is typically only 1% of total hemoglobin. On the other hand, in pigs and horses, the hemoglobin of the fetus is indistinguishable from that of the adult, and replacement of fetal blood by adult blood in humans does not seem to compromise survival of the fetus. Thus, **HbF may be more of a physiologic luxury than a necessity in mammals.**

In addition to variations in the hemoglobin molecule of individual animals (HbF versus HbA), there are also variations between species in the protein (globin) part of the molecule, but not the heme fraction.

Fetal Versus Adult Erythropoietin Production

During fetal life, the major site for EPO production (as for erythropoiesis) is the liver. As the neonate matures, EPO production is taken over by the kidneys. The liver is thought to retain the capacity to produce about 15% of the EPO in adults. Because of this relatively low amount, when renal mass is significantly reduced by disease in adults, the liver cannot adequately compensate—EPO production falls and anemia develops.

Although erythropoietin-releasing tumors that result in polycythemia have been described in animals, the majority of problems related to EPO and thus erythropoiesis result from **decreased** production.

The major factor controlling EPO production is the Po_2 of blood perfusing the kidneys. Decreased renal blood flow, cardiopulmonary disease, decreased hemoglobin production, hemorrhage, high altitude, and hypotension are all examples of factors that cause renal hypoxemia (see **Part A**). Anemia due to decreased EPO production is therefore a major factor to consider in patients with renal failure or any of the above conditions. Placental lactogen and testosterone are also known to be physiologic stimuli for EPO production, and catecholamine-producing tumors (i.e., pheochromocytomas) and thyroxine-producing tumors are also known to stimulate EPO release (see Chapters 46 and 50, respectively). Besides the presence of EPO, erythropoiesis also requires appropriate levels of growth hormone, thyroxine, and cortisol (in both males and females).

The principal site for EPO inactivation is the liver, and the hormone has a circulating half-life of about five hours. However, the increase in circulating red cells that it triggers takes about two to three days to appear (because red cell maturation is a relatively slow process).

The factors stimulating erythropoietin production, as well as the primary effects of the hormone in bone marrow and the small intestine, are shown in **Part A.**

Synthetic Erythropoietin

The gene for erythropoietin has been cloned (like that for somatotropin), and recombinant EPO produced in culture is now therapeutically available. As the structure for EPO has apparently been fairly well conserved across species, either intravenous or subcutaneous *recombinant human erythropoietin alfa (rHuEPO alfa or epogen)* has been reported to be effective in the treatment of anemic domestic animals. However, some dogs and cats with chronic renal failure have been reported to develop anti-rHuEPO antibodies, and therefore exhibit a blunted response to therapy. Anti-rHuEPO antibody production has not been reported in humans.

43 Natriuretic Peptide

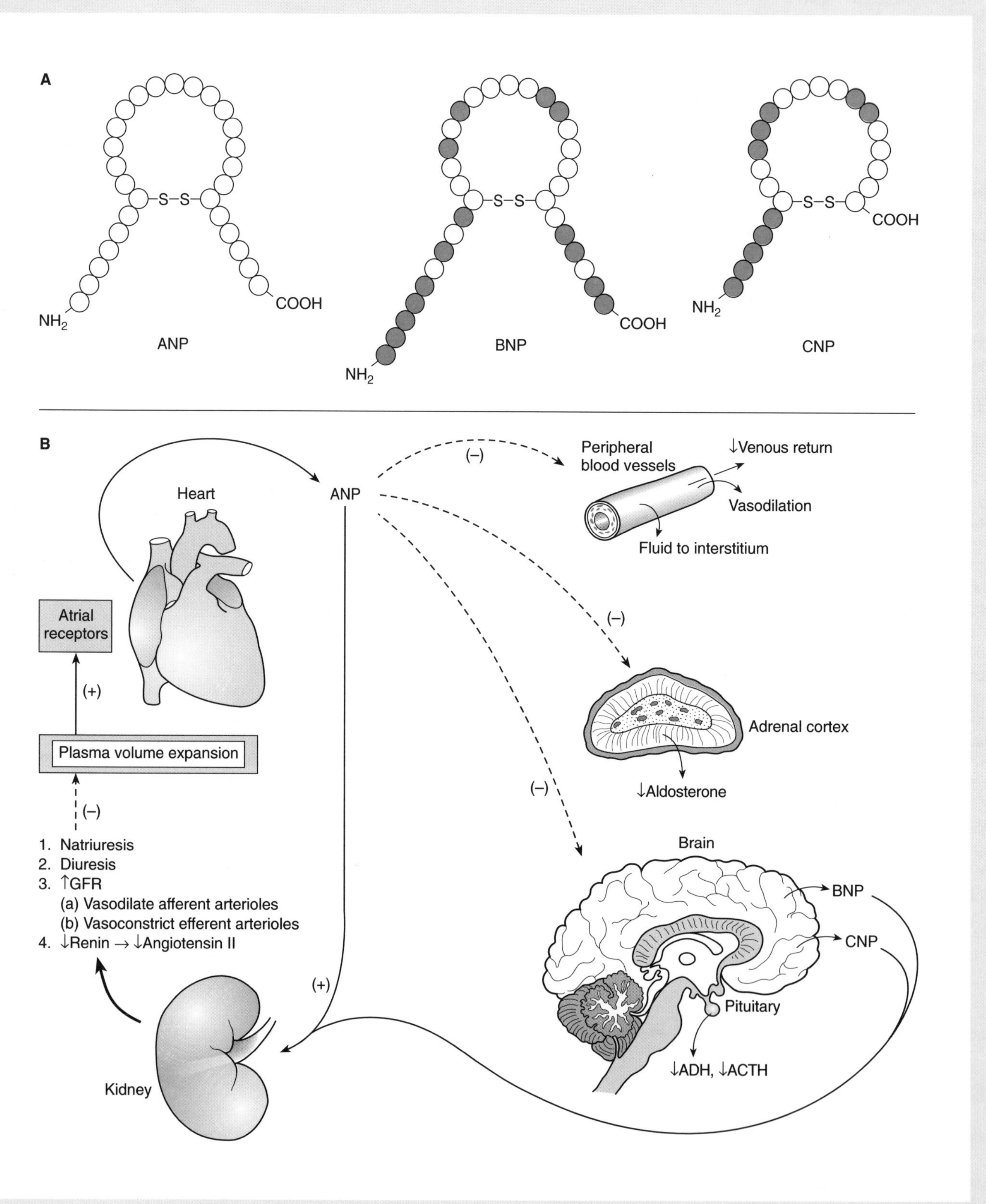
A
S–S
NH2
COOH
ANP
S–S
NH2
COOH
BNP
S–S
NH2
COOH
CNP
B
Heart
ANP
(–)
Peripheral blood vessels
↓Venous return
Vasodilation
Fluid to interstitium
Atrial receptors
(+)
Plasma volume expansion
(–)
1. Natriuresis
2. Diuresis
3. ↑GFR
(a) Vasodilate afferent arterioles
(b) Vasoconstrict efferent arterioles
4. ↓Renin → ↓Angiotensin II
(–)
Adrenal cortex
↓Aldosterone
(–)
Brain
BNP
CNP
Pituitary
↓ADH, ↓ACTH
(+)
Kidney

Overview

- The mammalian heart and brain produce (anti-aldosterone) natriuretic peptides in response to plasma volume expansion.
- The primary effects of ANP are natriuresis and diuresis.
- ANP decreases vascular smooth muscle responsiveness to angiotensin II.
- ANP, BNP and CNP work through the cGMP second messenger system.
- Bioassayable ANP-like activity has also been noted in nonmammalian vertebrates.

Mechanical stretch of the atrial wall caused by blood volume expansion is known to result in the secretion of a peptide hormone into blood that reduces vascular volume. This hormone, produced in atrial myocytes and known as *atrial natriuretic peptide (ANP),* is 28 amino acids in length, has a characteristic 17-amino-acid ring formed by a disulfide bond between two cysteines (**Part A**), and is cleaved from a storage precursor molecule that has 151 amino acid residues including a 24-amino-acid signal peptide. It was first reported in 1981 by DeBold and coworkers, who found that intravenous administration of atrial extracts to rats caused natriuresis and diuresis, and it has been found in all mammals examined to date.

Ultrastructurally, myocytes of mammalian atria (but not those of ventricles) resemble typical protein secretory cells. They possess secretory-like granules that increase in number in animals undergoing water deprivation and sodium deficiency. Because atria also appear to possess fluid volume receptors, they are an ideal site for the synthesis and release of a substance that can participate in fluid volume regulation.

Atrial stretch is directly correlated with a positive Na^+ balance and, hence, volume expansion. In order to counteract these effects, ANP reduces both Na^+ and fluid levels in blood through its actions on blood vessels, the hypothalamus, the adrenal cortices, and the kidneys (**Part B**). In general, **ANP acts through antagonizing the actions of aldosterone, ADH, and angiotensin II,** as well as other components of the renin–angiotensin system.

Physiologic Actions of ANP

Renal actions of ANP include increasing the glomerular filtration rate (GFR) and, therefore, the filtered load of Na^+. It does this by vasodilating afferent arterioles, vasoconstricting efferent arterioles, and possibly increasing glomerular membrane permeability. Receptors for ANP are found on glomerular mesangial cells, where ANP-stimulated relaxation presumably increases the effective surface area for filtration. Atrial natriuretic peptide also decreases renin secretion by juxtaglomerular (JG) cells of afferent arterioles, which has the indirect effects of decreasing plasma angiotensin II and III concentrations, reducing peripheral resistance, and decreasing aldosterone secretion. Inhibition of NaCl reabsorption by the collecting ducts also occurs due to the presence of ANP. Although this effect may be augmented by reduced aldosterone levels, ANP has been found to act directly on cells of medullary collecting ducts through its second messenger, *cyclic guanine monophosphate (cGMP).* Through cGMP, ANP apparently inhibits Na^+ channels from opening in apical membranes, thereby reducing NaCl reabsorption. Atrial natriuretic peptide also reduces the ability of ADH to act on medullary collecting ducts. Through these combined influences on renal function, **ANP causes natriuresis and diuresis.**

At the level of the hypothalamus and pituitary, ANP inhibits ADH secretion from the neurohypophysis and ACTH secretion from the adenohypophysis. Atrial natriuretic peptide also decreases the responsiveness of the adrenocortical zona glomerulosa to stimuli that normally increase aldosterone release (e.g., increased K^+ and angiotensin II).

This peptide also causes relaxation of vascular smooth muscle, which in turn causes a decline in arterial blood pressure. There is a reduction in venous return to the heart and, therefore, a reduction in cardiac output following ANP release. The ability of ANP to decrease intravascular volume is achieved not only through its renal effects, but also through its ability to facilitate transport of intravascular fluid into interstitial fluid spaces. Through arteriolar vasodilation, an increase in capillary hydrostatic pressure occurs, thus allowing filtration pressure to overcome reabsorption pressure. The actions of ANP on vascular smooth muscle occur in large part through its ability to decrease responsiveness of vascular smooth muscle tissue to various vasoconstrictor substances, particularly angiotensin II.

Part B summarizes the physiologic actions of ANP.

Other Natriuretic Peptides

Natriuretic peptides have also been isolated from brain tissue, where they exist in two forms that are somewhat different from circulating ANP. *Brain natriuretic peptide (BNP),* which has 32 rather than 28 amino acid residues, has been isolated from porcine, but not human, brain tissue (see **Part A:** dark circles represent amino acids different from those of ANP). An additional *CNS natriuretic peptide (CNP),* which is present in human brain but not heart tissue, has only 22 amino acid residues (see **Part A**).

These peptides may be present in neural pathways that project from the hypothalamus to areas of the brain stem concerned with neural regulation of the cardiovascular system. In general, their CNS effects are thought to be opposite to those of angiotensin II and appear to be involved with lowering blood pressure.

The systemic actions of BNP and CNP are thought to be similar to those of ANP, and are brought about through the cGMP second messenger system as well.

Natriuretic Peptides in Nonmammalian Vertebrates

Bioassayable ANP-like activity has been demonstrated in atria of teleosts (bony fishes), birds, amphibians, and reptiles (snakes, lizards, and turtles). Although natriuretic peptide–like activity was not found in the brains of rainbow trout, it was found in the brains of two marine species. Avian and amphibian ANP-like peptides have been shown to decrease aldosterone release. Therefore, it is likely that this peptide system for reducing blood pressure and volume has been conserved across species lines.

44 Adrenal Medulla: I

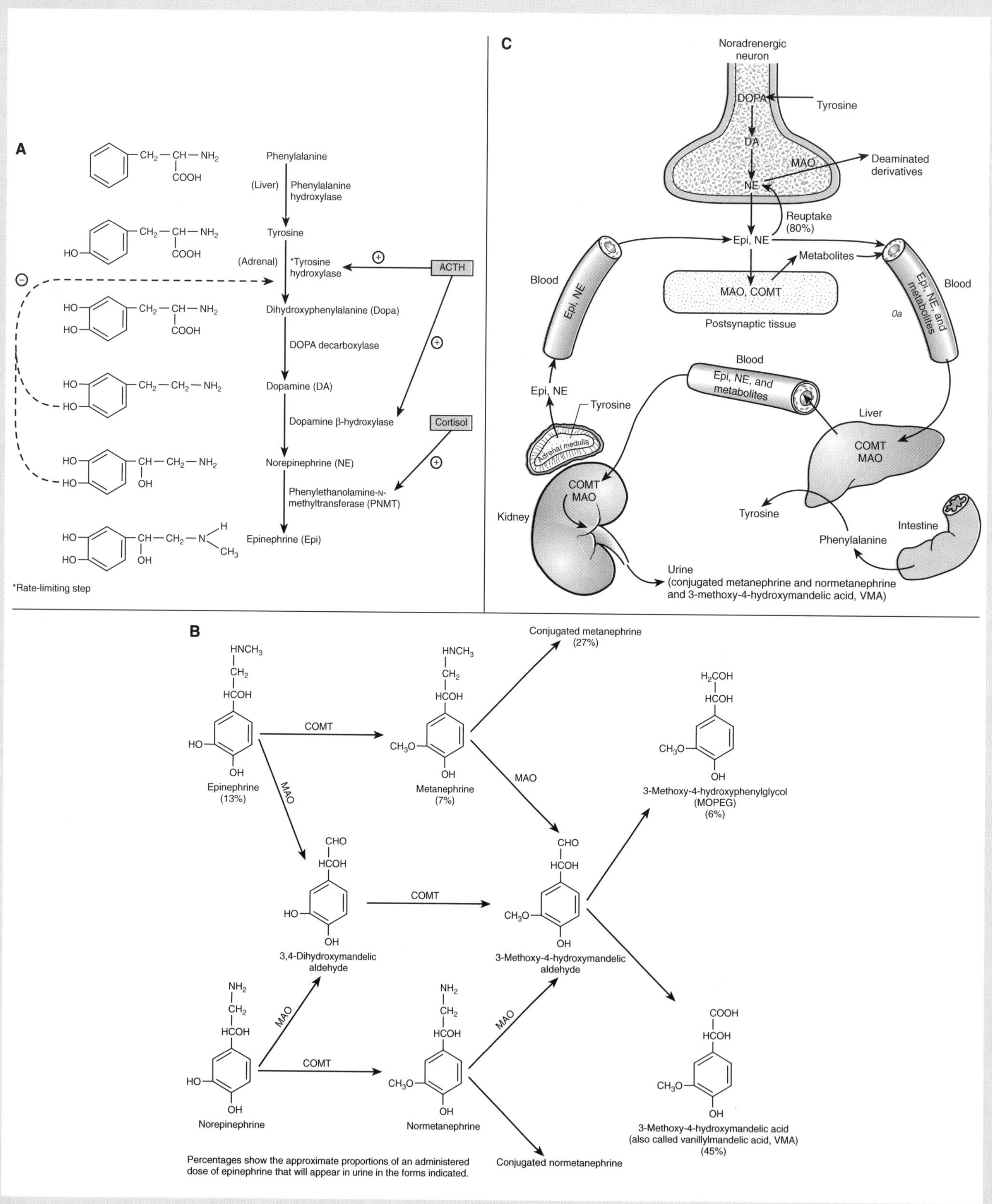
A
Phenylalanine
(Liver) Phenylalanine hydroxylase
Tyrosine
(Adrenal) *Tyrosine hydroxylase
ACTH
Dihydroxyphenylalanine (Dopa)
DOPA decarboxylase
Dopamine (DA)
Dopamine β-hydroxylase
Cortisol
Norepinephrine (NE)
Phenylethanolamine-N-methyltransferase (PNMT)
Epinephrine (Epi)
*Rate-limiting step
C
Noradrenergic neuron
DOPA
Tyrosine
DA
MAO
Deaminated derivatives
NE
Reuptake (80%)
Epi, NE
Metabolites
MAO, COMT
Postsynaptic tissue
Blood
Epi, NE
Epi, NE, and metabolites
Blood
Epi, NE, and metabolites
Epi, NE
Tyrosine
Adrenal medulla
Liver
COMT MAO
Kidney
COMT MAO
Tyrosine
Intestine
Phenylalanine
Urine
(conjugated metanephrine and normetanephrine and 3-methoxy-4-hydroxymandelic acid, VMA)
B
Conjugated metanephrine (27%)
COMT
MAO
Epinephrine (13%)
Metanephrine (7%)
3-Methoxy-4-hydroxyphenylglycol (MOPEG) (6%)
3,4-Dihydroxymandelic aldehyde
3-Methoxy-4-hydroxymandelic aldehyde
Norepinephrine
Normetanephrine
3-Methoxy-4-hydroxymandelic acid (also called vanillylmandelic acid, VMA) (45%)
Conjugated normetanephrine
Percentages show the approximate proportions of an administered dose of epinephrine that will appear in urine in the forms indicated.

Overview

- Catecholamines are synthesized from amino acids.
- The stress hormones, ACTH and cortisol, can increase catecholamine biosynthesis.
- Circulating catecholamines are inactivated by MAO and COMT.
- MOA inhibitors are used to treat depression.
- VMA is the most plentiful catecholamine metabolite found in urine.

The medulla of the mammalian adrenal gland is a modified sympathetic ganglion. It consists of cholinergic sympathetic preganglionic nerve endings as well as modified chromaffin cells that are homologous to postganglionic sympathetic adrenergic neurons. Chromaffin cells secrete *norepinephrine (NE)* and/or *epinephrine (Epi)* directly into blood when the sympathetic nervous system is activated. Although the adrenal medullae are not essential to life, the cortices are (because they produce aldosterone and cortisol). Therefore, the medullae may be regarded as endocrine luxuries for animals, available to reinforce the effects of generalized sympathetic nervous system discharge.

Adrenal glands of nonmammals fail to exhibit the anatomical medullary-to-cortical relationships characteristic of mammals. Avian adrenal glands, for example, consist of a mixture of cortical and chromaffin cells with no distinct cortex and medulla found, and cardiac chromaffin cells have been claimed to represent the homologue of the adrenal medulla in lungfishes. Nonetheless, both NE and Epi are produced by chromaffin-cells of nonmammals, and their physiologic actions are thought to be similar to those described for mammals.

Fetal and neonatal adrenals secrete predominantly NE, followed by a gradual increase in the proportion of Epi secreted. The percentage of adrenal catecholamine secreted as NE in mature dogs and primates is reported as being 0% to 20%; rodents, 2% to 50%; rabbits, 8% to 13%; carnivores (i.e., cats), 27% to 60%; ungulates (hoofed mammals), 15% to 50%; and whales, 83%.

Catecholamine Biosynthesis

Catecholamines are synthesized by hydroxylation and decarboxylation of the amino acids *phenylalanine* and *tyrosine* (**Part A**). Phenylalanine, an essential amino acid, is first hydroxylated into tyrosine, largely by the liver, and then converted to *dihydroxyphenylalanine (dopa)* by the rate-limiting enzyme *tyrosine hydroxylase* in catecholamine-producing cells. Dihydroxyphenylalanine is next decarboxylated to *dopamine (DA)* by dopa hydroxylase, and the DA thus formed is transported into granular vesicles, where it is converted into NE by the enzyme *dopamine β-hydroxylase.* Both tyrosine hydroxylase and dopamine β-hydroxylase are activated by the pituitary "stress" hormone, ACTH, and negative feedback regulation of tyrosine hydroxylase is thought to be exerted by both DA and NE.

Methylation of NE to form Epi occurs through the action of *phenylethanolamine-N-methyltransferase (PNMT).* Because the venous effluent of the adrenal cortex normally passes through the adrenal medulla, the concentration of glucocorticoids (e.g., cortisol) present in this effluent may be 100 times that found in systemic arterial blood, particularly under conditions of physiologic stress. Cortisol is a known activator of PNMT, which enhances conversion of NE to Epi, thus helping to assure adequate levels of this humoral mediator during times of stress.

Catecholamine Degradation

Circulating NE and Epi are inactivated by the enzymes *catecholamine-O-methyltransferase (COMT)* and *monoamine oxidase (MAO),* predominantly in the liver (**Part B**). Catecholamine-*O*-methyltransferase is a cytosolic enzyme found in many tissues of the body, which catalyzes addition of a methyl group, usually in the 3 position (meta) on the benzene ring of the catecholamines, with S-adenosylmethionine acting as the methyl donor. Monoamine oxidase is an oxidoreductase that deaminates monoamines. It is located in mitochondria of many tissues, but occurs in highest concentrations in the liver, stomach, kidney, and intestine. Two isozymes of MAO have been described. The MAO-A isozyme is found in neural tissue, while the MAO-B isozyme is found in extraneural tissues. Inhibitors of MAO are effective in treating depression.

Although a number of catecholamine metabolites have been found in blood and urine, only a few have diagnostic significance because they are found in readily measurable amounts. Metanephrines represent the methoxy derivatives of epinephrine and norepinephrine, and small amounts of these are normally conjugated to sulfates and glucuronides by the liver, returned to the circulation and excreted in urine (**Part C**). The *O*-methylated deaminated product of the metanephrines is 3-methoxy-4-hydroxymandelic acid (also called vanillylmandelic acid, VMA), which is generally the most plentiful catecholamine metabolite found in urine. Urinary levels of metanephrine, normetanephrine, their sulfate and glucuronide conjugates and more importantly, VMA are useful in screening patients for pheochromocytoma, a usually benign, well-encapsulated, intermittently-secreting vascular tumor of adrenomedullary chromaffin tissue (see Chapter 46).

Tyrosine is formed from phenylalanine by phenylalanine hydroxylase, an irreversible reaction. Thus, whereas phenylalanine is a nutritionally essential amino acid, tyrosine is not (provided the diet contains adequate amounts of phenylalanine). The phenylalanine hydroxylase complex is a mixed-function oxygenase present in the mammalian liver but absent from other tissues. Tyrosine is used by catecholamine-producing tissues (e.g., neurons and the adrenal medulla) as a substrate for biogenic amine synthesis. In neural tissue, approximately 80% of the norepinephrine secreted is taken back up across presynaptic membranes for further secretion.

45 Adrenal Medulla: II

D

Pharmacologic Agent	Adrenergic receptor subtype α_1	α_2	β_1	β_2
Antagonists				
Propranolol	−	−	+	+
Yohimbine	+	±	−	−
Butoxamine	−	−	−	+
Phentolamine	±	+	−	−
Terazosin	+	−	−	−
Metoprolol	−	−	+	−
Agonists				
Clonidine	−	+	−	−
Isoproterenol	−	−	+	+
Phenylephrine	+	−	−	−
Ritodrine	−	−	−	+

+ = major binding; ± = weak binding; − = no binding.

E

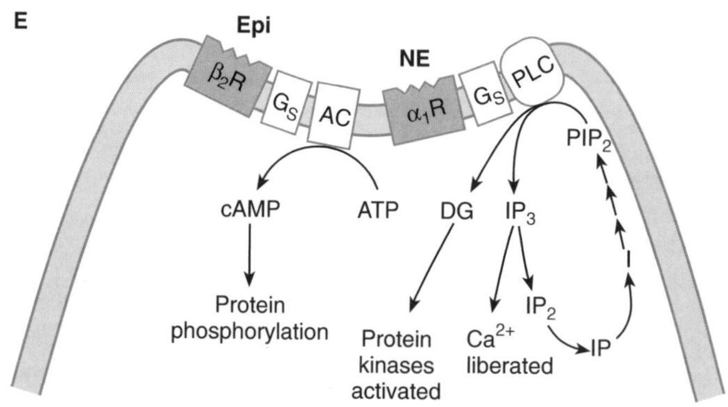

R = receptor
G_S = stimulatory G-protein
PLC = phospholipase C
AC = adenyl cyclase
DG = diacylglycerol

F

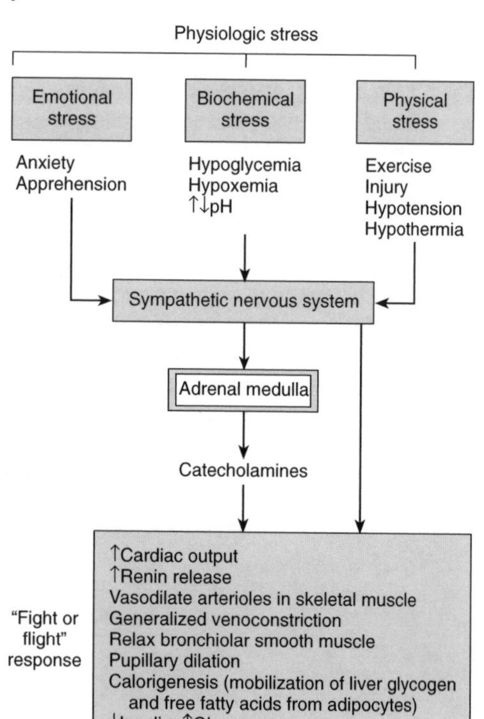

G

Organ or Tissue	Adrenergic Receptor	Responses or Effect
Adipose tissue	β_1, β_3	Increased lipolysis
Blood vessels	α_1, α_2	Vasoconstriction
	β_2	Vasodilation
Bronchioles	β_2	Dilation
Eye		
Iris radial muscle	α_1	Constriction (mydriasis—dilated pupil)
Ciliary muscle	β_2	Relaxation for far vision
GI tract		
Motility and tone	α, β_2	Decreased
Sphincters	α_1	Contraction
Heart	β_1	Increased force and rate of contraction
Kidney		
Juxtaglomerular cells	β_1	Increased renin release
Bladder		
Detrusor	β_2	Relaxation
Sphincter	α_1	Contraction
Ureter	α_1	Increased motility and tone
Liver	α_1, β_2	Increased glycogenolysis and gluconeogenesis
Most other tissues	β_2	Increased calorigenesis
Pancreas		
Acini	α	Decreased secretion
Islets	α_2	Decreased insulin* and glucagon secretion
	β_2	Increased insulin and glucagon* secretion
Pineal gland	β_2	Increased melatonin synthesis and secretion
Skin (apocrine glands)	α_1	Increased sweating
Spleen capsule	α_1	Contraction
	β_2	Relaxation
Uterus	α_1	Contraction of myometrial smooth muscle
	β_2	Relaxation of myometrial smooth muscle

* Primary effect in pancreatic islet tissue.

Overview

- α_1-Adrenergic receptors work through the Ca^{2+} messenger system and β-adrenergic receptors work through the cAMP messenger system.
- α_2-Adrenergic receptors are largely found on presynaptic membranes of NE-secreting neurons.
- β_3-Adrenergic receptors may be present in brown adipose tissue.
- Sympathetic nervous system activation results in a fight-or-flight response.
- Blood catecholamine levels increase in hypoglycemic shock.

Adrenergic Receptors

The response of effector organs and tissues to adrenergic nerve stimulation or to circulating catecholamines depends on the type of plasma membrane receptor stimulated. Generally, there are two basic types of adrenergic receptors: alpha (α) and beta (β). The α-adrenergic receptors are further subdivided into α_1 and α_2 receptors, as are β receptors (β_1 and β_2). Both α_1 and α_2 receptors respond more to NE than to Epi, while β_2 receptors respond more to Epi than NE and β_1 receptors respond to NE and Epi equally. Various pharmacologic agonists and antagonists of the adrenergic receptors are presented in **Part D.**

Activation of β-adrenergic receptors results in an increase in adenyl cyclase activity, leading to an increase in intracellular cAMP (see Chapters 3 and 4). The manner in which α_1-adrenergic receptors mediate their intracellular effects is through increasing Ca^{2+} permeability, thus leading to transient increases in the cytoplasmic Ca^{2+} concentration (**Part E**). Stimulation of α_2-receptors causes a decrease in the activity of adenyl cyclase, thus decreasing intracellular levels of cAMP.

Factors Stimulating Adrenomedullary Catecholamine Release

Adrenomedullary catecholamine release is brought about through generalized discharge of the sympathetic nervous system in response to emergency or stressful situations. Physiologic stress can be conveniently subclassified as either emotional, biochemical, or physical (**Part F**). Anxiety and apprehension, for example, bring about *emotional stress;* acute hypoglycemia, hypoxemia, and derangements in acid-base balance can bring about *biochemical stress;* and certainly injury, exercise, hypotension, and hypothermia can induce *physical stress.*

The Sympathoadrenal Response

When the sympathetic nervous system is activated, the combined sympathoadrenal responses resemble those of severe stress and anger. They generally increase the ability to fight or avoid a predator, and in so doing utilize primary catabolic pathways (i.e., glycogenolysis, lipolysis, etc.). The collective response, therefore, is frequently referred to as the "fight or flight" response (depicted in **Part F**), and animals may generally look angry or frightened when exhibiting this response.

One easy way to mimic various physiologic aspects of the fight or flight response is to inject catecholamines directly into the circulation. Catecholamines, when administered intravenously at physiologic levels, produce a marked tachycardia with an increase in cardiac output and an overall fall in peripheral vascular resistance. This latter effect varies in different segments of the circulation. For example, in the skin and splanchnic vascular beds (where α_1-adrenergic receptors predominate), catecholamines constrict arterioles, but they dilate arterioles in skeletal and cardiac muscle (where β_2-adrenergic receptors predominate). Catecholamines dilate the pupil and relax ciliary muscle of the eye (which favors far vision), relax bronchiolar smooth muscle (making it easier to breathe), and increase the rate and depth of respiration (a central effect that increases minute volume, thus leading to a fall in alveolar CO_2). Catecholamines also relax visceral smooth muscle of the gut, with the exception of sphincters, which are constricted. Both actions tend to delay passage of intestinal contents (**Part G**).

Catecholamines stimulate cellular metabolism and have a strong calorigenic effect. In general, mammalian (white) adipose tissue is unresponsive to most lipolytic hormones apart from the catecholamines, thyroxine, and cortisol. Under normal physiologic conditions, it is likely that catecholamines are the main lipolytic stimulus, providing needed energy to blood in the form of free fatty acids. Brown adipose tissue is characterized by a well-developed blood supply and a high content of mitochondria and cytochromes. Metabolic emphasis is placed on oxidation of both glucose and fatty acids, which is important because brown adipose tissue is a site of heat production in newborn animals. Catecholamines are important inducers of nonshivering thermogenesis in brown adipose tissue, perhaps acting through recently proposed β_3 receptors.

Another important function of the adrenal gland is to help maintain the blood glucose concentration by secreting both cortisol and catecholamines (see Chapters 33–36). When the blood glucose concentration is lowered acutely (e.g., in hypoglycemic shock), Epi is released to force breakdown of liver glycogen in order to restore the blood glucose concentration. Both epinephrine and cortisol also stimulate hepatic gluconeogenesis. This is particularly important to ruminant animals and carnivores, which store only modest amounts of hepatic glycogen. In muscle tissue, the glycogenolysis stimulated by epinephrine results in an increase in lactate formation; glucose formation is not stimulated, because muscle tissue lacks the enzyme glucose-6-phosphatase. The lactate, however, can be used by liver tissue as a gluconeogenic substrate.

Catecholamines normally reduce pancreatic insulin output, yet increase glucagon secretion. Glucagon, like the catecholamines, is a potent stimulator of hepatic glycogenolysis and gluconeogenesis.

Juxtaglomerular (JG) cells of the kidney are stimulated by catecholamines to produce renin, which initiates the renin–angiotensin system (see Chapters 39 and 40). In response to hypovolemic shock, the catecholamines thus help to restore blood pressure and volume.

Additional actions of the catecholamines are presented in **Part G.**

46 Pheochromocytoma

A

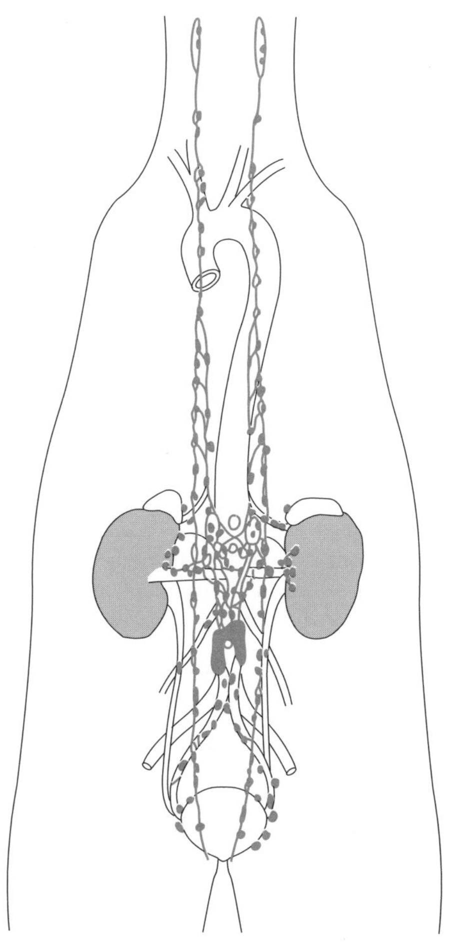

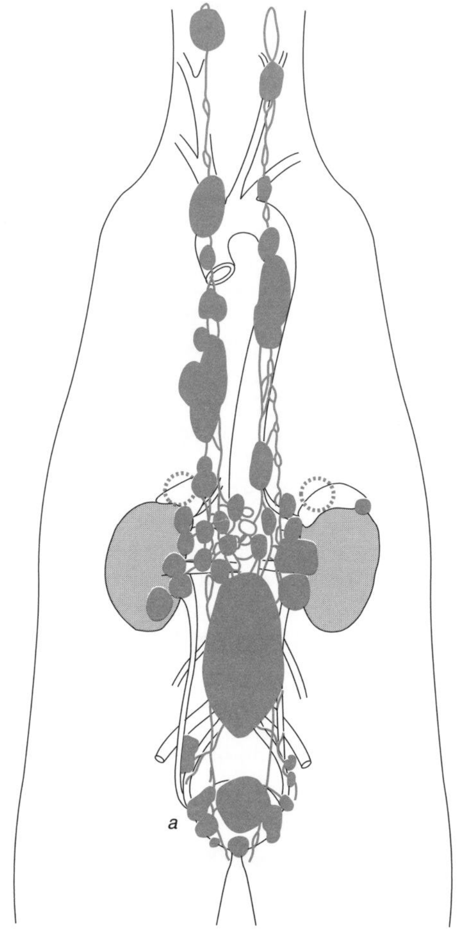

B

Stimuli Causing Paroxysmal Catecholamine Release from a Pheochromocytoma
Activity
Postural change
Exertion
Mating
Eating
Urination and defecation
Emotional stress
Trauma and pain
General anesthesia and barbiturates
Hormones/drugs (e.g., glucagon, ACTH, and histamine)

C

Signs and Symptoms of Pheochromocytoma	
Physical	**Blood**
Generalized weakness	↑Serum alkaline phosphatase (SAP)
Tremor	↑Alanine aminotransferase (ALT)
Anxiety and nervousness	Hypercholesterolemia
Panting	Hyperglycemia
Tachycardia	Ketoacidosis
Mydriasis	↑Red blood cell (RBC) mass
Pale mucous membranes	
Muscle wasting	**Urine**
Nausea, vomiting, and abdominal pain	PU/PD
Weak bowel sounds	Proteinuria
↑BMR	↑VMA excretion
Hypertension (sustained or paroxysmal)	↑Normetanephrine and metanephrine excretion
↑Systolic and diastolic blood pressure	Glucosuria
	Ketonuria

Source: Part A modified from Page LB, Copeland RB. In: Dowling HF, et al., eds. Disease-a-month (January). St. Louis: Year Book, 1968:7.

Overview

- Pheochromocytomas are catecholamine-secreting tumors.
- Pheochromocytomas are slow maturing and potentially fatal.
- Most pheochromocytomas are noninnervated.
- EPO release is sometimes stimulated by catecholamine-secreting tumors.
- Urinary VMA levels are increased in patients with pheochromocytoma.

A pheochromocytoma is a catecholamine-secreting tumor arising from chromaffin cells of the sympathoadrenal system. Over 90% are located in the abdomen, and 90% of those arise within the adrenal glands. The other 10% of abdominal pheochromocytomas are extra-adrenal. Although this tumor type reportedly occurs with a higher incidence in older dogs, there appears to be no breed or gender predisposition.

Most mammalian chromaffin cells are localized within the adrenal medulla and arise from neuroectoderm. Those few that are not associated with the adrenal gland are generally associated with sympathetic ganglia and normally regress early in postnatal development. However, if they do not regress, they sometimes become sites of tumor formation (i.e., paragangliomas). **Part A** shows the anatomic distribution of chromaffin tissue (paraganglia) in the newborn (*left*), as well as reported locations of paragangliomas (*right*), with the most common locations being the aortic bifurcation and the bladder wall.

Pheochromocytoma most often leads to secondary hypertension in animals, but if diagnosed properly it can be effectively treated by resection of the tumor. If left undetected, however, this condition is potentially fatal. Unfortunately, pheochromocytoma is reportedly diagnosed during life in fewer than half of the animal patients in whom it is later found at necropsy, and in 30% to 60% of human patients in whom it is found at autopsy.

Most pheochromocytomas are slow maturing and somewhat independent of physiologic stress. Therefore, they tend to release catecholamines into the circulation in a sporadic, uncontrolled fashion. A high incidence of metastasis at the time of necropsy has been reported in dogs, along with entrapment and compression of major blood vessels.

Catecholamine Release

Although the precise mechanism of catecholamine release from a pheochromocytoma remains largely undefined, it is apparent that most pheochromocytomas are noninnervated; therefore, catecholamine release may not be initiated by neural impulses. Rather, alterations in blood flow to the tumor site, various physical activities, direct pressure, and/or a variety of chemicals or drugs may initiate secretion (**Part B**). While some tumors tend to secrete excessive amounts of catecholamines (both norepinephrine and epinephrine) continuously, others do so episodically.

Signs and Symptoms

Although many of the signs and symptoms reported for pheochromocytoma are associated with other, more common disorders (e.g., hyperthyroidism), several are specifically predictable and result from a lack of normal feedback control on catecholamine release (**Part C;** see also Chapters 44 and 45). Findings on physical exam can be variable, however, and directly related to tumor activity.

An important action of thyroxine is to augment the response of adrenergic effectors to the catecholamines. An increased *basal metabolic rate (BMR)* accords with hyperthyroidism but could also be a manifestation of the calorigenic action of excess catecholamines. Generalized hypermetabolism produced by excess thyroxine causes autoregulatory vasodilation to increase blood flow to tissues, producing a lowered diastolic pressure, an increased cardiac output, and a wide pulse pressure. Patients with pheochromocytoma, in contrast, would be expected to have elevated diastolic pressures.

Increases in red blood cell mass may be due to catecholamine-stimulated erythropoietin release from kidneys or an erythropoietin-like peptide produced by the tumor itself. High catecholamine levels suppress insulin release and stimulate hepatic glycogenolysis and gluconeogenesis. The resulting hyperglycemia may result in glucosuria.

Catecholamine inhibition of pituitary vasopressin release via a nonpressor interaction with arterial baroreceptors has been described and could help to explain the polyuria and polydipsia that develops in these patients. Biochemical confirmation of excessive catecholamine production is generally found in either plasma or urine via assay for norepinephrine, epinephrine, normetanephrine, metanephrine, total urinary catecholamines (free plus conjugated), and/or vanillylmandelic acid (VMA) (see Chapters 44 and 45).

A *clonidine suppression test* may also be useful in diagnosing this disease. Clonidine is an α_2-agonist that works presynaptically to inhibit norepinephrine release. In animals with increased catecholamine release due to neurogenic stimulation rather than a tumor, clonidine should reduce plasma catecholamine levels. Patients with pheochromocytoma, on the other hand, should fail to respond to this suppression test.

A *glucagon stimulation test* may also be employed in patients who have infrequent symptoms and signs. Following intravenous injection, patients with pheochromocytoma should manifest a substantial increase in plasma catecholamines and a rise in blood pressure (which could be hazardous). Imaging studies may also be required to determine whether the tumor is adrenal or extra-adrenal.

47 Phasic Response to Trauma

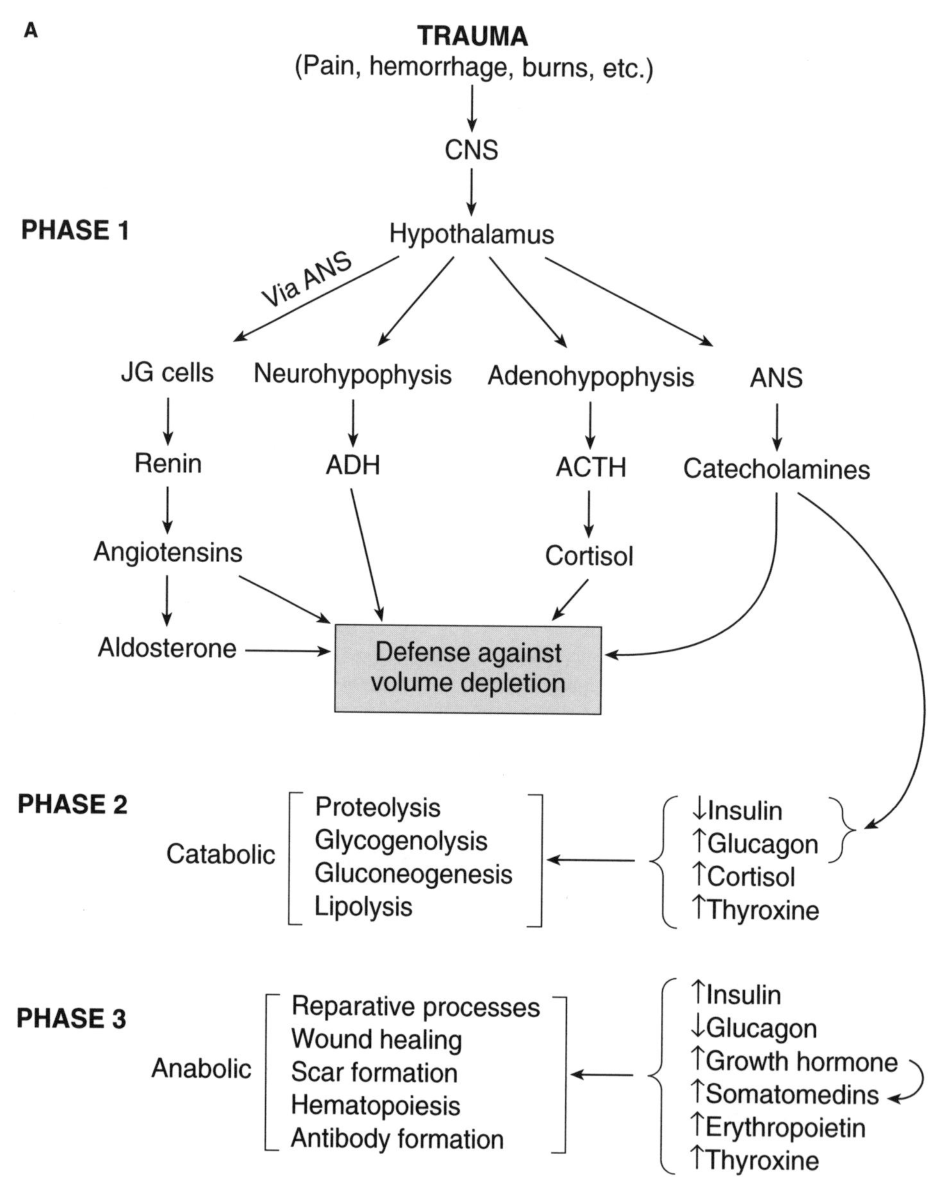

Overview

- Phase 1 of the response to trauma helps to ensure continued blood supply to vital organs.
- Phase 2 is the catabolic phase that redistributes stored substrates for energy purposes.
- Phase 3 is the anabolic reparative phase.

Physiologic trauma (i.e., hemorrhagic shock, pain, burns, severe infections, hypoxemia, invasive surgery, extreme cold exposure, etc.) evokes compensatory responses in the organism that involve several endocrine glands. One of the earliest detectable changes following trauma is a depletion of cholesterol and ascorbic acid in the adrenal glands, which is associated with increased output of adrenal steroids (i.e., cortisol and aldosterone). A negative nitrogen balance is characteristic of the early response, which can sometimes be reversed by force-feeding carbohydrate. The sequence of compensatory physiologic events following trauma cannot occur in the absence of the hypophysis (pituitary); therefore, hypophysectomized or adrenalectomized animals have been found to be notoriously vulnerable to traumatic stresses such as those enumerated above.

It is not surprising that the pituitary–adrenal axis is activated by such a wide variety of potentially lethal stimuli. From a teleologic perspective, it seems likely that the general reaction by which fat and labile protein are catabolized as a result of injury (or even in anticipation of injury) provides energy and amino acids for the healing process. It also appears to this author that the pituitary–adrenal response to trauma may be primitive and independent of nutrition, as a wounded animal is necessarily reduced in its capacity to feed itself.

Part A summarizes the phasic response to physiologic trauma (see Chapters 9, 25, 26, 33–36, 38–40, 42, 44, 45, 48, 49, 52–54 for additional explanations).

Phase 1

The immediate responses to trauma are mediated primarily by way of the hypothalamus. These responses are largely concerned with ensuring continued blood supply to vital organs, particularly the heart, lungs, and brain. Other tissues, such as skeletal muscle (approximately 50% of body weight), kidneys, the GI tract, and reproductive organs, are not accorded the same high priority. Major compensatory efforts appear to be a defense against fluid volume depletion and hypotension, and in this exercise the CRH–ACTH–adrenal glucocorticoid axis collaborates with catecholamines, ADH, and the renin–angiotensin–aldosterone system in maintaining a blood pressure and volume compatible with life. Over a relatively short period of time following hemorrhage (minutes to hours), these endocrine control systems stimulate lifesaving compensatory fluid shifts from intracellular and interstitial spaces to vascular spaces. These compensatory fluid shifts have a tendency to modestly decrease hematocrit and the plasma protein concentration.

Phase 2

The next phase in the physiologic response to trauma is largely **catabolic** and involves redistribution of stored substrates for energy purposes. During this phase, glucocorticoids (e.g., cortisol) collaborate with hormones of the thyroid gland and endocrine pancreas (decreased insulin and increased glucagon) and with biogenic amines of the sympathetic nervous system and adrenal medulla in bringing about decreased utilization of glucose yet increased utilization of fatty acids by the body. These hormones also cause mild muscle protein breakdown in order to provide the liver with needed gluconeogenic substrates and, therefore, a sustained output of glucose (through both glycogenolysis and gluconeogenesis). Adipose tissue lipolysis is driven during this phase largely by cortisol, thyroxine, and the catecholamines. Insulin secretion is inhibited by catecholamines (see Chapter 54), and glucagon secretion is stimulated by both cortisol and the catecholamines (see Chapter 55).

The duration of phase 2 is dependent on several factors (e.g., the type and severity of trauma, acute versus chronic injury, age, and nutritional status). The sooner an animal can be effectively and appropriately fed, and thus regain its nitrogen balance (i.e., move from a negative to a positive nitrogen balance), the sooner it will move into phase 3.

Phase 3

Once metabolic stabilization has been achieved and the animal can begin effectively assimilating needed nutrients through either alimentation or parenteral feeding, the **anabolic** repair process (phase 3) begins. The hormonal mix and the pool of energy-yielding substrates and protein precursors together provide a metabolic climate favorable to protein synthesis and cell proliferation. This is achieved by increasing the roles of insulin, erythropoietin, and thyroid hormones (T_4 and T_3), with important additional contributions from growth hormone and the liver-derived growth factors (i.e., somatomedins—discussed in Chapter 9).

48 Thyroid: I

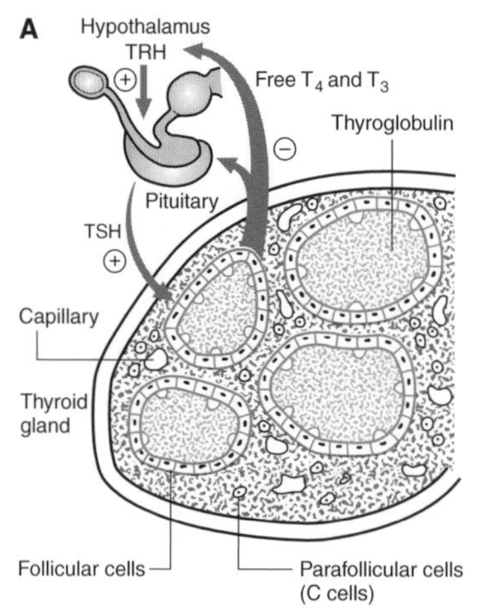

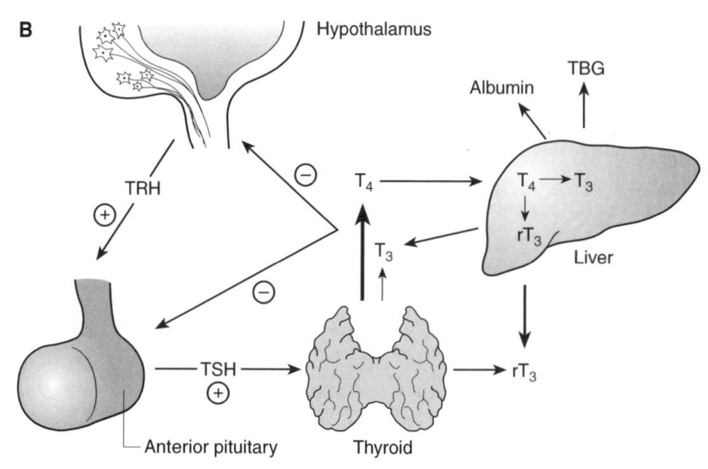

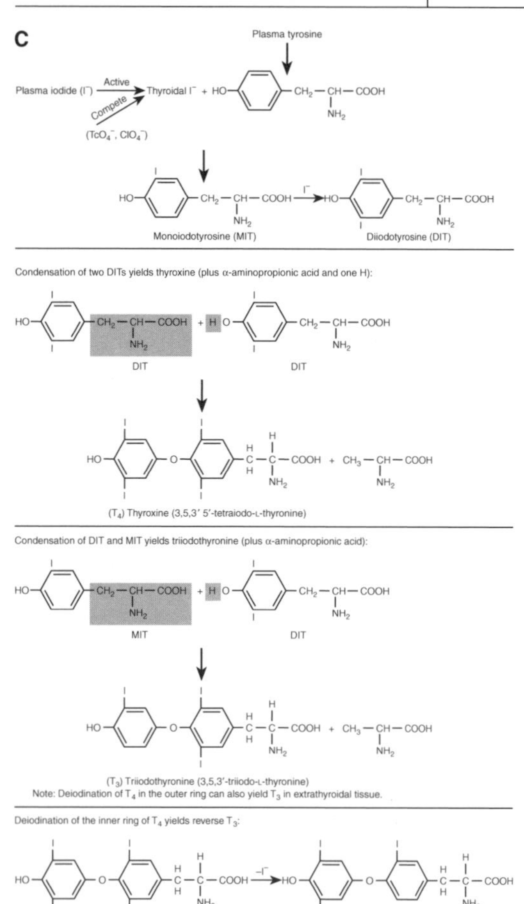

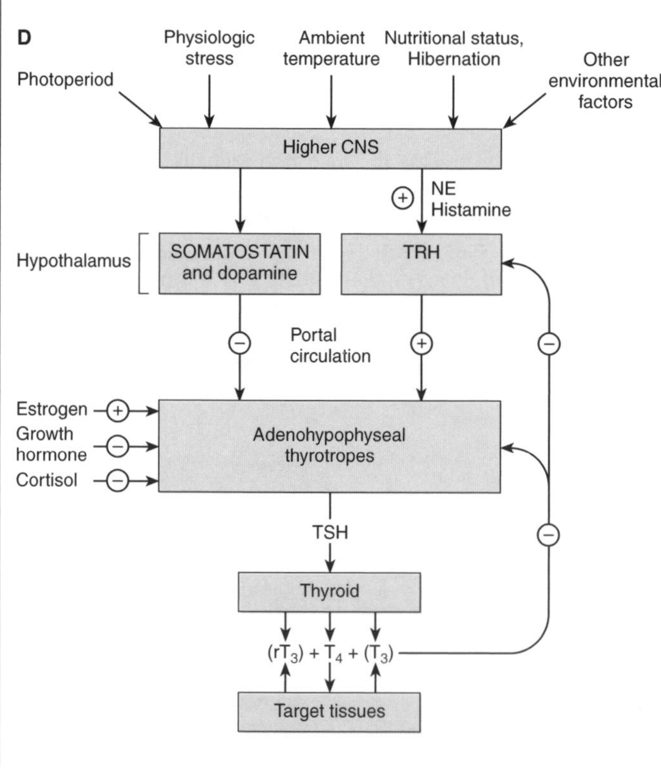

Source: Part A modified from Chastain CB, Ganjam VK. Clinical endocrinology of companion animals. 1st ed. Philadelphia, PA: Lea & Febiger, 1986:116.

Overview

- Thyroxine is synthesized from tyrosine and iodide (I^-).
- Hypothalamic TRH stimulates TSH release from the anterior pituitary which in turn controls thyroid gland activity.
- The liver can inactivate T_4 by converting it to rT_3.

The thyroid gland is present in all vertebrates and is unique among endocrine glands in that it stores its secretory products (the thyroid hormones) extracellularly. It is among the most highly vascularized of endocrine glands in mammals and appears to be one of the oldest phylogenetically.

The thyroid gland is innervated by sympathetic, postganglionic nerve fibers and, therefore, responds to sympathetic activation. *Follicular cells* of the thyroid synthesize and secrete the thyroid hormones (thyroxine, T_4; triiodothyronine, T_3; and reverse T_3, rT_3) mainly in response to the presence (or absence) of *thyroid-stimulating hormone (TSH),* while *parafollicular cells* (otherwise known as "clear," or C cells), which are scattered in the interstitium, synthesize and secrete *thyrocalcitonin* (see Chapters 29 and 30). *Thyroglobulin* is a glycoprotein synthesized by follicular cells and secreted into the colloid by exocytosis (**Part A**). It binds thyroid hormones until they are secreted. Thyroglobulin enters blood as well, and plasma levels increase in hyperthyroidism and some forms of thyroid cancer. However, the function of thyroglobulin (if any) in plasma remains obscure.

Biosynthesis of Thyroid Hormones

Thyroid hormone biosynthesis occurs within the follicular lumen of the thyroid gland in conjunction with thyroglobulin (**Part A**). In response to physiologic need, *TSH-releasing hormone (thyrotropin-releasing hormone, TRH)* from the hypothalamus stimulates release of TSH from thyrotropes of the anterior pituitary (**Part B**). This latter hormone is required for the uptake of iodide and further thyroid hormone synthesis within follicular cells of the thyroid. Although vertebrates require a continuous source of iodine for thyroid hormone synthesis, iodine deficiency is rare today among most domestic animals because adequate amounts are generally present in their diets.

Iodine is converted to iodide (I^-) before being absorbed from the small bowel. Iodide then circulates in plasma, largely bound to plasma proteins (though some is free). Iodide is actively removed from plasma by thyroid follicular cells, with thyroid-to-plasma ratios normally remaining around 25:1. The thyroid gland normally contains about 90% of total body I^- stores. Monovalent anions such as perchlorate (ClO_4^-) and pertechnetate (TcO_4^-) compete with I^- for uptake, and they are also concentrated by thyroidal follicular cells against a gradient. Technetium-labeled pertechnetate is used clinically to monitor thyroid activity via thyroid scans and is useful in hyperthyroid animals.

Although T_4 is the major thyroid hormone produced by the thyroid gland, it acts as a prehormone to T_3, the more active intranuclear form in target tissues (see Chapter 4). Reverse T_3 is the inactive form produced mainly in the liver and kidney by deiodination of T_4 (**Parts B** and **C**). Lesser amounts are produced by the thyroid gland.

Peripheral production of T_3 decreases and that of rT_3 increases during periods of sustained catabolism (e.g., starvation, anorexia, fever, burns, severe illness, or hibernation). This is thought to be a beneficial response to caloric restriction, serious illness, or stress that conserves energy through a reduction in the BMR.

Secretion, Plasma Transport, and Turnover of Thyroid Hormones

Thyroxine and (to a lesser extent) T_3 circulate bound to plasma proteins. The exact proteins and their binding affinities vary with species. *Thyroid hormone–binding globulin* (*TBG;* see **Part B**), a glycoprotein synthesized by the liver, binds T_4 with high affinity. It is present in relatively high amounts in humans and large domestic animals but much lower amounts in dogs and cats. *Albumin* appears to be a more important plasma binding protein for small animals. During pregnancy, estrogen stimulates hepatic synthesis of TBG and decreases its clearance. Therefore, total plasma thyroid hormone levels are generally increased in the maternal circulation; however, free T_4 and T_3 levels usually remain unchanged.

Although the ratio of T_4-to-T_3 secretion from the thyroid of the dog is about 4:1, circulating levels are about 20:1. This is due to differences in serum binding (T_4 is more tightly protein bound) and perhaps a larger intracellular compartmentalization for T_3. Increased plasma protein binding of T_4 also means that the turnover rate of T_4 in dogs is slower than that of T_3.

Thyroid hormones are lipophilic, metabolized primarily via deiodination or conjugation in the liver to sulfate and glucuronides, and excreted in bile. Approximately 45% of T_4 is deiodinated to T_3 and rT_3, and 55% is excreted in bile. Lesser amounts are removed via deamination, decarboxylation, and urinary excretion. Most of the hormone that appears in the glomerular filtrate is reabsorbed by renal tubules.

Only about 15% of T_4 and T_3 in the dog is reabsorbed from the gut following biliary excretion, compared to 79% to 100% in humans. This comparatively low reabsorption rate explains why dogs have a higher production rate and replacement requirement for thyroxine than humans.

Regulation of Thyroid Hormone Secretion

Thyrotropin-releasing hormone (TRH) was the first releasing factor to be identified, purified, and synthesized. More than 80% of TRH is extrahypothalamic, appearing in the higher brain centers, spinal cord, GI tract, retina, pancreatic islets, reproductive tract, and placenta. However, the highest single concentration is hypothalamic. TRH is a tripeptide (Glu-His-Pro) whose release is inhibited in hot environments and stimulated in cold environments. Physiologic stress, photoperiod, and nutritional status, among other factors, also indirectly control TRH release (**Part D**).

TSH is synthesized by basophilic thyrotropes of the adenohypophysis and is a glycoprotein of 211 amino acids. It has a chain length similar to those of LH, FSH, and CG. TSH is usually not used clinically, because it is a protein and because T_4 administration is more effective. The plasma half-life of TSH is about 60 minutes.

TSH maintains the structure, growth, and secretory activity of the thyroid by enhancing activity of the hexose monophosphate shunt (NADPH is needed for I^- reutilization), glycolysis, protein synthesis, tricarboxylic acid (TCA) cycle activity, and oxygen consumption. It also enhances thyroidal I^- uptake from plasma, thus increasing T_4 and T_3 synthesis. The response to TSH is reportedly greater in females than in males.

Thyroid hormone secretion is regulated via a classic physiologic negative feedback scheme involving the hypothalamic–pituitary–thyroid axis (**Part D**). There is also some intrathyroidal autoregulatory control. Note from **Part D** the negative feedback effects of T_4 and T_3 on hypothalamic TRH release and the release of TSH from adenohypophyseal thyrotropes. Somatostatin and dopamine (ostensibly from the hypothalamus) inhibit TSH release, while norepinephrine (released in response to stress) and histamine from higher brain centers stimulate TRH release. The pituitary response to TRH is reduced by cortisol and growth hormone and enhanced by estrogen.

49 Thyroid: II

E

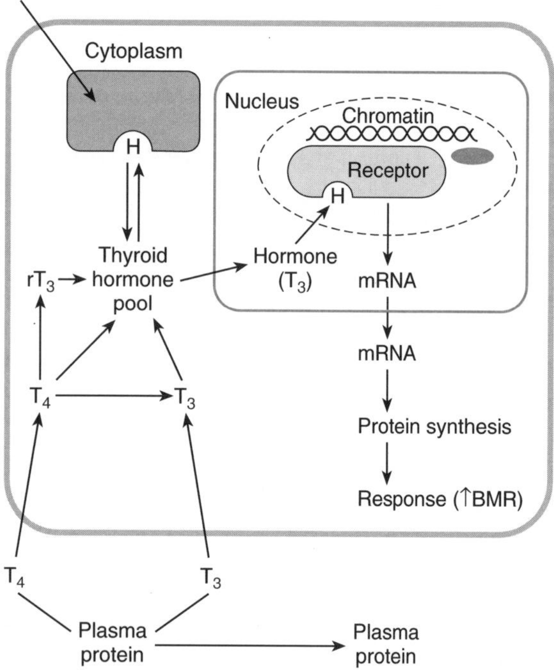

F

Metabolic Effects of Thyroid Hormones
Calorigenic
General
↑O_2 consumption
↑BMR
↑Heat dissipation
Panting
Sweating
↑β-adrenergic receptors
Cutaneous vasodilation
↑Cardiac output
Body temperature, increased
Uncouple oxidation from phosphorylation in brown adipose tissue
Neonates
Arousal from hibernation
Protein synthesis
Stimulated
Pre-adolescent growth and development
Inhibited
Hyperthyroidism
Carbohydrate metabolism—provide more glucose
↑Effects of diabetogenic hormones (GH, cortisol, glucagon, and epinephrine)
↑Gluconeogenesis and glycogenolysis
↑Intestinal carbohydrate absorption
Lipid metabolism—provide more fatty acids
↑Lipolysis (synergistic with epinephrine)
↑β-Oxidation
↑Hepatic ketogenesis
↑Hepatic triglyceride synthesis
↑Hepatic LDL-receptor synthesis
↑Cholesterol clearance
Interactions with catecholamines—↑β-adrenergic receptor synthesis
↓Diastolic pressure
↑Lipolysis in fat tissue
Skeletal muscle—maintain muscle protein synthesis
Muscle weakness occurs in both hyper- and hypothyroidism
Heart—↑β-adrenergic receptor synthesis
↑Chronotropic behavior
↑Ionotropic behavior
Skin
Maintain protein synthesis and turnover
Maintain hair coat and sebaceous gland activity
Bone
Maintain growth and epiphyseal closure
Erythrocytes
Support erythropoiesis
↑2,3-Diphosphoglycerate (2,3-DPG) synthesis
Brain
↑Fetal brain development, synapse formation, and myelination
Kidney—maintain renal response to aldosterone
↑Na^+ pump in distal nephron
GI tract—maintain smooth muscle growth, development, and activity
Segmentation and peristalsis
Reproductive tract
Maintain gonadotropin output from the adenohypophysis

G

Tissues Not Affected by Thyroid Hormones
Nerves (adults)
Adenohypophysis
Lymph nodes
Spleen
Lungs
Testes
Uterus
Retinas

H

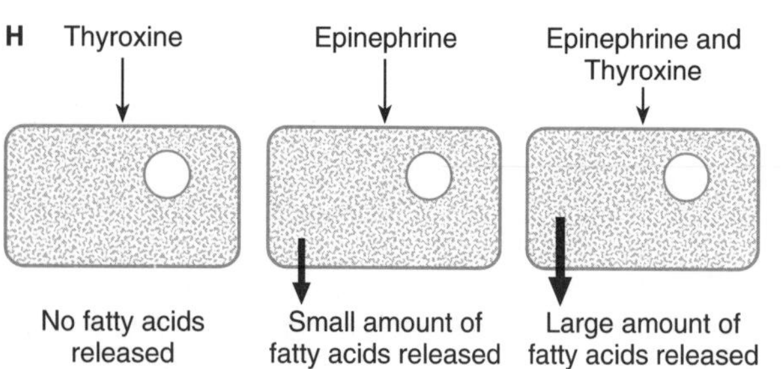

Source: **Part H** modified from Vander AJ, Sherman JH, Luciano DS. Human physiology, the mechanisms of body function. 3rd ed. New York: McGraw-Hill, 1980:200.

As discussed in Chapter 5, major effects of thyroid hormones are produced via changes in the synthesis and activity of regulatory proteins in target cells, including key metabolic enzymes, hormones, and receptors. These occur via the regulation of specific gene expression at the nuclear level and the subsequent induction of specific RNA synthesis. Nuclear activation occurs via binding of T_3, the most biologically active form of thyroid hormone, to specific high-affinity receptor sites (**Part E**).

Specific responses to thyroid hormones vary between species and tissues. They are often under multihormonal regulation, frequently by glucocorticoids, and may be affected by other factors such as carbohydrate, fat, and protein intake. Binding sites for T_3 have also been identified in the plasma membranes of some cells (such as erythrocytes, thymocytes, placental cells, carcinoma cells, and several other cell lines). After binding, T_3 is internalized by endocytic vesicles similar to peptides. The physiologic importance of this binding is unknown, but it may mediate stimulation of carbohydrate and amino acid transport into cells. Binding sites for T_3 have also been found on mitochondria.

Metabolic Effects of Thyroid Hormones

The metabolic effects of thyroid hormones are summarized in **Part F.**

Calorigenic Actions

General Stimulation of oxygen consumption, which results in an increase in the BMR, may be the single most important effect of thyroid hormones. Thyroid hormones increase oxygen consumption in most tissues, with the notable exception of those listed in **Part G.**

Enhanced mitochondrial oxidation results in energy, which is stored in the form of ATP or released as heat (thereby maintaining body temperature). Heat-dissipating mechanisms (such as panting and sweating) are also activated (**Part G**). Peripheral resistance is decreased due to cutaneous vasodilation brought about by an increase in β-adrenergic receptor synthesis. The enhanced cardiac output, which also occurs due to increased β-adrenergic receptor synthesis, also helps to dissipate heat.

Body Temperature Body temperature is maintained via a variety of mechanisms. In nonprimate mammals, however, thyroid hormones play a key role in maintaining body temperature in cold environments. Under the stimulus of cold or a drop in core body temperature, hypothalamic TRH-secreting neurons secrete increased amounts of TRH, thus resulting in adenohypophyseal TSH release and subsequent thyroid hormone secretion from follicular cells of the thyroid gland (see Chapter 48).

Thyroxine (T_4) also uncouples oxidation from phosphorylation in brown adipose tissue, which is important to newborn animals and those arousing from hibernation. The resulting nonshivering thermogenesis helps to assure survival.

Protein Synthesis Nitrogen excretion is increased and weight is lost if food intake is not increased in hyperthyroidism. In the hypothyroid state, small doses of hormone will cause a positive nitrogen balance, while large doses may cause catabolism. Thyroid hormones stimulate the synthesis of many structural proteins, enzymes, and hormones and, therefore, play an important role (with insulin, GH, and the somatomedins) in pre-adolescent growth and development.

Carbohydrate Metabolism In general, thyroid hormones act to provide more glucose, primarily via enhancement of the effects of the diabetogenic hormones (i.e., epinephrine, GH, cortisol, and glucagon). Hepatic glucose production is increased via gluconeogenesis and glycogenolysis, and carbohydrate absorption from the GI tract is also enhanced.

Lipid Metabolism Thyroid hormones provide more fatty acids for oxidation and ketogenesis, an important component of their calorigenic action. Hepatic triglyceride synthesis is also stimulated following fatty acid and glycerol mobilization from adipose tissue. Thyroxine increases the sensitivity of hormone-sensitive lipase (also called adipolytic triglyceride lipase) to the lipolytic actions of the catecholamines (i.e., epinephrine; see **Part H**), while decreasing sensitivity of this adipose tissue enzyme to the antilipolytic action of insulin. Thyroxine, like estrogen and insulin, also helps to maintain hepatic low-density lipoprotein (LDL)-receptor synthesis and, thus, removal of cholesterol from the circulation.

Interactions with Catecholamines The actions of thyroid hormones and catecholamines are intimately related, with many signs and symptoms of thyroid disease being similar to those of increased catecholamine discharge (see Chapter 46). As previously noted, thyroid hormones increase the number of β-adrenergic receptors in myocardial tissues, skeletal muscle, smooth muscle, adipose tissue, and lymphocytes, and they decrease myocardial α-adrenergic receptors. Apparently, changes in catecholamine levels themselves do not play a similar role.

Specific Organs and Tissues

Skeletal Muscle

Thyroid hormones are essential for normal muscle growth, skeletal maturation, and mental development. This is in part due to the effects of T_3 on protein synthesis and to its potentiation of the actions of growth hormone. Muscle weakness is present in both hypo- and hyperthyroidism.

Heart

As stated previously, β-adrenergic receptors are increased in hyperthyroidism, thus increasing sensitivity to the inotropic and chronotropic effects of the catecholamines.

Skin

Thyroid hormones maintain protein synthesis in skin, as well as patency of hair follicles and sebaceous glands.

Bone

In the absence of normal levels of thyroid hormones, bone growth is slowed and epiphyseal closure is delayed.

Erythrocytes

Thyroid hormones support erythropoiesis. There is a mild anemia in hypothyroidism and a slight polycythemia in hyperthyroidism due to related changes in protein turnover and oxygen needs. Thyroid hormones stimulate erythrocytic 2,3-diphosphoglycerate (2,3-DPG) synthesis and activity, which decreases the affinity of hemoglobin for oxygen, and thus increases delivery of oxygen to tissues.

Brain

Slow mentation and reflexes occur in hypothyroidism, while irritability and restlessness occur in hyperthyroidism. Glucose and oxygen consumption do not seem to be involved. Adequate thyroid hormone levels are critical in the fetus for brain development, normal synapse formation, and myelination. Fetal hypothyroidism causes cretinism (see Chapter 51).

Kidney

Hypothyroidism leads to excessive renal Na^+ loss and hyponatremia. The renal response to aldosterone is depressed because thyroid hormones are needed to maintain Na^+/K^+ ATPase activity in distal renal tubular cells.

GI Tract

Normal thyroid hormone levels are important for maintaining synthesis and smooth muscle activity of the GI tract. Constipation occurs in hypothyroidism (see Chapter 51), and diarrhea occurs in hyperthyroidism (see Chapter 50).

Reproductive Tract

Thyroid hormones are required for normal reproductive function in both males and females. It is thought that they exert their effects at the hypothalamic level and, thus, affect gonadotropin release from the anterior pituitary.

50 Hyperthyroidism

A Physical Signs of Hyperthyroidism in Cats

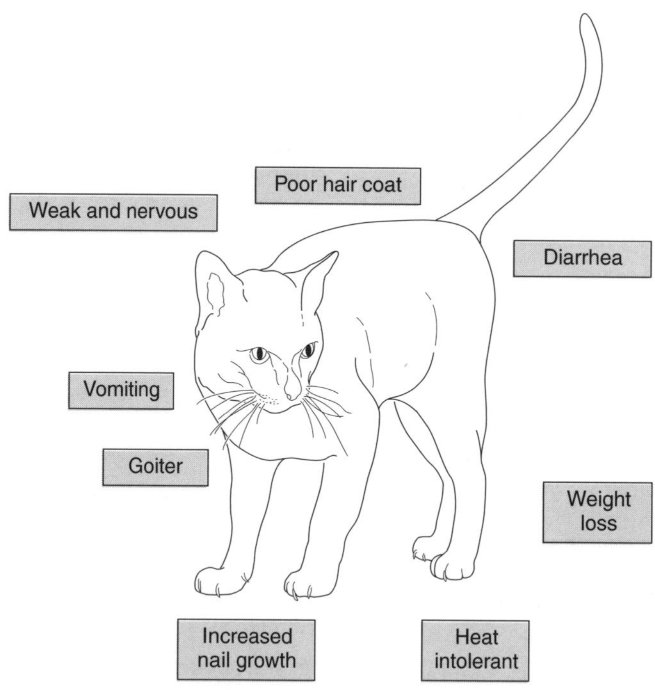

B

Signs and Symptoms of Hyperthyroidism

Physical	Blood
PU/PD	Erythrocytosis
↑BMR	Leukocytosis
Vomiting and diarrhea (dehydration)	Eosinopenia
Polyphagia (usually)	Lymphopenia
Weakness (muscle wasting)	↑T_4 and T_3
Reduction in dermal fat	↓TSH
Thin (and sometimes cachectic)	↑ALT
Nervousness, restlessness, and aggressiveness	↑AST
Tachycardia, left ventricular hypertrophy	↑AP
Poor hair coat/alopecia (patchy)	↑LDH
Heat intolerant	↑Creatinine
Panting	↑BUN
Shivering	Hyperglycemia
Small goiters (cats), larger goiters (dogs)	Hypocholesterolemia
Increased nail growth	↑Free fatty acids
	Hyperphosphatemia
	Hypernatremia (mild) and hypokalemia
	Hyperbilirubinemia

Overview

- Hyperthyroidism is the most common endocrinopathy affecting older cats.
- Enlarged thyroid glands may be palpable.
- Hyperthyroid animals are generally heat-intolerant and may exhibit GI disturbances (e.g., vomiting and diarrhea).
- Disorders that can mimic hyperthyroidism include renal and cardiac failure, diabetes mellitus, liver disease, maldigestion/malabsorption, and neoplasia.

The term *thyrotoxicosis* refers to an excess of thyroid hormones, generally due to thyroid hypersecretion. Although TRH-secreting tumors of hypothalamic nuclei or TSH-secreting basophilic tumors of the anterior pituitary could conceivably cause thyrotoxicosis, most tumors in domestic animal species are of primary thyroidal origin.

Hyperthyroidism, caused by autonomous growth and function of thyroid follicular cells, was first reported as a clinical entity in humans in 1913, and in cats in 1979. Most feline thyroid tumors are reportedly functional, noninvasive, and relatively small, while those in dogs are more often nonfunctional, invasive, and large. Although thyroid tumors account for only 1% to 4% of canine neoplasms, more than 90% are reportedly malignant. Only 10% to 20% of thyroid tumors in dogs are reported to be hypersecreting.

Hyperthyroidism (i.e., the clinical entity resulting from excessive production and secretion of thyroid hormones) is **therefore more often seen in cats than in dogs, and it is postulated to be the most common endocrinopathy affecting older cats (Part A).**

Signs and Symptoms

The signs and symptoms of hyperthyroidism are listed in **Part B.** Disorders that can mimic hyperthyroidism include renal and cardiac failure, diabetes mellitus, liver disease, maldigestion/malabsorption, and neoplasia.

Most animals with thyrotoxicosis show signs of weight loss and an unkempt hair coat. They are generally restless, aggressive, and difficult to handle. Enlarged thyroid glands may be palpable, and the muscle wasting that accompanies this disease may eventually lead to periods of weakness.

Increased calorie utilization generally leads to increased appetite and food intake. However, the GI hypermotility brought about by high titers of thyroid hormones frequently leads to vomiting and diarrhea. The glomerular filtration rate appears to be increased in many hyperthyroid animals, and high titers of thyroid hormones may decrease the concentrating ability of the nephron. Therefore, medullary washout can occur, leading to polyuria and secondary polydipsia (PU/PD). Vomiting and diarrhea also cause dehydration, which again increases thirst. The cause of azotemia (increased BUN and serum creatinine) in animals with thyrotoxicosis is not as well understood. It has been postulated that increased protein catabolism may contribute. Azotemia is more likely to occur following treatment for the hyperthyroid state, and therefore renal function should be carefully assessed before, during, and following therapy.

Alterations in respiratory function (e.g., panting, decreased vital capacity, and pulmonary compliance) are thought to result from a combined increase in carbon dioxide production and decrease in respiratory muscle strength. Tachycardia results from an increase in β-adrenergic receptor synthesis in heart muscle, and most animals with hyperthyroidism eventually develop left ventricular hypertrophy. The decrease in peripheral resistance that accompanies increased β-adrenergic receptor synthesis in arterioles, as well as the increases in tissue metabolism and oxygen requirements that occur, contributes to this hypertrophy. Hyperthyroidism thus results in a high cardiac output state in which vascular resistance is low. This in turn results in compensatory volume overload. The principal cardiac reaction is dilatation in response to the overload, and then hypertrophy in response to the dilatation.

The stress response to hyperthyroidism is reflected in the combined blood count (CBC), which typically shows erythrocytosis, mature leukocytosis, eosinopenia, and lymphopenia. The erythrocytosis most likely results from both a direct effect of thyroid hormones on bone marrow function and an increase in erythropoietin secretion.

Animals with primary hyperthyroidism (i.e., resulting from an autonomous, hyperactive thyroid gland) are expected to have increased levels of both free and bound T_4 and T_3 in the circulation and decreased levels of TSH. Increases in the plasma concentrations of several enzymes have been noted in cats (i.e., alanine aminotransferase, ALT; aspartate aminotransferase, AST; alkaline phosphatase, AP; and lactate dehydrogenase, LDH). Fatty liver infiltration, with some necrosis evident, is common in hyperthyroid cats, thus giving rise to an elevation in liver enzymes as well as a mild hyperbilirubinemia. However, as only ALT is liver-specific in cats, it is possible that other tissues may also be contributing to elevations in AP, LDH, and AST in this species (e.g., heart muscle, kidney, and bone tissue).

Because thyroid hormones increase the basal metabolic rate (BMR) and help to provide more glucose (see Chapter 49), hyperthyroidism can result in heat intolerance and hyperglycemia. Hepatic LDL-receptor synthesis is increased by thyroid hormones, thereby making it easier for the liver to clear cholesterol from the circulation. Thus, hypocholesterolemia may be seen in hyperthyroidism. Because thyroid hormones also enhance the lipolytic effects of the catecholamines, fat depletion occurs and the plasma free fatty acid level rises.

Hyperthyroidism causes excessive skeletal Ca^{2+} resorption, which in turn decreases serum PTH and 1,25-DHC levels (see Chapters 29 and 30). As a result, Ca^{2+} absorption from the intestinal tract is compromised, as is its reabsorption from the renal filtrate. Consequently, excessive amounts of Ca^{2+} are lost in both urine and feces (although serum levels remain largely unchanged). With low serum PTH levels, however, renal tubular reabsorption of PO_4^{3-} is increased, resulting in excessive PO_4^{3-} retention (i.e., hyperphosphatemia).

As the renal response to aldosterone is enhanced by thyroid hormones, hyperthyroidism leads inexorably to increased Na^+ retention and renal K^+ excretion. The ensuing hypokalemia leads to a decrease in neuromuscular irritability (see Chapter 32) and sometimes to ventroflexion of the head.

51 Hypothyroidism

A

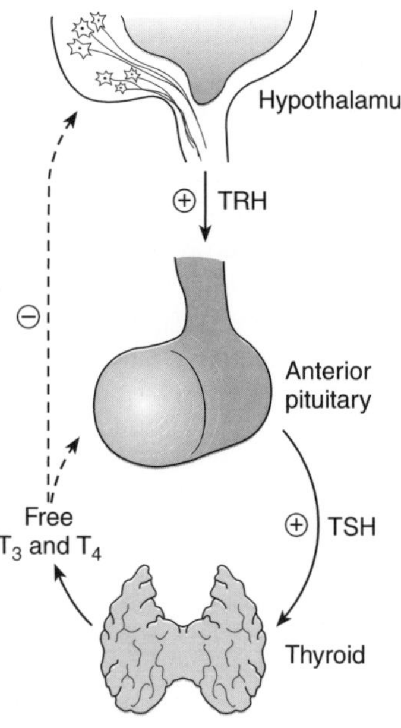

Hypothalamic lesion = *Tertiary hypothyroidism* with increase in TSH after administering TRH

Pituitary lesion = *Secondary hypothyroidism* with no increase in TSH after administering TRH

Thyroid lesion = *Primary hypothyroidism* with no increase in T_4 after administering TSH

B

Canine Breeds with a Predisposition to Hypothyroidism

Great Dane
Cocker Spaniel
Dachshund
Irish setter
Shetland sheep dog
Airedale
Boxer
Miniature schnauzer
Poodle
Pomeranian
*Golden retriever
*Doberman pincher

*Reportedly a higher incidence.

C

Signs and Symptoms of Hypothyroidism

Metabolic rate
- ↓BMR
- Dullness
- Lethargy
- Unwillingness to exercise
- Cold intolerance
- Weight gain

Skin and hair coat
- Dry, scaly skin
- Seborrhea
- Coarse, dull hair coat
- Alopecia (bilateral)
- Changes in hair coat color
- Hyperpigmentation
- Myxedema

Eyes
- Corneal lipid deposits
- Corneal ulceration
- Uveitis

Skeletal (congenital hypothyroidism)
- Disproportionate dwarfism
- Short, broad skull
- Epiphyseal dysgenesis

CNS
- Mental retardation (cretinism) decreased myelin formation
- Circling, head tilt
- Facial nerve paralysis, ↓facial sensation
- Ataxia
- Depression, irritability, seizures

Neuromuscular
- Lower motor neuron paresis/paralysis
- Decreased spinal reflexes
- Muscle weakness

Cardiovascular
- Bradycardia
- Decreased blood volume and pressure

Gastrointestinal
- Constipation
- Loss of appetite

Renal
- Increased urinary Na^+ excretion

Reproductive organs (female)
- Prolonged interestrus intervals
- Failure to cycle, infertility
- Galactorrhea
- Weak or still-born young

Reproductive organs (male)
- Low libido
- Testicular atrophy, infertility
- Hypospermia
- Azoospermia

Blood
- $\downarrow T_4$, $\downarrow T_3$
- Anemia
- Hypertriglyceridemia
- Hypercholesterolemia (and atherosclerosis)
- Hyponatremia

Overview

- Hypothyroidism is more common in dogs than cats.
- Most cases of hypothyroidism in dogs are classified as acquired primary hypothyroidism.
- Hypothyroidism decreases the number of β-adrenergic receptors.
- Untreated neonatal hypothyroidism results in irreversible cretinism.

Hypothyroidism is common in dogs, yet comparatively rare in cats. Iatrogenic (i.e., veterinarian-induced) hypothyroidism occurs more often than naturally acquired hypothyroidism in cats, and is secondary to bilateral thyroidectomy for the treatment of hyperthyroidism, ablation of the thyroid with ^{131}I, or an overdosage of antithyroid drugs.

More than 95% of canine cases are classified as *acquired primary hypothyroidism,* which results in compensatory increases in both TRH and TSH because the typical negative feedback of thyroid hormones on the hypothalamus and pituitary is lacking (**Part A**). Antibodies against the TSH receptor have been found in human patients and lead to thyroid gland atrophy. As TRH is a stimulator of prolactin release from the anterior pituitary, primary hypothyroidism may lead to galactorrhea (i.e., excessive or spontaneous flow of milk irrespective of nursing) in sexually intact bitches. Destruction of the thyroid in animals has been reported to result from lymphocytic thyroiditis, idiopathic thyroid atrophy, or (rarely) neoplastic invasion. *Secondary hypothyroidism* (decreased TSH) is seen in humans but is uncommonly recognized in dogs (probably due to inadequate assay for TSH) (see **Part A**). Causes of acquired secondary hypothyroidism in dogs include pituitary neoplasia and pituitary malformations such as cystic Rathke's pouch. *Tertiary hypothyroidism* (decreased TRH) has not been documented in dogs (see **Part A**).

Rare cases of hypothyroidism due to peripheral resistance to thyroid hormones have been decribed in humans. Affected individuals reportedly have abnormal thyroid hormone receptors or postreceptor defects. Consequences of hypothyroidism are most severe when the condition occurs in infancy. Untreated neonatal hypothyroidism results in irreversible *cretinism,* a congenital syndrome characterized by mental retardation and growth failure. Cretinism does occur in dogs, but it is rarely diagnosed because it usually results in early death. This syndrome is, unfortunately, remarkably common in humans, occurring once in every 8500 births.

Canine breeds with a predisposition for hypothyroidism are listed in **Part B.**

Signs and Symptoms

In spite of the wide spectrum of functional deficiencies associated with hypothyroidism, onset of the disease is reportedly slow and the manifestations are subtle, so that owners of domestic animals may not recognize the extent of illness until it reaches a rather advanced stage. Once thyroid hormone therapy is instituted, however, a dramatic improvement in overall physiologic status can be expected.

Characteristic signs of hypothyroidism include loss of appetite, lethargy, obesity, constipation, hypercholesterolemia, bradycardia, coarse hair coat, and bilateral alopecia (**Part C**). The intestinal musculature is among the many functional systems in which activity is conditioned by the presence of thyroid hormones. Hyperthyroidism is characterized by hypermotility and a tendency toward diarrhea, while hypothyroidism leads to decreased motility and constipation.

Myxedema, represented by the deposition of large amounts of mucopolysaccharides in the skin (particularly evident over the eyes and shoulders), takes up Na^+ in the form of increased tissue fluid as well as Na^+ directly bound to the chondroitin sulfuric acid in mucopolysaccharides. The loss of Na^+ would be compensated by renal conservation were it not for the fact that an additional route for Na^+ loss is the kidneys. Normal activity levels of the tubular Na^+ pumps and, more specifically, the active transport mechanism stimulated by aldosterone are dependent on adequate titers of thyroid hormones (see Chapter 49). With thyroid deficiency, the aldosterone Na^+ conservation mechanism is impaired, and Na^+ wastage occurs. Renal loss of Na^+, which carries significant water osmotically, can substantially deplete the extracellular fluid volume (if left unchecked), including the blood volume. This lowered blood volume, together with a decreased response to the noradrenergic vasoconstrictor mechanism, can bring about significant hypotension. Although the renal response to aldosterone is suppressed in hypothyroidism, the renal response to ADH is apparently maintained.

Hypothyroidism has a tendency to decrease the number of β-adrenergic receptors in heart muscle, as well as sarcolemmal calcium ATPase activity, Na^+/K^+ ATPase activity, and calcium channel function. Therefore, hypothyroidism causes impaired myocardial conductivity and action. Thyroid hormones, along with insulin and estrogen, also increase the number of hepatic LDL receptors. Therefore, hypothyroidism, like diabetes mellitus, results in a decreased ability to clear LDL and, therefore, cholesterol from the circulation, which can result in atherosclerosis. Impaired mental states associated with atherosclerosis and cerebral myxedema can be signs of hypothyroidism. Other effects of atherosclerosis including retinopathy and renal failure have been described in hypothyroid beagles.

Because thyroid hormones are essential for normal musculoskeletal growth and development, juvenile-onset hypothyroidism results in stunted growth.

52 Endocrine Pancreas: I

A

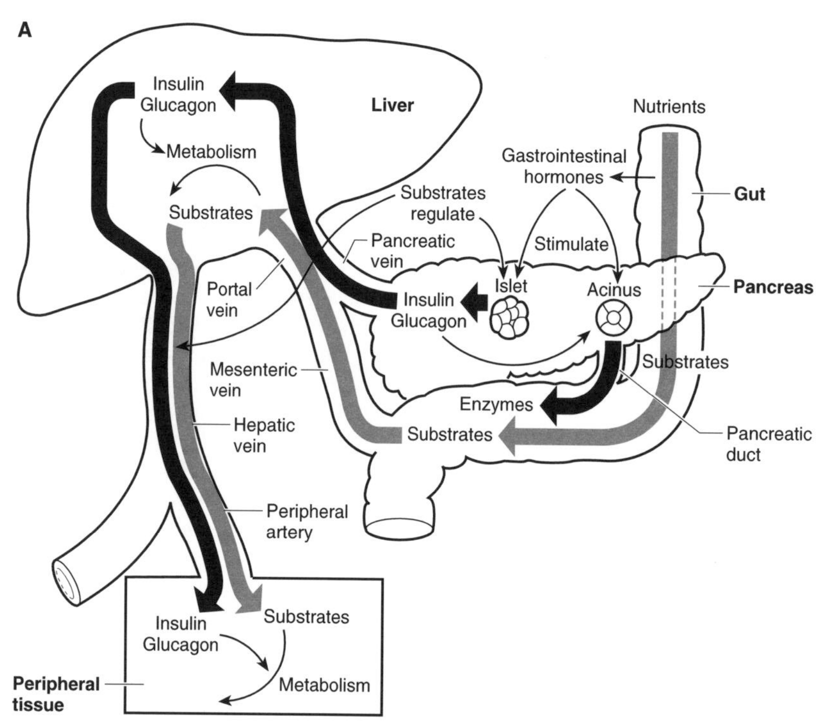

B

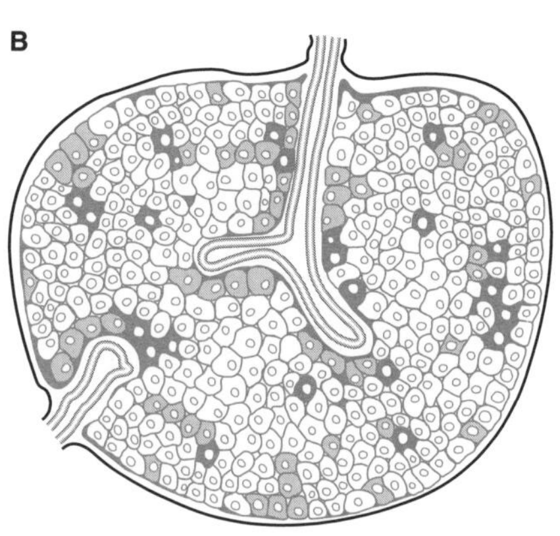

Islet cell type	%	Hormone
α	20	Glucagon
β	80	Insulin
Δ	1–5	Somatostatin
PP	1–2	Pancreatic polypeptide

C

Regulators	*Insulin Release (β Cell)*	*Glucagon Release (α Cell)*	*Somatostatin Release (Δ Cell)*
Hormones			
Enteric (glucagon-like peptide-1 [GLP-1], gastric inhibitory polypeptide [GIP], gastrin, CCK)	↑	↓	↑
Insulin	↓	↓	—
Somatostatin (octreotide)	↓	↓	↓
Glucagon	↑	—	↑
Amylin and pancreastatin	↓	—	—
Cortisol	—	↑	—
Growth hormone	—	↑	—
GABA	—	↓	—
Catecholamines	↓ (α-Adrenergics)	↑ (β-Adrenergics)	—
Neural			
α-Adrenergic	↓	↓	—
β-Adrenergic	↑	↑	—
Vagal	↑	↑	—
Nutrients			
Glucose	↑	↓	↑
Amino acids	↑	↑	↑
Free fatty acids	—	↓	—
Volatile fatty acids	↑ (ruminants)	—	—
Ketone bodies	↑	↓	—

Source: Part A modified from Berne RM, Levy MN. Principles of physiology. 1st ed. St. Louis: Mosby, 1990:505. **Part B** modified from Niewoehner CB. Endocrine pathophysiology. 1st ed. Madison, CT: Fence Creek, 1998:118, 119.

Overview

- The endocrine pancreas is composed of nests of cells known as the islets of Langerhans.
- Insulin and glucagon are the primary endocrine messengers secreted by the pancreas.
- Certain tissues in the body are uniquely dependent upon glucose as an energy source.
- The normal blood glucose concentration varies among animal species.

Multicellular organisms, unlike unicellular organisms, utilize a storage and release system for nutrients that permits intermittent rather than continual uptake. Insulin, secreted from specialized islet cells in the pancreas, is the primary hormone involved with energy storage, and its action is opposed by several *counter-regulatory hormones,* namely glucagon, cortisol, epinephrine, and growth hormone. In the absence of insulin, each acts on insulin-sensitive tissues including liver, muscle, and adipose tissue to release energy-rich nutrients in the form of glucose, lactate, amino acids, and/or free fatty acids (FFAs). Also, hormone-like products of islet cells (including somatostatin, pancreatic polypeptide, pancreastatin, and amylin) may play subsidiary roles in metabolic regulation.

The liver plays an important role as a site for storage of glucose as glycogen, synthesis of triglyceride from fatty acids and glucose, and conversion of nutrients released from extrahepatic storage sites into forms more easily utilized by cells. Glucose can be oxidized by virtually all living cells and is the primary source of energy for those lacking mitochondria (hence the inability of these cells to oxidize lipid). Although free fatty acids and ketone bodies may be oxidized by tissues containing mitochondria, the brain retains an absolute requirement for glucose and fails to function properly when glucose supplies fall below 1 mg/kg/min. The brain's dependency on glucose is protected by the counter-regulatory hormone system, which generally prevents glucose concentrations from falling below the critical limit, which would lead to serious brain dysfunction.

Ruminants are thought to be somewhat less dependent on the insulin–glucagon scheme than carnivores and omnivores, primarily because they are less dependent on tissue oxidation of glucose and more dependent on volatile fatty acids as a source of energy. Glucose accounts for only about 10% of ruminant tissue carbon dioxide production, whereas in carnivores and omnivores, 20% to 50% of carbon dioxide production is generally derived from carbohydrate. Nonetheless, blood glucose is important to all animals, and the physiologic roles of insulin and glucagon must be kept in mind when evaluating metabolic disorders.

Insulin and glucagon are secreted directly into portal blood; hence, the liver is the first organ subjected to the effects of these hormones before they are distributed to extrahepatic sites (**Part A**). This is quite different from the pharmacologic situation, in which insulin is injected into peripheral parts of the body and slowly finds its way to the liver in a diluted form.

Secretion of insulin and glucagon is coordinated with secretion of exocrine pancreatic enzymes, with secretion of both being stimulated by entry of nutrients into the GI tract and by GI hormones. Within the liver, these hormones, acting through second messengers that activate various hepatic enzymes, affect metabolism of ingested substrates. Islet hormones (particularly insulin) that pass through the liver with digested substrates affect disposition of these substrates by peripheral tissues. The substrates in turn feed back negatively on pancreatic islets to modulate further secretion of insulin and glucagon.

The normal blood glucose concentration, which varies among animal species from 25 mg/dL in the goat to 160 mg/dL in the pigeon, is maintained within a fairly narrow range, with fluctuations kept to a minimum. In the dog, for example, a blood glucose concentration of around 100 mg/dL is maintained, with daily fluctuations of only 10% to 20%. This minimal fluctuation could not be maintained if there were no precise control mechanisms, as the ingestion of a large carbohydrate meal (or strenuous exercise or starvation) would certainly cause greater fluctuations.

Islets of Langerhans

The endocrine pancreas is composed of nests of cells known as the islets of Langerhans, which are distributed throughout the exocrine pancreas (**Part B**). There are approximately one million islets in the porcine pancreas, many of which contain several hundred cells. The endocrine pancreas has great reserve capacity; however, like neurons, islet tissue has little regenerative capacity. Over 70% must usually be lost before hyperglycemia can develop.

There are four basic cell types within the islets, each producing a different primary secretory product. Insulin-secreting B cells (β cells) are located centrally and normally comprise 80% of total islet tissue. Glucagon-secreting A cells (*α cells*) comprise almost 20% of islet tissue and are located mainly in the periphery. Somatostatin-secreting D cells (*Δ cells*) are located between these two cell types and are few in number. Pancreatic polypeptide–secreting F cells (or *PP cells*) are located mainly in islets of the posterior lobe and receive a different blood supply.

Islets are more highly vascularized than exocrine pancreatic tissue. Blood flow proceeds from the center of the islet to the periphery, thereby allowing insulin to inhibit glucagon release. Blood from the islets then drains into the hepatic portal vein. Islet tissue is also abundantly innervated by the autonomic nervous system, with parasympathetic activation increasing both insulin and glucagon output, and sympathetic activation increasing glucagon while decreasing insulin output (**Part C**).

53 Endocrine Pancreas: II

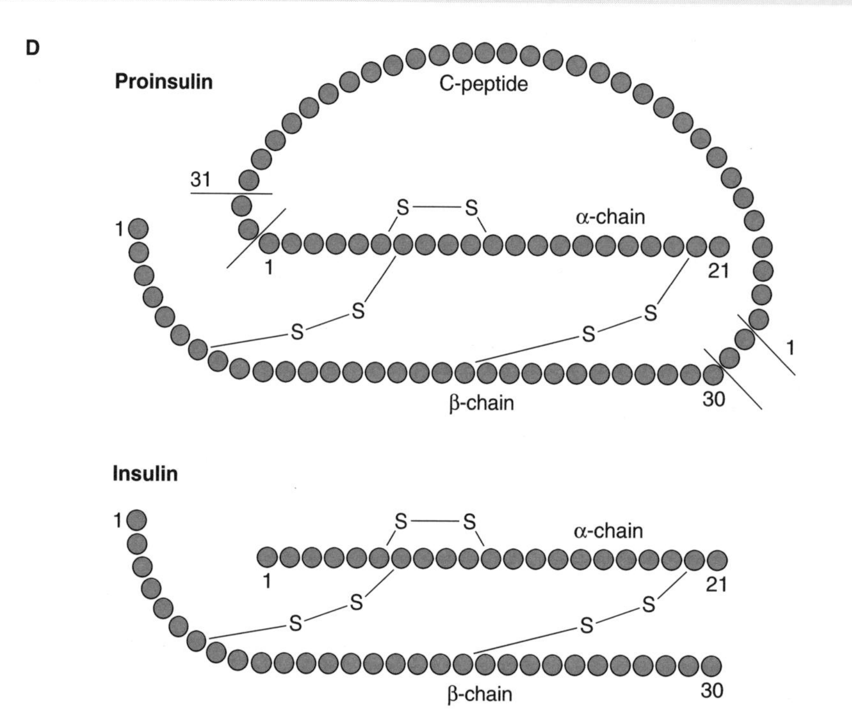

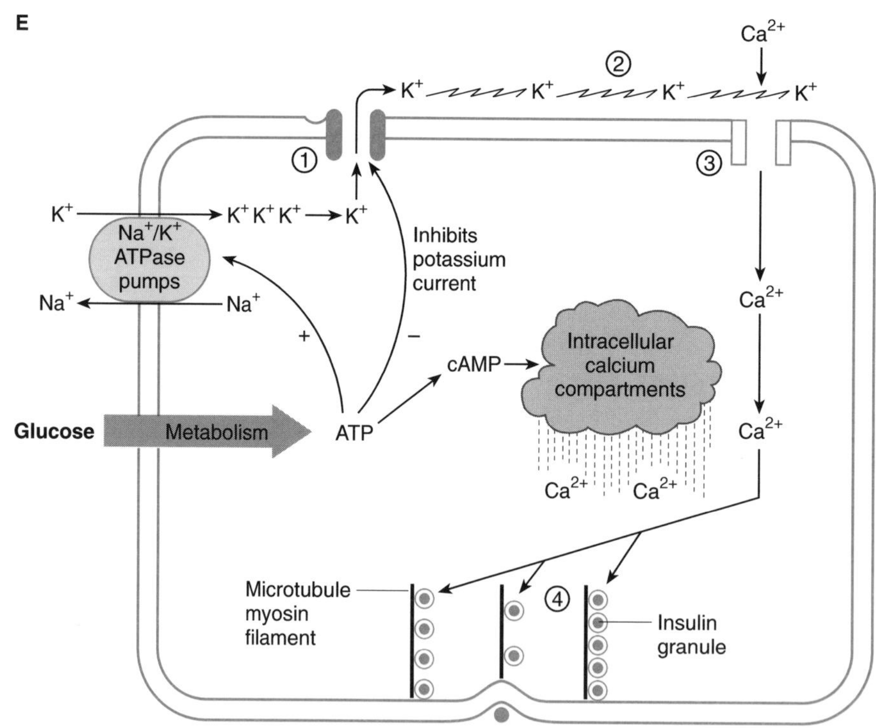

Source: Part D modified from Niewoehner CB. Endocrine pathophysiology. 1st ed. Madison, CT: Fence Creek, 1998:119. **Part E** modified from Kavam JH. Type II diabetes and Syndrome X. Endocrinol Metab Clin North Am 1992;21:339.

Overview

- Glucose is the primary secretagogue for insulin.
- K^+ efflux across insulin-secreting β cells influences insulin release.
- Ca^{2+} is involved in insulin release.
- Islet amyloid isolates pancreatic β cells.

Insulin Synthesis and Secretion

Insulin, like other peptide hormones, is synthesized as a larger molecule. This *proinsulin* includes a signal peptide that helps direct its folding and movement through the Golgi but is removed before storage in secretory granules. The connecting peptide is cleaved from proinsulin in secretory granules, thus forming two separate molecules, insulin and C-peptide. This connecting peptide is reported to be metabolically inert but is released in equimolar amounts with insulin, thus serving as a marker for insulin production by β cells.

Part D shows the structures of proinsulin, C-peptide, and insulin, with slashes representing cleavage sites and the numbers representing the respective amino acid positions of cleavage and bridge sites.

Insulin is a protein consisting of two chains that are designated α and β, having 21 and 30 amino acids, respectively, and are connected by two disulfide bridges (see **Part D**). Differences in amino acid sequence between species are small; for example, cattle, sheep, horses, dogs, and whales differ only in positions 8, 9, and 10 of the α-chain. Consequently, biologic activities of insulin are not highly species specific.

Insulin-like growth factor-2 (IGF-2) immunoreactivity has been reported in association with pancreatic β cells, whereas IGF-1 immunoreactivity has been found in association with glucagon-secreting α cells (see Chapter 9). Both may influence islet cell function in a paracrine fashion.

Glucose is the primary secretagogue for insulin. It enters β cells via a glucose transporter that has low affinity for glucose, thereby allowing a graded response. Once in β cells, metabolites of glucose, rather than glucose itself, are thought to stimulate insulin release. Phosphorylation of glucose by glucokinase, an enzyme with low affinity (high *Km*) for glucose, may act as a glucose sensor in β cells. Normally, K^+ efflux (process *1* in **Part E**) polarizes the β-cell membrane and prevents Ca^{2+} entry by closing a voltage-dependent channel (process *2*). However, when glucose is taken up by β cells, metabolic factors like ATP are thought to inhibit K^+ efflux, thus depolarizing the cell and allowing Ca^{2+} to enter (process *3*). Insulin-containing secretory vesicles attached to microtubules are expelled in the presence of Ca^{2+} (process *4*).

Although glucose is the most potent secretagogue for insulin, amino acids ingested with a meal, FFAs, volatile fatty acids, ketone bodies, glucagon, certain enteric hormones, and vagal stimulation also cause release (see **Part C**).

Pancreatic β cells are also known to synthesize and secrete *pancreastatin,* a 49-amino-acid peptide, and *amylin,* a 37-amino-acid peptide. Pancreastatin is co-secreted with insulin and may participate in autofeedback regulation because it inhibits insulin release. Other compounds known to inhibit insulin release include insulin itself, α-adrenergics, somatostatin, and amylin.

Amylin Secretion by β Cells

Islet amylin (or amyloid) initially forms intracellularly in β cells, then accumulates extracellularly after exocytosis or cell death. It is stored and co-secreted with insulin from secretory granules. Although amylin is reportedly secreted from β cells of all species studied to date, only a few species reportedly develop amyloid deposits in association with diabetes mellitus—namely humans, other primates, and cats. Overproduction of amylin has been reported in dogs with insulinomas but not in those with diabetes. Most diabetic dogs apparently experience islet cell destruction by the time of diagnosis; therefore, they are less likely to develop islet amyloidosis. Islet amyloid surrounds β cells, isolating them from adjacent pancreatic tissue and blood capillaries, and is believed to act as a barrier to the diffusion of nutritive substances and glucose. Because amylin inhibits insulin secretion and stimulates muscle glycogenolysis, it may also play an important role in the control of insulin secretion and in the modulation of glucose homeostasis. Amylin is anorectic, shares a common amino acid sequence with calcitonin, and may be associated with diabetic hypertension.

54 Insulin

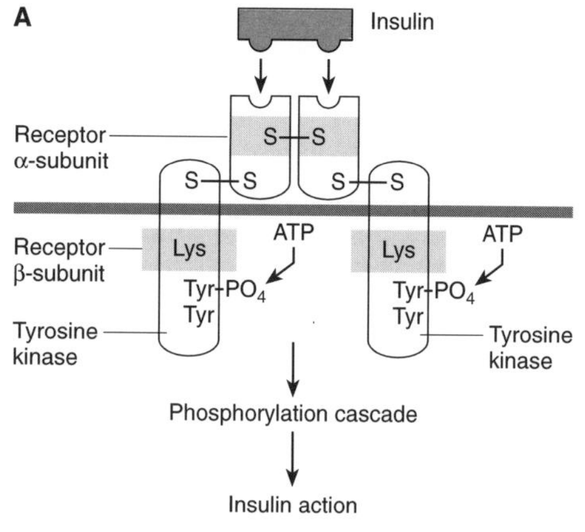

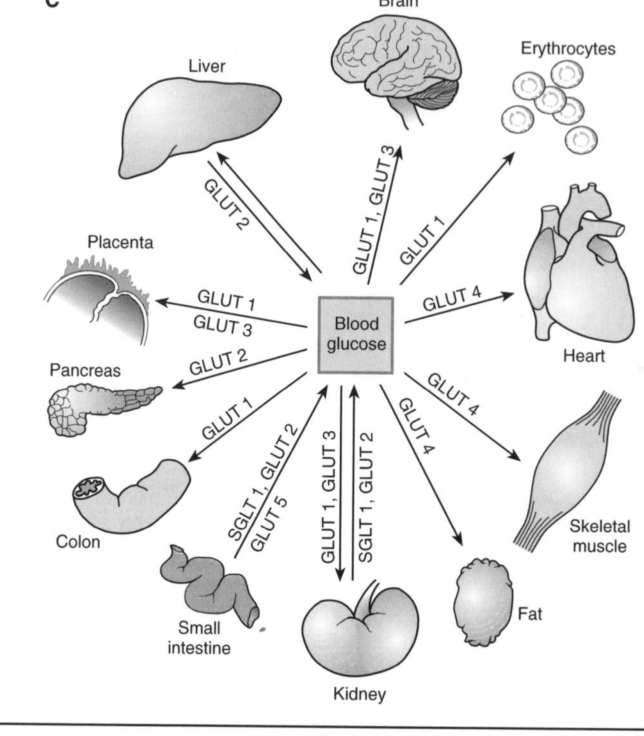

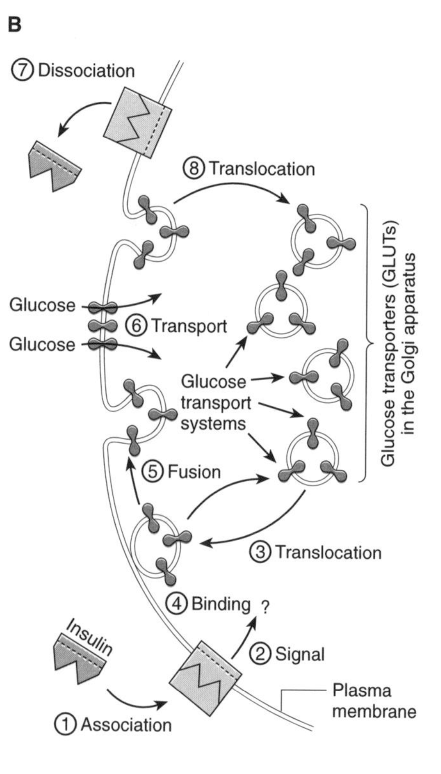

D Endocrine Regulation of Fuel Metabolism

Tissue	*Insulin*	*Glucagon*	*Catechol-amines*	*Cortisol*	*Growth hormone*
Liver					
Fuel storage					
Glycogenesis	↑	↓	↓	↑	—
Lipogenesis	↑	↓	—	—	—
Protein synthesis	↑	↓	↓	↓	↑
Fuel breakdown					
Glycogenolysis	↓	↑	↑	—	—
Gluconeogenesis	↓	↑	↑	↑	↑
β-Oxidation/ketogenesis	↓	↑	↑	↑	↑
Proteolysis	↓	—	—	—	—
Muscle					
Fuel storage					
Glucose uptake (glycogenesis)	↑	—	↓	↓	↓
Amino acid uptake (protein synthesis)	↑	—	—	↓	—
Fuel breakdown					
Glycogenolysis	↓	—	↑	—	—
Proteolysis	↓	—	—	↑	—
Adipose					
Fuel storage					
Lipoprotein lipolysis	↑	—	—	—	—
Glucose uptake	↑	—	—	—	—
Fatty acid esterification	↑	—	—	—	—
Fuel breakdown					
Lipolysis of stored triglyceride	↓	—	↑	↑	↑

Source: Part A modified from Niewoehner CB. Endocrine pathophysiology. 1st ed. Madison, CT: Fence Creek, 1998:121. **Part B** modified from Kamieli E, et al. Insulin-stimulated translocation of glucose transport systems in the isolated rat adipose cell. J Biol Chem 1981;256:4772.

Mechanism of Action

The glycoprotein receptors for insulin are found on the surface of target cells in liver, muscle, and fat tissue; that is, on classic insulin-sensitive tissues responsible for energy homeostasis. In addition, insulin can mediate anabolic effects in other nonclassic target tissues, such as the ovary, via interaction with insulin receptors or by cross-reactivity with IGF-1 receptors. The insulin receptor is a tetrameric structure consisting of two α-subunits and two β-subunits held together by disulfide bonds. The α-subunits are extracellular in location and contain the insulin-binding site, which is rich in cysteine residues. The β-subunits span the plasma membrane and anchor the receptor to the cell, and they contain specific tyrosine residues that are autophosphorylated by the receptor when insulin binds to the α-subunit. This autophosphorylation turns the receptor into a tyrosine kinase, which phosphorylates other cellular proteins, thereby mediating the effects of insulin on cellular metabolism (**Part A**). Numerous target cell enzymes are ultimately activated or inactivated, resulting in a shift in the metabolism of glucose, for example toward glycogen and pyruvate.

Although it is not precisely known how binding at the cell surface is translated into the constellation of effects described for insulin, we may speculate that the rate of glucose transport across the plasma membrane of muscle and adipose cells determines the rate of phosphorylation of glucose and its further metabolism. Data indicate that in adipocytes the carrier-mediated facilitated diffusion of glucose is accomplished by moving glycoprotein *glucose transporters (GLUTs)* from the Golgi fraction to the plasma membrane. This transporter translocation is temperature and energy dependent.

The GLUT translocation process is summarized in **Part B.** Insulin binds with its plasma membrane receptor (process *1* in **Part B**), which in turn brings about an intracellular signal (process *2*; mechanism unknown) that causes the translocation of GLUT 4 (process *3*) from an inactive pool in the Golgi fraction. These transporters are moved and bound (process *4*) to active sites on the plasma membrane, where fusion (process *5*) to this membrane brings about facilitated diffusion of glucose into the cell (process *6*). Following removal of insulin from its binding sites on plasma membrane receptors (process *7*), the GLUT 4 transporters are translocated back to the Golgi (process *8*).

The hepatic cell represents a notable exception to this scheme. Insulin does not promote facilitated diffusion of glucose into hepatocytes, but rather indirectly enhances net inward flux by converting intracellular glucose to glucose-6-phosphate through activation of glucokinase. Rapid phosphorylation keeps the free glucose concentration low in hepatocytes, thus allowing entry of the nonpolar glucose molecule by simple diffusion down its concentration gradient. Insulin also promotes entry of amino acids into cells, particularly in muscle, and enhances uptake of K^+, Mg^{2+}, nucleosides, and inorganic phosphate—actions independent of insulin's effects on glucose entry.

One Na^+-dependent glucose transporter (SGLT 1) isoform and five GLUT transporter isoforms have been identified in various tissues (**Part C**). The SGLT 1 transporter is responsible for secondary active transport of glucose out of the intestine and renal tubules, whereas the five GLUT transporters are responsible for the facilitated diffusion of glucose. Four are found in **insulin-independent** tissues: *GLUT 1* is responsible for basal glucose uptake in erythrocytes, the placenta, the kidneys, the colon, the blood–brain barrier, etc.; *GLUT 2* is the β-cell glucose sensor and also transports glucose out of intestinal cells, the liver, and renal tubular epithelial cells; *GLUT 3* is responsible for basal glucose uptake in neurons, the placenta, the kidneys, and other organs; and *GLUT 5* participates in the dietary absorption of glucose in the jejunum. The *GLUT 4* transporter has been identified in **insulin-dependent** tissue, namely muscle and fat. Transport activity of GLUT 4 appears to be increased through activation of protein kinase C (PKC).

Glycogen synthase in liver is activated by a specific phosphatase that removes key phosphate residues previously added by cAMP-dependent protein kinase A (PKA) in response to hormones such as glucagon and epinephrine. Some actions of insulin are apparently mediated through a phosphoinositol IP_3 kinase, and others continue to be elucidated. These multiple downstream events in the action of insulin are referred to collectively as *postreceptor insulin actions.*

Lipoprotein lipase (LPL), anchored to the capillary endothelium by proteoglycan chains of heparan sulfate, has been found in the heart, adipose tissue, spleen, lungs, renal medulla, aorta, diaphragm, lactating mammary gland, and neonatal liver. This important enzyme, needed for the clearance of triglyceride from circulating chylomicrons (CMs) and very-low-density lipoprotein (VLDL), hydrolyzes the ester bonds of triglyceride, and its activity is greatly increased by insulin. Many of the macrovascular, atherosclerotic effects of diabetes mellitus are due to the lack of LPL stimulation by insulin.

Major Effects of Insulin on Liver, Muscle, and Fat Tissue

Insulin promotes fuel storage in the liver by stimulating glycogen synthesis and storage (**Part D**). It inhibits gluconeogenesis and glycogenolysis, thereby reducing hepatic export of glucose to the circulation, and promotes formation of precursors for fatty acid synthesis by stimulating glycolysis. Moreover, insulin stimulates hepatic lipogenesis, leading to increased synthesis and secretion of VLDL, which delivers triglyceride from the liver to fat tissue for storage. Insulin also inhibits hepatic fatty acid β-oxidation and the production of ketone bodies, which are water-soluble alternative fuel produced only in the liver that can be used by the brain and fetus when glucose supplies are low (e.g., starvation).

Although hepatic uptake of glucose is important, uptake by muscle generally accounts for the majority of insulin-stimulated glucose disposal (see **Part D**). However, insulin's effect on K^+ entry into muscle cells is greater than its effect on glucose entry. Insulin promotes muscle glucose storage by stimulating glycogen synthesis and inhibiting glycogen catabolism. It also promotes muscle protein synthesis.

Insulin stimulates fat storage by stimulating LPL activity (see **Part D**). The FFAs cleaved from the triglyceride contained in circulating CMs and VLDL enter adipocytes, where they become available for triglyceride resynthesis. Insulin-stimulated glucose uptake by adipocytes via upregulation on the GLUT 4 transporter increases intracellular levels of glycerol-3-phosphate, the activated triglyceride backbone needed for fat storage. Insulin also inhibits lipolysis by decreasing the activity of hormone-sensitive lipase, the enzyme in adipocytes that hydrolyzes fatty acids from stored triglyceride. Together, these effects of insulin result in increased fat storage.

Degradation of Insulin

Insulin has a circulatory half-life of about three to five minutes and is catabolized in both the liver and the kidney. The liver is commonly believed to catabolize approximately 50% of insulin on its first pass. In contrast, both C-peptide and proinsulin (see Chapters 52 and 53) are catabolized only by the kidney and, therefore, have half-lives three to four times longer.

55 Glucagon

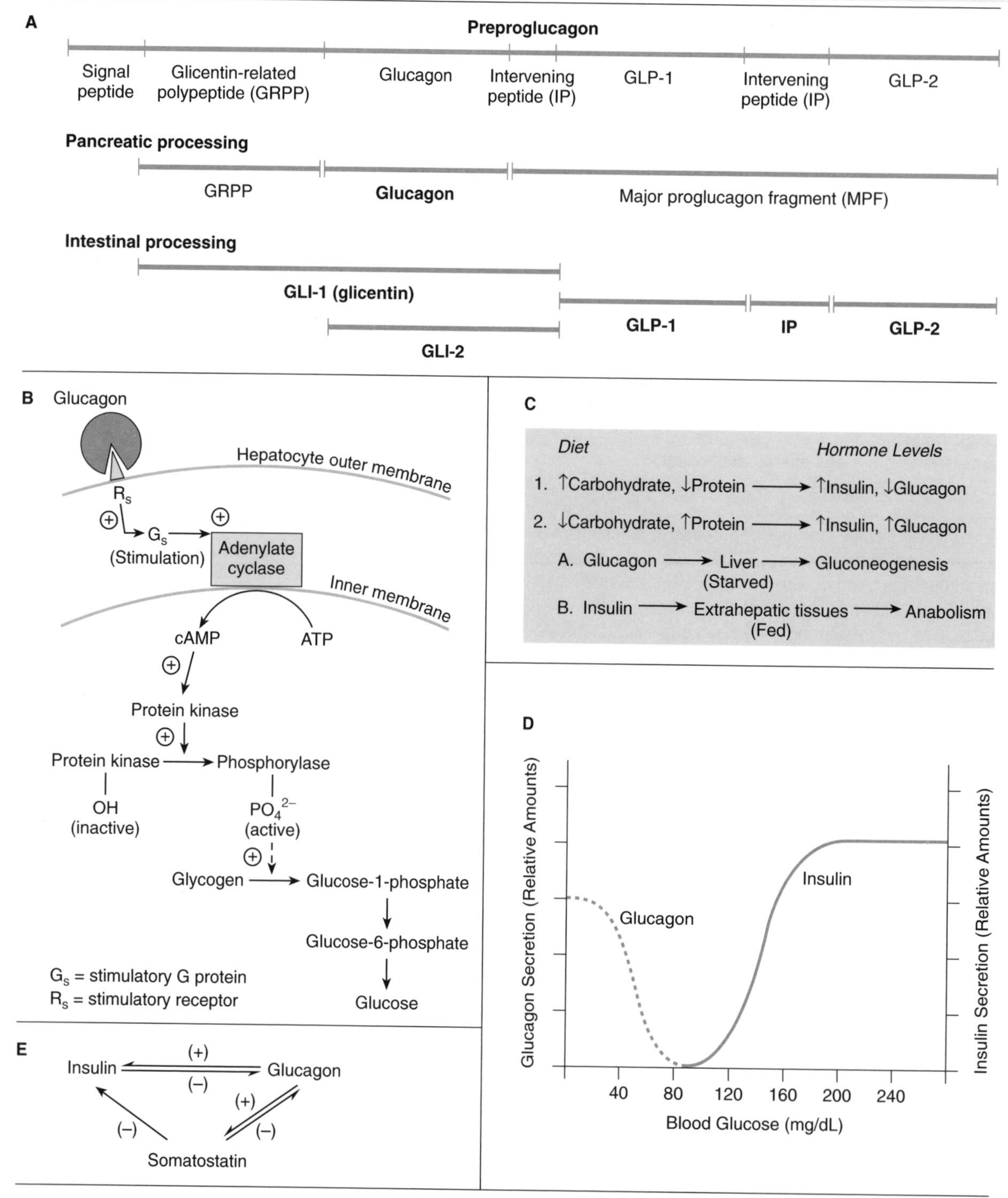

Source: Part A modified from McPhee SJ, et al. Pathophysiology of disease. 2nd ed. Appleton and Lange, 1997:428. **Part D** modified from Marliss EB et al. Normalization of glycemia in diabetics during meals with insulin and glucagon delivery by the artificial pancreas. Diabetes 1977;26:663. **Part E** modified from Ganong WF. Review of medical physiology. 18th ed. Stamford, CT: Appleton & Lange, 1997:323.

Overview

- The primary target organ for glucagon is the liver.
- Glucagon works through cAMP.
- Insulin inhibits glucagon release, however, glucagon stimulates insulin release.

Synthesis and Metabolism

Glucagon, a 29-amino-acid peptide, is derived from a much larger precursor protein, *preproglucagon.* This precursor molecule is proteolytically processed to form several biologically active peptides (**Part A**). Preproglucagon and the smaller proglucagon are synthesized in the pancreas, GI tract, and brain. However, only pancreatic α cells have been shown to cleave glucagon from proglucagon. Other biologically active peptides derived from preproglucagon, such as *glucagon-like peptides (GLP-1 and GLP-2)* and *glucagon-like immunoreactivity peptides* (GLI-1 and GLI-2), are primarily synthesized by the GI tract in response to a meal. Of these, a metabolite of GLP-1 is reported to be a more potent stimulator of insulin release than glucagon, and it may be the most important enteric hormone associated with postprandial insulin release (see Chapter 54, **Part D**). Glucagon-like peptide-1 decreases glucagon secretion from pancreatic α cells, and GLP-2 binds glucagon receptors, though with only 10% potency. The physiologic roles of these glucagon-related peptides are currently under investigation.

Degradation

The circulatory half-life of glucagon is similar to that of insulin—about three to six minutes. Like insulin, glucagon is metabolized in the liver and kidney; however, the liver is thought to account for only 25% of glucagon clearance (compared to 50% for insulin—see Chapter 54).

Mechanism of Action

Glucagon's major target organ is the liver, where it binds to cell surface receptors (**Part B**). Interaction of the receptor with a stimulatory G (G_s) protein then activates adenylate cyclase. Cyclic-AMP (cAMP), generated by adenylate cyclase, activates protein kinase A (PKA), which then phosphorylates various enzymes.

Effects of Glucagon on the Liver

Glucagon counters the effects of insulin on the liver by promoting output rather than input of glucose. This occurs through stimulation of both glycogenolysis and gluconeogenesis. Glucagon stimulates β-oxidation of fatty acids and thus promotes ketone body formation, providing alternative fuel for the brain when glucose supplies are low. Glucagon also stimulates hepatic uptake of amino acids, which are then used as gluconeogenic substrates (see Chapter 54, **Part D**).

The plasma glucagon concentration reaches a peak on the third day of starvation, then decreases thereafter as FFAs and ketone bodies become major sources of energy.

Effects of Glucagon on Extrahepatic Tissues

Because glucagon lowers serum triglyceride and FFA concentrations while stimulating lipolysis, it may increase muscle uptake and catabolism of FFAs; however, it functions mainly at the level of the liver. Few effects of glucagon on extrahepatic tissues have been described in mammals.

The Insulin/Glucagon Ratio

The ratio of insulin to glucagon plays an important role in controlling the level of cAMP in liver cells and, thereby, the rate of glucose synthesis or biotransformation. In addition, in felines ingesting meals containing fat and protein (but little or no carbohydrate), and in ruminant animals in which little or no glucose is absorbed from the GI tract, insulin is still released at a rate greater than basal (**Part C**). Increasing concentrations of amino acids initiate this insulin release, while the lack of incoming glucose and the presence of glucogenic amino acids maintain glucagon release. Therefore, extrahepatic tissues receive the "fed" signal to take up circulating fuels (such as amino acids and fatty acids), yet the liver remains in the starvation mode (i.e., the gluconeogenic mode) in order to maintain the blood glucose concentration. Thus, whether the liver is gluconeogenic or glycogenic-glycolytic is a function of the ratio of insulin to glucagon. In the absence of amino acid, if sufficient carbohydrate is absorbed from the GI tract to displace the need for hepatic glucose production, then the rise in glucose concentration is sufficient to increase β-cell insulin release and thus suppress α cells from releasing glucagon. As a result, hepatic glucose production is suppressed (**Parts C** and **D**). In addition, this slight increase in the blood glucose concentration markedly synergizes β cells to produce even more insulin as a response to increased amino acids, so that the insulin/glucagon ratio increases even more.

Somatostatin

Somatostatin, a 14-amino-acid peptide, is also formed by the proteolytic cleavage of a preprohormone that is synthesized in the pancreas, GI tract, and brain (as well as other tissues). Unlike the situation for glucagon, however, all of these tissues apparently retain the ability to cleave the preprohormone and prohormone to form somatostatin.

Somatostatin was originally discovered in the hypothalamus as a factor responsible for the inhibition of growth hormone (somatotropin) release—hence its name. Only later was it appreciated that Δ cells of the pancreas also produce and secrete somatostatin. Unlike most prohormones, however, prosomatostatin, a 28-amino-acid peptide, is more potent than its derivative. *Octreotide,* a synthetic 8-amino-acid analogue of somatostatin used clinically, is also more potent than somatostatin. The half-life of somatostatin has been reported as less than three minutes.

Several of the same secretagogues that stimulate insulin release also stimulate somatostatin release. These include glucose, amino acids, certain enteric hormones, and glucagon (see Chapters 52 and 53, **Part E**). Somatostatin acts as a paracrine agent to inhibit both insulin and glucagon release and, therefore, to modulate their output. Glucagon, however, stimulates insulin release in a paracrine fashion, while insulin inhibits glucagon release (**Part E**).

Summary

Insulin is anabolic, increasing the storage of glucose, fatty acids, and amino acids, while glucagon is catabolic. These two major pancreatic hormones are reciprocal in their overall action, and they are also reciprocally secreted in most circumstances. Insulin excess causes hypoglycemia, which leads to convulsions and coma, while insulin deficiency (either absolute or relative) causes diabetes mellitus, a complex and debilitating disease that can be fatal if left untreated. Glucagon deficiency causes hypoglycemia, and glucagon excess can worsen diabetes. Excess pancreatic production of somatostatin causes hyperglycemia and other manifestations of diabetes. Other counter-regulatory hormones such as cortisol, growth hormone, and epinephrine also play important roles in the regulation of carbohydrate, fat, and protein metabolism.

56 Diabetes Mellitus

A

Heterogenic Causes of Diabetes Mellitus in Animals
Genetic predisposition
Pancreatic injury
Trauma
Neoplasia
Infection
Autoantibodies
Inflammation
Drugs
Hormone-induced β-cell exhaustion
Growth hormone
Thyroid hormones
Cortisol
Catecholamines
Progestins
Target tissue insensitivity
Decreased number of insulin receptors
Defective insulin receptors
Defect in postreceptor effects
Dyshormonogenesis of insulin

B

Normal animal

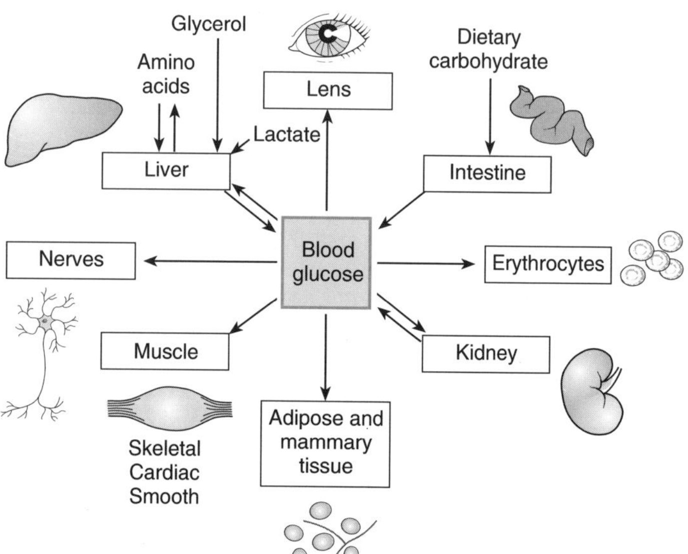

Diabetic Animal (Absence of Insulin)

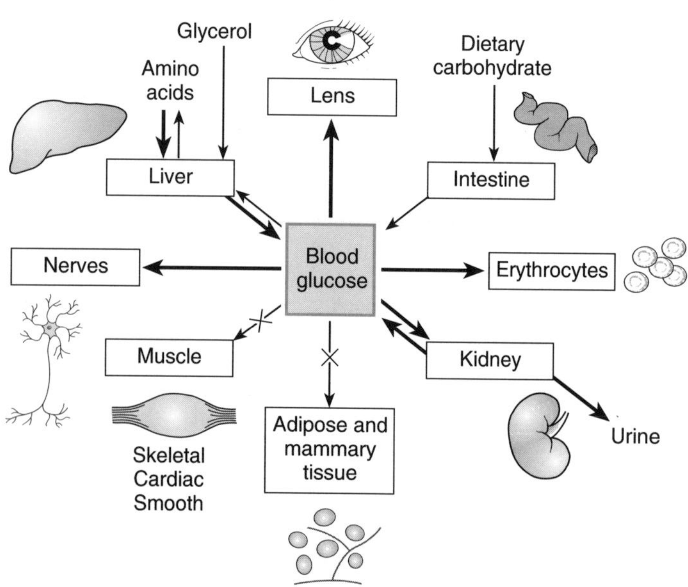

Tissues in Which Insulin Facilitates Glucose Uptake
Skeletal muscle
Cardiac muscle
Smooth muscle
Adipose
Mammary

Tissues in Which Insulin Does Not Facilitate Glucose Uptake
Nerves (except in part of the hypothalamus)
Kidney tubules and glomeruli
Intestinal mucosa
Erythrocytes (RBCs)
Lens
Blood–brain barrier
Pancreatic β cell

Overview

- Diabetes mellitus is a common endocrine disorder of dogs and cats.
- The liver and kidneys continue producing glucose in hyperglycemic, diabetic animals.
- Most diabetic animals are hypoinsulinemic, and therefore require insulin replacement therapy.

The term *diabetes,* meaning *syphon* or *running through,* was used by the Greeks over 200 years ago to describe the striking urinary volume excreted by certain subjects. *Mellitus,* meaning *sweet,* distinguishes this urine from the large quantities of *insipid* urine produced by patients suffering from ADH deficiency (see Chapters 25 and 26).

Sweet urine was first described in the 17th century, but in England the illness had long been called the "pissing evil." Because of marked weight loss despite a large food intake, the body's substance was believed to be dissolving and pouring out through the urinary tract (a view that is not far from the truth). In 1889, experimental diabetes mellitus (DM) was produced in dogs by surgical removal of the pancreas, and 32 years later Banting and Best discovered insulin.

Diabetes mellitus is characterized by a persistent hyperglycemia that most typically results from an absolute or relative deficiency of insulin. It is a commonly recognized endocrine disease in cats (with an approximate incidence of 1 in 800), and the second most common endocrine disorder in dogs (approximately 1 in 200). Diabetes mellitus is rare in birds, horses, and other domestic animals.

Canine DM most frequently occurs in small breeds (e.g., the dachshund and poodle), but all breeds are affected. German shepherds, cocker spaniels, collies, and boxers, however, appear to have a significantly decreased risk. The age of onset is usually 8 to 9 years, and affected intact and neutered female dogs outnumber males by two- to fourfold. The diabetogenic effect of progesterone or progesterone-induced hypersecretion of growth hormone during metestrus has been cited as a potential cause of DM in sexually intact female dogs (see Chapter 10).

In contrast, feline DM is apparently more common in males than females. Most affected cats are sexually altered (as is the usual feline hospital population). Domestic shorthairs are the most frequently affected breed, but again the incidence may not exceed that of the general hospital population. The usual age of onset is more than 9 years.

Most avian species tolerate pancreatectomy well, except the owl, which is carnivorous and suffers severely from pancreatectomy. Pancreatectomy in some birds (e.g., ducks) is followed by a lowering of the blood glucose concentration. This is undoubtedly associated with the fact that the avian pancreas contains about ten times as much extractable glucagon as the mammalian pancreas. Little work has been done on metabolic disturbances following pancreatectomy or naturally occurring DM in domestic animals (except the dog).

Excess glucagon must be considered a possible cause of DM. In humans, some diabetic patients have elevated levels of glucagon, which could come from pancreatic α cells or an enteric source. The ensuing hyperglycemia may lead to β-cell exhaustion. In this regard, β cells of most species are so susceptible to injected growth hormone (GH) that one wonders if overproduction of endogenous GH could also be a cause of DM.

Cattle that have recovered from viral foot-and-mouth disease have a high incidence of DM, and the incidence of DM in humans (2% to 10% of the American population) is thought to be higher than that in most domestic animal species.

Although not enough research has been done to allow classification of all conditions that may contribute to the onset of DM in domestic animals, it is thought that the multiplicity of biochemical manifestations observed stems from five general heterogenic causes: 1) genetic predisposition, 2) pancreatic injury, 3) hormone-induced β-cell exhaustion, 4) target tissue insensitivity, and 5) dyshormonogenesis of insulin (**Part A**).

Diabetes arises through two etiologically distinct routes. *Type I diabetes* in humans most commonly results from immunologically mediated destruction of pancreatic β cells and usually requires replacement therapy with insulin. Type I diabetes is also referred to as *insulin-dependent diabetes mellitus (IDDM),* or *juvenile diabetes* in humans. *Type II diabetes* appears to result from a combination of alterations in insulin sensitivity and insulin secretion. It can be treated with dietary therapy or oral hypoglycemic agents and infrequently requires exogenous insulin. Type II diabetes in humans is therefore referred to as *non-insulin-dependent diabetes mellitus (NIDDM)* or *adult-onset DM.*

Dogs with DM (mostly middle-aged to old dogs) have been classified in two major groups:

1. **A minority of cases that are hyperinsulinemic** have elevated growth hormone levels and mild clinical signs (mainly ketotic).
2. **A majority of cases that are hypoinsulinemic.** This group has been further divided into two subgroups:
    a. Those that are **mildly ketotic.**
    b. Those that are **severely ketotic.**

Dogs in group 1 are similar to type II human diabetics, while dogs in group 2 are similar to type I human diabetics.

Glucose Intolerance in Diabetes

Glucose intolerance in diabetic animals is in part due to reduced entry of glucose into insulin-sensitive tissues (**Part B**). In the absence of insulin, the entry of glucose into skeletal, smooth, and cardiac muscle as well as adipose and mammary tissue is decreased. Intestinal absorption of glucose remains unaffected because mucosal cells are insulin insensitive, and proximal tubular reabsorption of glucose from the renal filtrate remains unaffected. However, as the renal threshold for reabsorption is reached (at a concentration of about 180 mg/dL), glucose begins to appear in urine. As the plasma glucose concentration rises, glucose also cannot be kept out of insulin-insensitive tissues. Therefore, intracellular glucose concentrations rise in glomerular renal tubular epithelial cells, erythrocytes, nerve cells (including those of the brain), and the lens. All are affected pathophysiologically.

The liver and kidney, both gluconeogenic organs, continue producing glucose from glycerol and incoming glucogenic amino acids under the effects of the diabetogenic hormones (glucagon, epinephrine, growth hormone, and cortisol), particularly in times of stress.

Perhaps the best way to appreciate what insulin means to the economy of the body is to consider in detail the biochemical and physiologic manifestations of acute insulin withdrawal. When insulin is withdrawn acutely from a severely diabetic patient, a remarkable sequence of intricately interconnected events begins and, if there is no intervention, the inevitable outcome will be coma and death. These events involve not merely carbohydrate metabolism, but fat and protein metabolism and electrolyte and fluid balance as well. The repercussions of insulin withdrawal appear in the CNS, as well as in the respiratory, cardiovascular, renal, and gastrointestinal systems. Insulin withdrawal, the focus of the next chapter, permits the unopposed action of the counter-regulatory diabetogenic hormones (which, unfortunately, elevate the plasma glucose concentration).

57 Acute Insulin Withdrawal: I

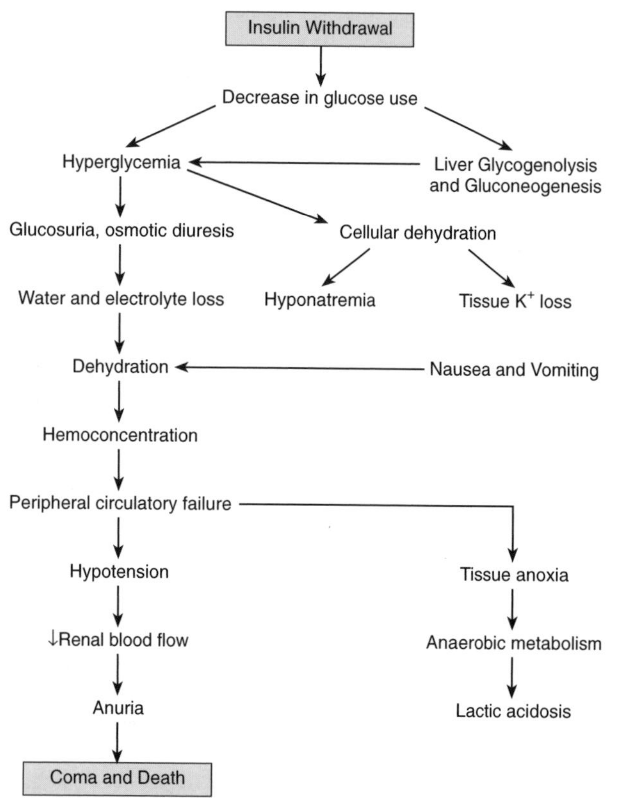

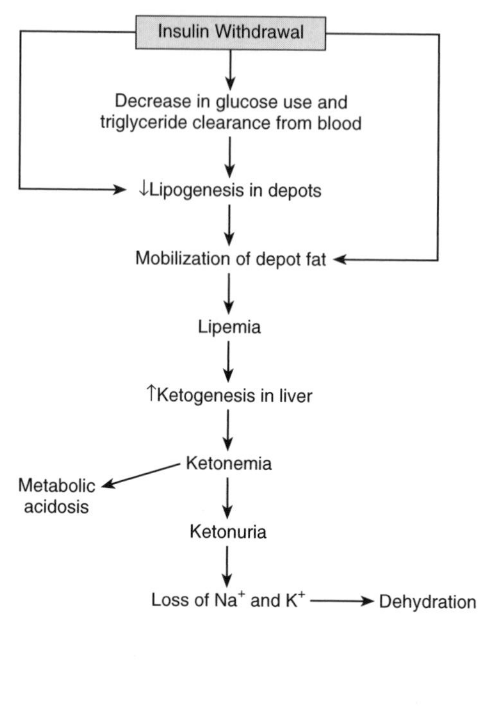

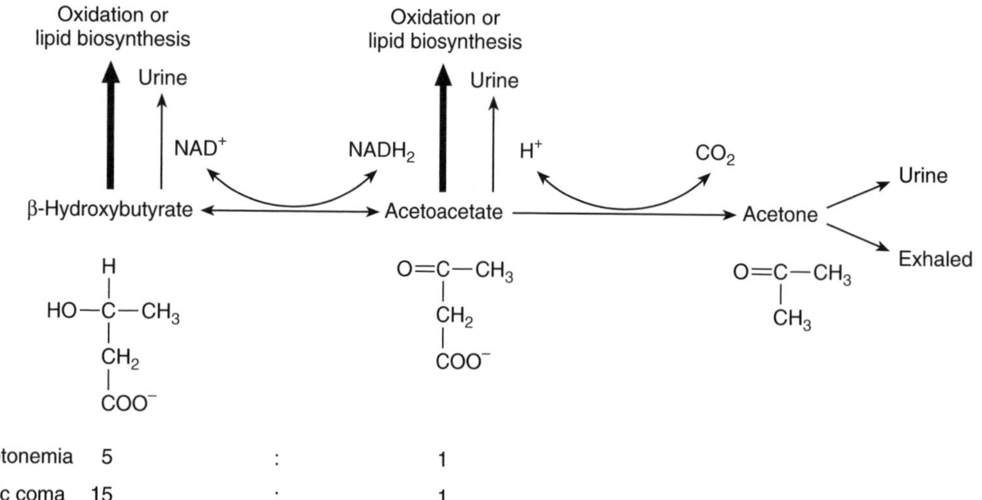

Source: Parts A and **B** modified from Tepperman J, Tepperman HM. Metabolic and endocrine physiology. 5th ed. St. Louis: Mosby Year-Book, 1987:282–284.

Overview

- Insulin withdrawal causes decreased glucose utilization.
- Glucosuria and ketonuria are common symptoms of uncontrolled diabetes mellitus.
- The insulinopenia of diabetes causes disorders in lipid metabolism.
- Acute insulin withdrawal can lead to a metabolic acidosis.

The effects of insulin deprivation in the diabetic patient form a ghastly caricature of the normal adaptation to starvation. Many of the same kinds of changes occur, but with inappropriately violent consequences. Moreover, it is often difficult to understand interrelationships among the many biochemical events that are essentially occurring simultaneously. For this reason, an arbitrary division of this topic into three segments has been made in this chapter, followed by a discussion of how all three processes are interrelated. This discussion will be concerned with the level of organization in the whole animal.

Carbohydrate Metabolism

The primary event that causes a disruption in normal carbohydrate metabolism is *relative insulin withdrawal* (**Part A**). In diabetic animals, this may not necessarily mean an absolute decrease in the amount of insulin the patient receives, but rather a sudden and unexpected increase in the insulin requirement. An attack of acidosis may be precipitated by an infection, physical trauma, or emotional distress, all of which tend to increase the need for insulin, or it may be initiated by the omission of insulin. Sometimes there is vomiting, which is then followed by inadequate food and water assimilation.

With insulin withdrawal, there is a decrease in glucose utilization by peripheral tissues, mainly by muscle and adipose tissue. This contributes to a developing hyperglycemia, and liver glycogenolysis also contributes to this condition. Hepatic gluconeogenesis from glycerol, lactate, and glucogenic amino acids also adds to the increase in blood sugar.

The plasma Na^+ concentration is generally low, owing to the hyperglycemic osmotic effect that draws intracellular water into extracellular spaces. The Na^+ concentration is thought to fall approximately 1.6 mmol/L for every 100-mg/dL increase in plasma glucose.

Total body stores of K^+ are reduced by diuresis and vomiting. However, acidosis, insulinopenia, and cellular dehydration due to hyperglycemia cause a shift in K^+ out of cells, thus maintaining normal or even elevated plasma K^+ concentrations. With administration of insulin and correction of the acidosis, the plasma K^+ concentration falls as K^+ moves back into cells. Without treatment it can fall to dangerously low levels, leading to potentially lethal cardiac arrhythmias. Therefore, K^+ supplementation is routinely given in the treatment of diabetic ketoacidosis.

When the plasma glucose concentration rises above the renal threshold for glucose (i.e., 180 mg/dL), *glucosuria* appears and an osmotic diuresis is instituted. This is the basis of the polyuria of diabetes, the first symptom of the disease to be recognized in antiquity. Loss of water and electrolytes in urine, especially combined with the fact that intake by ingestion has usually ceased, leads to dehydration and hemoconcentration. This, in turn, leads to peripheral circulatory failure because of the marked reduction in the effective circulating volume. One of the characteristic features of hypovolemic shock is hypotension followed by diminished renal blood flow, which may progress to the point of anuria. Generalized tissue anoxia, with a consequent shift to anaerobic metabolism, results in increasing concentrations of lactic acid in blood. Coma appears sometime after the appearance of peripheral circulatory failure, with death inevitable in the untreated diabetic. Hyperosmolality, not acidosis, is generally considered to be the cause of diabetic coma.

Lipid Metabolism

Oskar Minkowski, the man credited with describing the glucosuria associated with insulin withdrawal, is said to have tasted the urine of a pancreatectomized dog in 1889 because it attracted an inordinate number of flies. Had he smelled the urine instead, perhaps the emphasis on biochemical and physiologic disorders of insulin withdrawal initially would have been shifted toward disordered lipid metabolism instead of alterations in carbohydrate metabolism.

It is well known today that the insulinopenia of diabetes, and the subsequent decrease in glucose use by adipose tissue, results in retention of triglyceride-containing lipoproteins in blood (mainly chylomicrons and VLDLs), as well as large-scale mobilization of depot fat (**Part B**). Lipolysis may result in secondary hypertriglyceridemia as free fatty acids (FFAs) are synthesized back into triglycerides and then packaged by the liver into VLDLs, which are then exocytosed into blood.

The liver is flooded with long-chain FFAs, many of which can be oxidized only as far as the acetyl-CoA stage. The 2-carbon fragments then generate *acetoacetic acid* and *β-hydroxybutyric acid,* the two primary ketone bodies, which appear in hepatic venous blood in increasing amounts (**Part C**). The adult liver cannot oxidize ketone bodies, and, other than rumen epithelial cells, the liver is the only tissue in the body known to produce them.

Acetone is formed by the spontaneous decarboxylation of acetoacetate and is only detectable when the concentration of the latter is abnormally high (see **Part C**). Acetone is not further metabolized, but rather is excreted through the lungs and kidneys (where it accounts for the characteristic sweet or fruity smell on the breath and in the urine of severely diabetic patients).

The developing *ketonemia* has two prominent effects: 1) it leads to a progressive metabolic acidosis (because ketone bodies are strong acids), which in turn initiates the characteristic deep Küssmaul breathing that is one of the cardinal signs of diabetic ketoacidosis; and 2) as ketonemia exceeds the renal threshold for ketone body reabsorption, ketone bodies appear in urine. In the process of being excreted by the kidneys, ketone bodies, because they are anions, also pull Na^+ and K^+ with them. This means in effect that the ionic "skeleton" of extracellular fluid (i.e., Na^+) is diminished and, therefore, can "support" progressively smaller volumes of fluid.

Also of clinical relevance is the fact that, in diabetic coma, excessive hepatic β-oxidation of fatty acids can cause the concentration ratio of β-hydroxybutyrate to acetoacetate to rise from about 5 to as high as 15 due to decreases both in the mitochondrial NAD^+/NADH concentration ratio and in the intracellular pH (see **Part C**). Because a frequently used rapid test for ketonuria with *Clinistix* (Bayer Diagnostic) or similar material detects only acetoacetate (and acetone), it can sometimes result in serious underestimates of the extent of ketonuria.

Although diabetic ketoacidosis is common in the domestic animal hospital population, ketosis without acidosis and hyperosmolar nonketotic syndrome are also recognized. Concurrent diseases such as pancreatitis, pyometria, hyperadrenocorticism, pyelonephritis, renal, and/or heart failure are thought to be precipitating factors for these more severe forms of DM.

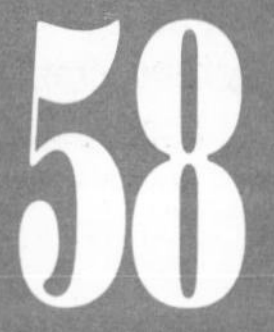

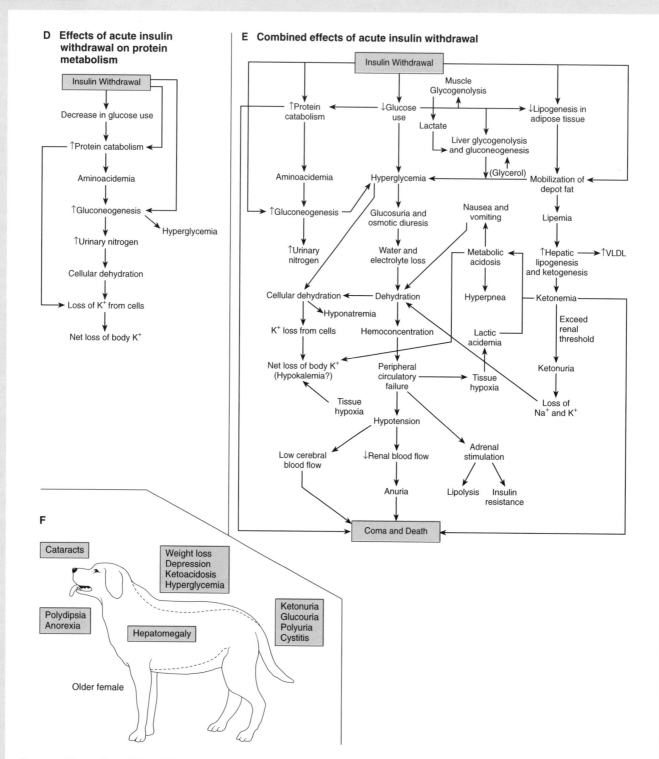

Acute Insulin Withdrawal: II

D Effects of acute insulin withdrawal on protein metabolism

Insulin Withdrawal
Decrease in glucose use
↑Protein catabolism
Aminoacidemia
↑Gluconeogenesis
Hyperglycemia
↑Urinary nitrogen
Cellular dehydration
Loss of K^+ from cells
Net loss of body K^+

E Combined effects of acute insulin withdrawal

Insulin Withdrawal
Muscle Glycogenolysis
↑Protein catabolism
↓Glucose use
↓Lipogenesis in adipose tissue
Lactate
Liver glycogenolysis and gluconeogenesis
Aminoacidemia
Hyperglycemia
(Glycerol)
Mobilization of depot fat
↑Gluconeogenesis
Glucosuria and osmotic diuresis
Nausea and vomiting
Lipemia
↑Urinary nitrogen
Water and electrolyte loss
Metabolic acidosis
↑Hepatic lipogenesis and ketogenesis
↑VLDL
Cellular dehydration
Dehydration
Hyperpnea
Ketonemia
Hyponatremia
K^+ loss from cells
Hemoconcentration
Lactic acidemia
Exceed renal threshold
Net loss of body K^+ (Hypokalemia?)
Peripheral circulatory failure
Tissue hypoxia
Ketonuria
Tissue hypoxia
Loss of Na^+ and K^+
Hypotension
Low cerebral blood flow
↓Renal blood flow
Adrenal stimulation
Anuria
Lipolysis
Insulin resistance
Coma and Death

F

Cataracts
Weight loss
Depression
Ketoacidosis
Hyperglycemia
Polydipsia
Anorexia
Hepatomegaly
Ketonuria
Glucouria
Polyuria
Cystitis
Older female

Source: Parts D and **E** modified from Tepperman J, Tepperman HM. Metabolic and endocrine physiology. 5th ed. St. Louis: Mosby Year-Book, 1987:282–284.

Overview

- Acute insulin withdrawal can lead to K^+ depletion.
- Withdrawal of insulin leads to protein catabolism and a net negative nitrogen balance.
- Therapy for the uncontrolled diabetic patient should be aimed at increasing the effective circulating volume facilitating nutrient uptake by muscle and adipose tissue and replacing lost electrolytes.

Protein Metabolism

Withdrawal of insulin and impaired use of glucose cause a decrease in protein synthesis and, therefore, have the effect of promoting net *protein catabolism,* at first in insulin-sensitive tissues and especially in muscle. This process is accompanied by a net negative nitrogen balance, as well as loss of K^+ into urine (**Part D**).

Besides an impairment in protein metabolism, there is interference with cell function by other effects of insulinopenia. For example, progressive water loss eventually causes intracellular dehydration, which favors catabolic processes and adds to the diffusion of intracellular electrolytes (e.g., K^+) into extracellular fluid. As long as urine flow continues, there is an opportunity for K^+ to be lost by the body in cumulatively dangerous amounts.

Summary

The foregoing discussion of the biochemical and physiologic manifestations of acute insulin withdrawal was used as an example to show how carbohydrate, lipid, and protein metabolism, as well as water and electrolyte balance, are interconnected. When all of these sequential events are united into a single diagram (**Part E**), the important points become obvious and intricate interrelationships are more readily appreciated.

Diabetic ketoacidosis develops when insulin levels are low. Early symptoms include weight loss, usually with increased appetite, thirst, and frequent urination (**Part F**). Initially plasma glucose levels rise, and once a concentration of about 180 mg/dL is reached, renal glucose reabsorptive mechanisms become saturated and glucose spills into urine, causing an osmotic diuresis. This stimulates thirst, which is compensated by taking in more fluid. As the condition worsens, excessive urinary loss of glucose and water leads to dehydration and stimulates release of catecholamines in order to maintain blood pressure and cardiac output (i.e., the early stages of hypovolemic shock). In the setting of low insulin levels, epinephrine secretion leads to lipolysis and release of FFAs from adipocytes. The FFAs are then taken up by the liver (which becomes increasingly engorged with fat), and in the presence of low insulin levels they are oxidized to ketone bodies in mitochondria. Although ketone bodies provide a critical source of energy for most tissues in the presence of intracellular glucopenia, their massive outpouring leads to their presence on the breath (acetone) and in the urine. Acetoacetate and β-hydroxybutyrate are strong acids and deplete the body's buffering systems, leading to metabolic acidosis. Excretion of these anions in urine results in a loss of balancing cations (Na^+ and K^+). The obligatory loss of Na^+ and water worsens the dehydration, causing catecholamines to rise to even higher levels. Growth hormone and cortisol also increase in response to this "metabolic stress," thus accelerating muscle and fat tissue breakdown, increasing hepatic glucose production, and further antagonizing the action of insulin. Glucagon is elevated due to the low insulin concentration. Thus begins a vicious cycle of tissue breakdown to release stored nutrients, poor uptake of those compounds, increased hepatic production of glucose and organic acids, and urinary loss of glucose, ketone bodies, water, and electrolytes. Eventually, acidosis leads to nausea and vomiting that preclude adequate oral intake of water; consequently, patients become quite ill.

Therapy generally should be aimed at increasing the effective circulating volume and replacing lost electrolytes (IV fluids), suppressing the massive gluconeogenesis and ketogenesis, and facilitating nutrient uptake by muscle, adipose tissue, and the liver (insulin). Acidosis can be reversed by administration of alkalinizing solutions. Because a lack of insulin has triggered the adverse effects being evaluated, insulin should be given by vein if shock is profound and the likelihood of insulin being picked up from a subcutaneous depot is small. In spite of the fact that the plasma glucose concentration may be high, depletion of muscle and liver glycogen stores most likely has been so extensive that carbohydrate should also be given in order to help replenish them.

Particular attention should be paid to the net K^+ deficit that has most likely developed. Infusion mixtures containing K^+ are recommended (with caution) in repairing the electrolyte disturbance. Efficacy of management can be assessed by tests of plasma glucose, K^+, and nonprotein nitrogen (i.e., BUN). Electrocardiographic tracings may also be helpful for the purpose of guiding K^+ administration.

Before this condition was as well understood biochemically and physiologically as it is today, results of treatment were reported as disappointing and mortality was high. These results demonstrate the importance of appropriate life-long insulin replacement therapy in the diabetic animal, as well as the catastrophic effects that might occur if insulin replacement therapy is discontinued.

59 Gastrointestinal Hormones: I

A Distribution of Peptides Along the Digestive Tract

Hormone	*Stomach*	*Pancreas*	*Small intestine*	*Large intestine*
Gastrin family				
Gastrin (G cells)	++	+	+	+
CCK (I cells)	–	–	++	+
Secretin family				
Secretin (S cells)	–	–	++	–
Glucagon (α cells)	++	++	+	–
GLI (L cells)	+	–	++	++
GIP (K cells)	–	–	++	–
VIP (D_1 cells)	++	++	++	++
Others				
Insulin (β cells)	–	++	–	–
Somatostatin (Δ_1 cells)	++	++	+	+
GRP	++	–	+	+
Motilin (EC_2 and M cells)	–	–	++	–
Neurotensin (N cells)	–	–	++	–
Substance P (EC_1 cells)	++	–	++	++
Guanylin	–	–	+	++
Pancreatic polypeptide (Δ_2F cells)	–	++	–	–

++ = present in large amounts; + = present; – = absent.

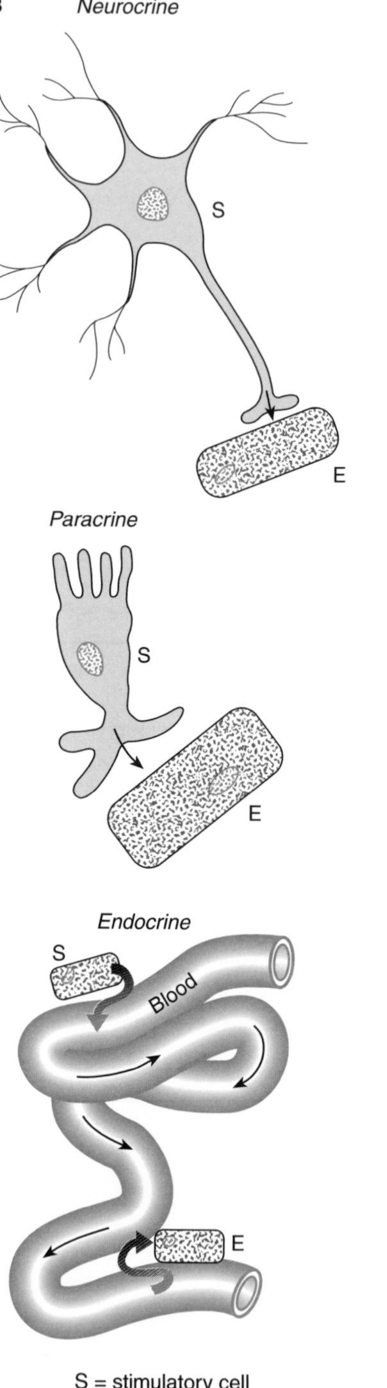

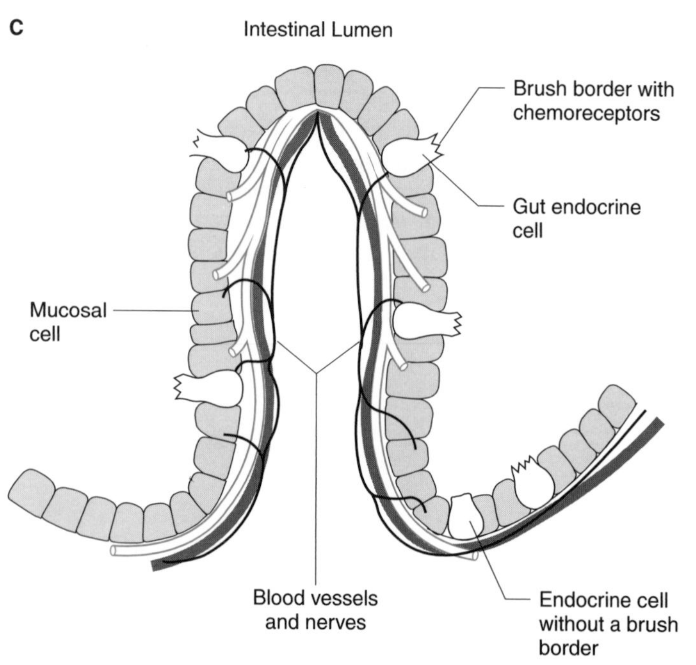

Source: Part C modified from Greenspan FS, Strewler GJ. Basic and clinical endocrinology. 5th ed. Stamford, CT: Appleton & Lange, 1997:577.

Overview

- Approximately 30 "new" gut peptides have been discovered over the past 25 years.
- Endocrine cells are found throughout the GI tract.
- Some GI peptides mimic the actions of others.
- The GI tract is the largest endocrine organ system of the body.

The gastrointestinal (GI) tract is the largest endocrine organ system of the body, and may secrete more hormones than all other organ systems combined. However, unlike other endocrine organs, which are more concentrated masses of endocrine tissue, endocrine cells of the GI tract are scattered throughout the pancreas and the mucosa of the stomach, small intestine, and colon (**Part A**).

Although William Bayliss and Ernest Starling are credited with initiating the "physiologic era" of gastrointestinal endocrinology with their discovery of secretin in 1902, the true "biochemical era" awaited the development of more modern laboratory techniques for the purification and analysis of extracts from the GI mucosa. Approximately 30 "new" GI peptides have been identified over the past 25 years in specialized endocrine cells of the GI tract, as well as in enteric neurons. Many of these peptides have also been identified in the central nervous system, thus leading to the concept of a brain-gut axis (see Chapter 63). The physiologic importance, however, of many of these newly discovered GI peptides remains to be elucidated.

Although disease states attributable to disorders of gut endocrine cells are rare among domestic animal species, certain neuroendocrine tumors are known to exist (see Chapters 62 and 63). With the exception of pancreatic insulin and diabetes mellitus, there are a few GI endocrine deficiency states that have been described, and animal models of GI hormone dysfunction are largely unavailable for study. However, naturally occurring animal models of thyroid and adrenal dysfunction, for example, do exist.

The principal stimulus for GI hormonal secretion is food in the lumen of the gut, yet hormone release is also affected by neural mechanisms and exposure to other hormones. Gastrointestinal hormones regulate digestive processes by influencing secretion, motility, and blood flow to the GI tract. Less evidence exists for direct hormonal control of absorptive processes.

Gastrointestinal peptides that regulate digestive processes may do so as endocrine, paracrine, or neurocrine agents (**Part B**). *Endocrines* are released into blood, which then allows them to reach all tissues (unless excluded from the brain by the blood–brain barrier); however, specific receptors that recognize and bind these peptides are present only on their target cells. *Paracrines* are released from endocrine cells and diffuse through extracellular fluid to their neighboring target cells. Their effects are limited by the short distances they diffuse. Nevertheless, these agents can affect large areas of the GI tract by virtue of the scattered and abundant distribution of cells containing them. A paracrine agent can also act on endocrine cells to influence their secretion. Some GI peptides are located in nerves and may act as *neurocrines* (or neurotransmitters). A neurocrine agent is released near its target cell and needs only to diffuse across a short synaptic gap. Neurocrines act to stimulate or inhibit release of other endocrine and/or paracrine agents.

Some peptides may possess more than one mode of delivery. Somatostatin, for example, is known to have endocrine actions (see Chapters 9 and 62), is present in neurons, and also exercises paracrine actions in the pancreas (see Chapter 55), as well as the gastric antrum and fundus (see Chapter 60). Because of their various modes of delivery (see **Part N,** Chapter 62), some investigators refer to these substances merely as GI regulatory peptides rather than hormones (a word first coined by William Hardy following the discovery of secretin by Bayliss and Starling).

Endocrine cells are scattered singly throughout the mucosa of the GI tract. Most have a broad base and narrow apex with a brush border that faces the intestinal lumen (**Part C**). These cells act as chemoreceptors, sensing luminal contents and then releasing their peptide hormones into adjoining blood vessels. Endocrine cells lacking a luminal brush border are presumably affected by neurocrine and paracrine agents.

When large doses of GI hormones are administered to animals, or when tumors of GI endocrine cells appear (see Chapter 63), certain GI peptides seem to mimic the actions of others through overlapping actions on each other's receptors. On the basis of structural similarity (**Part A**), several of the hormones fall into one of two families: the *gastrin family* (with the only two members being gastrin and cholecystokinin, CCK); and the *secretin family* (with the members secretin; glucagon; glicentin, GLI; vasoactive intestinal polypeptide, VIP; and gastric inhibitory polypeptide, GIP).

Although some of the GI regulatory peptides clearly possess endocrine activities (e.g., gastrin, secretin, CCK, somatostatin, and GIP), investigators have had difficulty delineating precise digestive regulatory activities of other GI neurocrine and paracrine agents. Difficulties have also arisen in measuring the concentrations of these locally acting agents at their presumed sites of action, and in effectively replicating those concentrations in experimental animal models.

Gastrointestinal Hormones: II

D

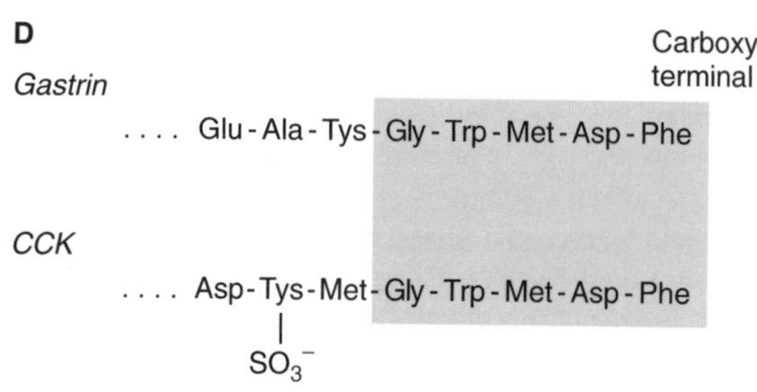

F

Control of Gastrin Release

Increase secretion
Primary
- Peptides and L-amino acids
- Vagal activation (GRP)
- Stomach distention

Secondary
- Epinephrine
- Calcium

Decrease secretion
Primary
- Luminal gastric pH <2.0
- Secretin
- Somatostatin

Secondary
- Calcitonin
- GIP
- VIP
- Glucagon

E

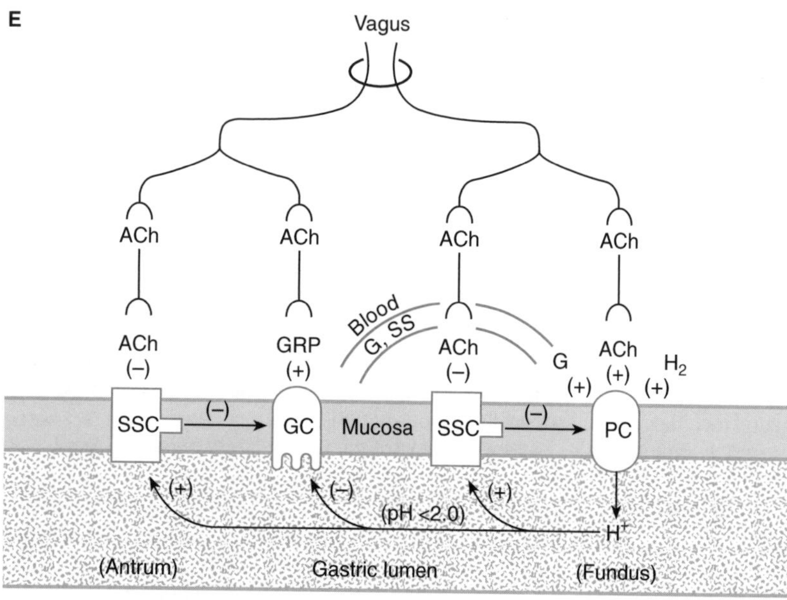

GC = gastrin-secreting cell
PC = parietal cell
H_2 = histamine
SSC = somatostatin-secreting cell

G

Actions of Gastrin

Physiologic
- ↑Gastric HCl secretion
- Trophic effect on gut
- ↑Gastric mixing
- ↑Pepsinogen secretion
- ↑Lower esophageal sphincter (LES) pressure
- ↓Ileocecal sphincter pressure
- ↑CT release

Pharmacologic
- ↑Exocrine pancreatic secretion
- ↑Insulin secretion
- ↑Biliary HCO_3^- secretion
- ↑Duodenal mucus and water secretion
- ↑Gallbladder contraction
- ↑Uterine contraction

Overview

- Only four amino acids in the gastrin molecule are responsible for its biologic activity.
- Protein digestion products, vagal activation, and stomach distention are primary stimulants for gastrin release.
- Somatostatin inhibits gastrin release.
- Bombesin stimulates gastrin release.
- Gastrin stimulates HCl secretion, and has a growth-effect of the gastric mucosa.

Gastrin

Edkins discovered a potent gastric acid secretagogue in extracts of the gastric antral mucosa in 1905, and named it "gastrin." By the early 1960s, gastrin had been isolated, sequenced and synthesized by Gregory and his co-workers.

Gastrin is primarily produced by G cells of the gastric antrum. Lesser amounts are produced throughout the small and large intestine. Gastrin is also found in the pancreas, pituitary gland, hypothalamus, medulla oblongata, and vagus and sciatic nerves.

Little gastrin (G17, indicating 17 amino acids) is the most abundant form. Big gastrin (G34) and mini gastrin (G14) exhibit similar biologic properties to G17, specifically because the entire spectrum of physiologic actions for gastrin is exhibited by the last four amino acids at the carboxyl terminus of all three forms. Gastrins obtained from the stomachs of pigs, cats, dogs, and sheep differ from each other and from human gastrin by one or two amino acid substitutions in the nonspecific part of the molecule. A synthetic gastrin (pentagastrin) is commercially available. Pentagastrin is stable and water-soluble and has the active tetrapeptide sequence, therefore giving it all the physiologic properties of the natural gastrins. Gastrin has a circulatory half-life of about two to three minutes and is inactivated primarily by the kidney and small intestine.

Gastrin and CCK have five identical carboxyl terminal amino acids (**Part D**). For CCK, eight carboxyl terminal amino acids are necessary for full biologic activity, whereas for gastrin only four are necessary. The biologic activities of gastrin and CCK are similar in that both stimulate gastric acid and pancreatic enzyme secretion and contract the gallbladder. However, their potency for eliciting these responses differs considerably. Gastrin is a strong stimulant of acid secretion, yet a weak stimulant of pancreatic enzyme secretion and gallbladder contraction. The relative potency of CCK for these actions is reversed. These differences are determined by the position of the tyrosine (Tys) moiety located near the carboxyl end of the molecule. In gastrin, Tys is the sixth amino acid from the carboxyl end, while in CCK it is the seventh (**Part D**). For CCK-like activity, the tyrosine must be sulfated.

Vagal efferents are directly facilitatory to gastric motility and secretion. Along with their effect on gastrin release, this accounts for the cephalic phase of gastric secretion, which is promoted by the sight, smell, taste, and chewing of food. Acid levels, sensed by gastrin-secreting as well as somatostatin-secreting cells, affect gastrin release, which partially controls acid secretion by parietal cells (**Part E**). Impulses reaching the antral gastric mucosa through vagal efferents stimulate gastrin release. The mediator for stimulation is thought to be *gastrin-releasing peptide (GRP;* also called *bombesin),* which is liberated from postganglionic parasympathetic neurons that directly innervate G cells. The primary mediator for inhibition is thought to be *somatostatin (SS),* which is liberated in a paracrine fashion in response to high concentrations of H^+ in the gastric lumen (i.e., pH <2.0—an example of negative feedback). Cholinergic input to SS-secreting cells apparently suppresses SS release, which leads to an increase in gastrin release (an example of stimulation by *disinhibition*, meaning the elimination of an inhibitory paracrine influence). Somatostatin-secreting cells in the acid-secreting fundic region of the stomach are closely coupled to parietal cells and are thought to function similarly to those in the antral region. Thus, GRP, acting directly on gastrin-secreting cells, and acetylcholine (ACh), acting mainly to eliminate the inhibitory paracrine influence of SS on these cells, are two important neurotransmitters regulating gastrin release. Other stimuli for gastrin release include products of protein digestion in the stomach, particularly L-amino acids; solutions of Ca^{2+} salts, including milk; epinephrine; and ethanol (particularly in dogs, which are confirmed "teetotalers") (**Part F**). Carbohydrates, fats, and caffeine do not release gastrin, but decaffeinated coffee does (an effect attributed to the peptides in the brew). Insulin-induced hypoglycemia or injection of 2-deoxyglucose is also known to stimulate gastrin release. This pathway is presumably mediated by neurons of the enteric nervous system, and may involve both arms of the autonomic nervous system as well.

Gastrin has a trophic (or growth) effect on the mucosa of the stomach, small intestine, and colon (**Part G**). Other major physiologic actions are to increase gastric HCl secretion, increasing mixing actions of the stomach, increase pepsinogen (proteolytic enzyme) secretion, close the lower esophageal sphincter (thus preventing gastroesophageal reflux), and decrease ileocecal sphincter pressure (part of the urge to defecate following a meal). In response to the presence of Ca^{2+} in the diet, gastrin releases calcitonin in an anticipatory fashion (see Chapters 29 and 30). Gastrin's pharmacologic actions, which are difficult to explain from a physiologic perspective, are seen only when blood levels are abnormally high (e.g., gastrinoma).

Gastrin can evoke acid secretion directly or indirectly by facilitating release of histamine from enterochromaffin (EC) cells of the gastric fundus (see Chapter 61). Prolonged hypergastrinemia is associated with enterochromaffin cell hyperplasia and, occasionally, EC cell carcinoid tumors (see Chapter 63).

61 Gastrointestinal Hormones: III

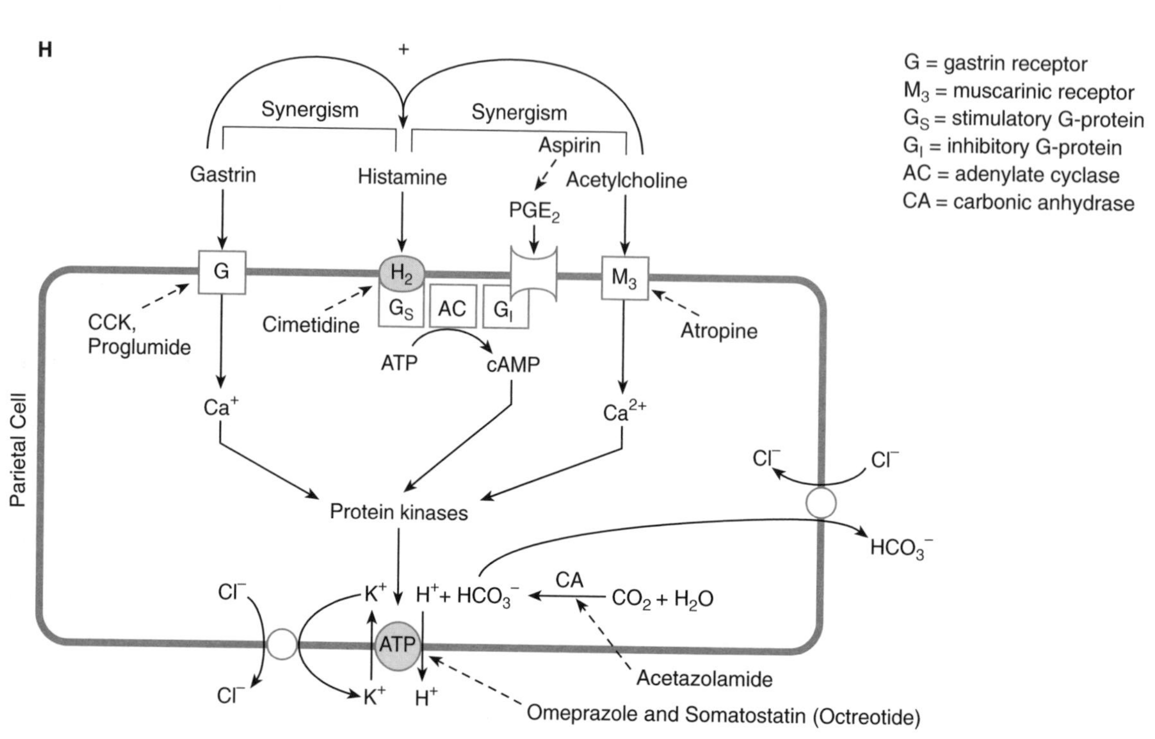

I

Stimulators of CCK Release	*CCK Actions*
Luminal fatty acids longer than 8 carbon atoms	Primary
Protein digestion products	↑Gallbladder contraction
Essential L-amino acids	↓Sphincter of Oddi pressure
	↑Pancreatic enzyme secretion
	↓Gastric emptying
	↑Pepsinogen secretion
	↓LES pressure (fatty meals)
	Secondary
	Trophic action on pancreas
	Synergistic with secretin (HCO_3^-)
	↑Insulin, glucagon, and CT secretion
	↑Satiety (present in brain)

J

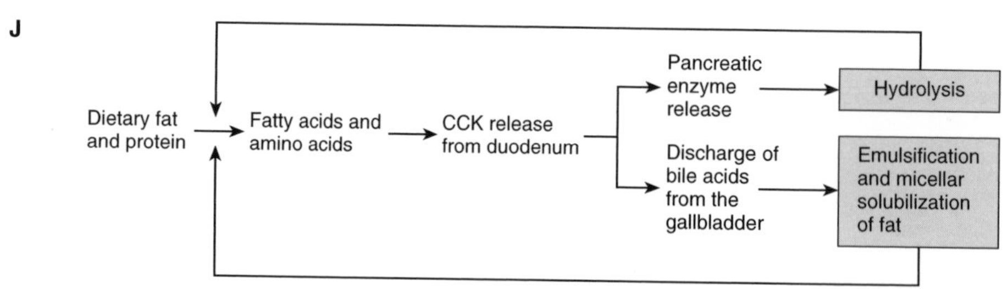

Overview

- Gastrin is synergistic with histamine on gastric HCl secretion.
- Drugs block gastric HCl release through different mechanisms.
- H^+/K^+ exchange is involved in parietal cell acid secretion.
- CCK causes gallbladder contraction, and the release of pancreatic digestive enzymes.

Control of Gastric HCl Secretion

Histamine, though not truly a hormone, is synthesized, stored (in large amounts), and released locally from the fundic mucosa. There is generally a continuous background concentration of histamine within gastric interstitial fluid, and its concentration increases when the gastric mucosa is injured. Histamine is found in *enterochromaffin (EC)* cells (i.e., mast cells), and both gastrin and ACh stimulate its release (**Part H**). Histamine, in turn, plays a central role (along with gastrin and ACh) in the direct stimulation of gastric parietal cell HCl secretion.

Synergism exists between gastrin and histamine, and between ACh and histamine, in stimulating parietal cell acid secretion. Hence, *cimetidine,* a drug that blocks histamine (H_2) receptors on parietal cells, blocks much of the effect of either elevated serum gastrin or abnormally high cholinergic discharge. Other, less well-understood roles of histamine include its ability to enhance gut motility (similar to prostaglandins), vasodilate arterioles of the digestive tract, enhance gastric pepsinogen release, and decrease pressure on the lower esophageal sphincter (LES).

The effects of histamine on gastric acid secretion are mediated through cAMP. Histamine combines with H_2 receptors on parietal cells, thereby stimulating adenylate cyclase to catalyze formation of cAMP. The cAMP then performs the function of stimulus–secretion coupling, thus making ATP available for Cl^- pumping, as well as for H^+/K^+ exchange. Therefore, net HCl secretion results. Histamine is methylated within the gastric mucosa, and most of the methylated derivatives are inactive.

Acetylcholine and parasympathomimetic drugs, such as carbachol, also stimulate parietal cell acid secretion, but not through cAMP. They stimulate release of intracellular Ca^{2+}, which in turn activates certain protein kinases, leading to enzyme phosphorylation/dephosphorylation. However, cAMP is required for the full stimulation of acid secretion. Therefore, ACh as a stimulant must partially rely on the simultaneous action of histamine.

Gastrin release from G cells in the antral mucosa stimulates acid secretion by combining with specific gastrin receptors on parietal cells. Like ACh, gastrin does not stimulate formation of cAMP, but works through mobilizing intracellular Ca^{2+} stores. Combination of gastrin with its receptors is competitively blocked by CCK, which shares gastrin's active *C*-terminal amino acid sequence (see Chapters 59 and 60, **Part D**). Because CCK is a much weaker stimulant of acid secretion than gastrin, CCK's net effect is to decrease gastrin-stimulated acid secretion by denying receptors to gastrin. Histamine also plays a central role in allowing for the maximal action of gastrin. Although histamine is a potent parietal cell secretagogue, gastrin is reported to be approximately 500 times more potent.

Acetazolamide inhibits acid secretion by inhibiting carbonic anhydrase, while *caffeine,* a phosphodiesterase inhibitor, enhances acid secretion (but not gastrin secretion) by increasing the half-life of cAMP. *Proglumide* blocks gastrin receptors, and prostaglandins inhibit acid secretion by inhibiting adenylate cyclase (through inhibitory G-protein) (see **Part H**). Nonsteroidal antiinflammatory drugs such as aspirin inhibit prostaglandin formation and, therefore, increase gastric HCl secretion. Somatostatin and *omeprazole,* a substituted benzimidazole, block H^+/K^+ ATPase, thereby reducing acid secretion.

Cholecystokinin

In 1928, Ivy and Oldberg observed that instillation of fat into the small intestine caused the gallbladder to contract. They postulated a hormonal mechanism and named their mediator *cholecystokinin (CCK).* In the early 1940s, Harper and Raper discovered a substance in extracts of the duodenal mucosa that stimulated secretion of enzyme-rich juice from the pancreas. They called the substance *pancreozymin (PZ).* In 1964, Jorpes and co-workers found that increasing the purification of a single extract from the small bowel proportionately increased its potency for gallbladder contraction and pancreatic enzyme secretion, indicating that the two actions were properties of a single hormone. For many years thereafter this hormone was appropriately called CCK-PZ; however, because Ivy and Oldberg discovered CCK first, theirs is the name used today.

Although CCK exists in three molecular forms (peptides of 39, 33, and 8 amino acids), the octapeptide is thought to be the most prevalent form. Like gastrin, CCK is probably synthesized as a precursor with 39 and then 33 amino acids, representing progressive steps in the reductive creation of CCK 8. The entire biologic activity of CCK resides in this carboxyl terminal 8-amino-acid sequence, and sulfation of tyrosine in position 7 is necessary for full biologic potency (see Chapters 59 and 60, **Part D**).

The physiologic actions of CCK are listed in **Part I.** In general, CCK causes exocrine pancreatic enzyme release to hydrolyze ingested macromolecules, as well as gallbladder contraction to provide needed bile acids for fat emulsification and micellar solubilization of the products of lipid digestion (namely long-chain fatty acids and monoglycerides) (**Part J**). Hypertrophy of the pancreas is produced by intraperitoneal injections of CCK 8, and the number of acinar, ductal, and β cells is increased. In the colon, gastrin and CCK are confined to neurons, where they may act as neurotransmitters. CCK also appears in the brain of many species. When an animal feeds, several mechanisms are activated that eventually result in satiety and in characteristic postprandial behavior such as grooming. Infusion of CCK suppresses feeding in rats and monkeys, and it is possible that CCK from the intestine or CNS nerve terminals is one of the satiety signals. Cholecystokinin has also been reported to block enkephalin receptors (like naloxone—see Chapters 7 and 8).

62 Gastrointestinal Hormones: IV

K

Properties of Secretin

Stimulate secretin release	Secretin actions
Primary	Primary
pH <4.5 in duodenum	↑Pancreatic HCO_3^- secretion
Secondary	↑Biliary HCO_3^- secretion
Peptides in duodenum	Secondary
Fatty acids in duodenum	↓Gastric motility
Amino acids in duodenum	↓Intestinal motility
	↓HCl secretion
Inhibit secretin release	↑Pepsinogen secretion
Nicotine	↑Insulin secretion
	Opposes trophic action of gastrin
	Synergistic with CCK (enzymes)

L

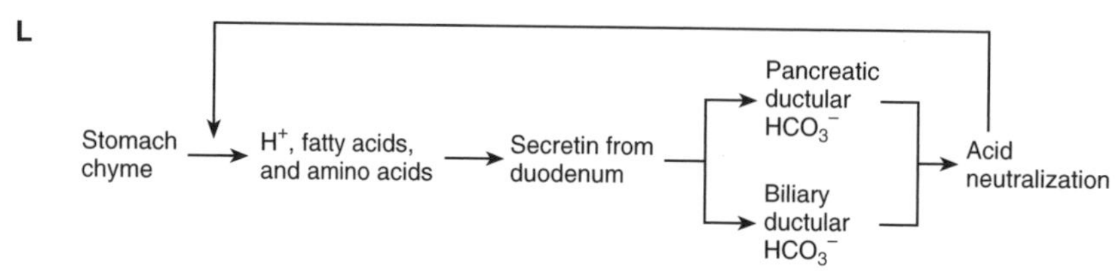

M

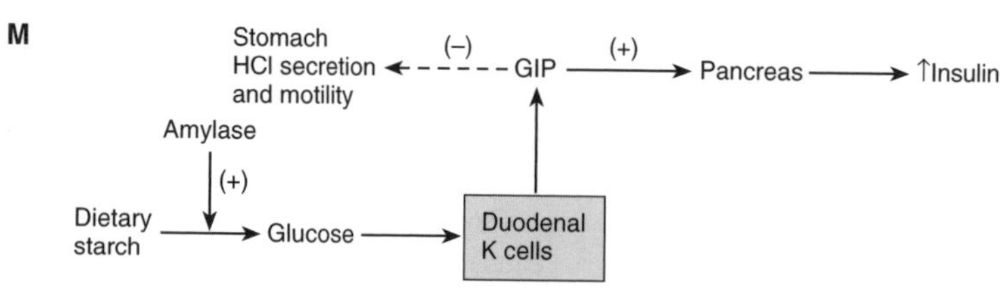

N

Major Actions of the GI Hormones

GI Hormone	Mode of Action	Major Action	Exist in both gut and brain?
Gastrin	E, (N)	Gastric acid and pepsinogen secretion	No
CCK	E, (N)	Gallbladder contraction, pancreatic enzyme secretion	Yes
Secretin	E	Pancreatic and biliary ductular HCO_3^- secretion	Yes
Glucagon	E, P	Enhances hepatic glycogenolysis and gluconeogenesis	Yes
GLI	(E), (N), (P)	Stimulates release of gastrin and CCK	No
GIP	E	Enhances glucose-mediated insulin release, inhibits HCl secretion	No
VIP	N, (P)	Smooth muscle relaxation, electrolyte secretion	Yes
Insulin	E	Enhances lipogenesis and cell membrane permeability to glucose	Yes
Somatostatin	E, N, P	Numerous inhibitory effects	Yes
GRP	N, (P)	Stimulates release of gastrin	Yes
Motilin	(E)	Initiates interdigestive intestinal motility	Yes
Neurotensin	E, (N), (P)	Inhibits GI motility and blood flow	Yes
Substance P	N, (P)	Increases intestinal motility	Yes
Guanylin	E, P	Increases Cl^- secretion into intestinal lumen	Yes
Pancreatic polypeptide	(E), (P)	Inhibits pancreatic HCO_3^- and enzyme secretion	Yes

E = endocrine; N = neurocrine; P = paracrine; ( ) = suggested, but not proven.

Source: Part G modified from Greenspan FS, Strewler GJ. Basic and clinical endocrinology. 5th ed. Stamford, CT: Appleton & Lange, 1997:576.

Overview

- Secretin is nature's antacid.
- Secretin was the first hormone discovered.
- Gastric inhibitory polypeptide stimulates insulin release.
- Guanylin increases intestinal Cl^- secretion.
- Nicotine inhibits secretin release.

Secretin

Secretin ("nature's antacid") holds the distinction in biology of being the first hormone discovered. In the afternoon of January 16, 1902, Bayliss and Starling found that when acid was placed in an intrinsically denervated loop of the upper small bowel of an anesthetized dog, the pancreas responded by secreting. "This cannot be a nervous reflex!", Starling exclaimed. "Then it must be a chemical reflex!" He then demonstrated that a crude extract of the intestinal mucosa also stimulated pancreatic secretion when given intravenously. Although in retrospect the experiment was far from conclusive, Starling's exclamation announced the birth of the science of endocrinology; he noticed that a specific stimulus acting on a specific receptor organ released a specific messenger that traveled by blood to a distant, specific target organ and elicited a specific response. In addition, the experiment by Bayliss and Starling demonstrated a negative feedback loop in which the stimulus evoked a response (HCO_3^- secretion) that ended in the elimination of the stimulus (H^+).

The amount of secretin normally released from the duodenum is proportional to the amount of acid entering, with secretion inhibited at a pH above 4.5. Secretin has a circulatory half-life of about four minutes, and its chief physiologic action is to stimulate bicarbonate release from pancreatic and biliary ductular cells (**Parts K and L**). Because it is synergistic with CCK, secretin also enhances pancreatic enzyme secretion and gallbladder contraction in the presence of CCK. Secretin opposes the trophic action of gastrin on the GI mucosa. It decreases gastric and intestinal motility, and it noncompetitively inhibits gastrin-stimulated acid secretion in dogs (probably a pharmacologic action). Secretin and glucagon share a common 14-amino-acid sequence; therefore, in pharmacologic amounts they mimic each other's actions (see Chapters 59 and 60, **Part A**).

Other GI Peptides

Glucagon is secreted by α cells of pancreatic islets as well as α cells of the GI mucosa. As discussed in Chapters 43 and 44, glucagon is thought to play a role in diabetic hyperglycemia. Glucagon-like immunoreactivity (GLI) peptide is also found in L cells of the large intestine (see Chapters 59 and 60, **Part A**).

Gastric inhibitory polypeptide (GIP) is a polypeptide of 43 amino acid residues and is produced by K cells of the small intestinal mucosa. Glucose and fat in the duodenum stimulate its release into the circulation. Gastric inhibitory polypeptide was so-named because it inhibits gastric secretion and motility; however, its more important role in metabolism may be its ability to stimulate insulin release (in an anticipatory fashion; **Part M**). Because of this important action, GIP is sometimes referred to as *glucose-dependent insulinotropic polypeptide*.

Vasoactive intestinal polypeptide (VIP) contains 28 amino acid residues and is found in nerves of the GI tract as well as D_1 cells. Tumors that secrete VIP, or VIPomas, are known to markedly stimulate intestinal electrolyte and water secretion, and hence cause diarrhea. Vasoactive intestinal polypeptide relaxes intestinal smooth muscle including sphincters, dilates peripheral blood vessels, and inhibits gastric HCl secretion. It is found in the brain as well as in several autonomic parasympathetic nerves.

Motilin is a 22-amino-acid peptide secreted by two specialized cell types within the duodenum. One is the EC_2 cell, and the other the M-cell (Chapters 59 and 60, **Part A**). Motilin contracts intestinal smooth muscle and appears to be an important regulator of interdigestive intestinal motility (i.e., the housekeeper that helps to sweep leftover luminal contents down the gut between meals).

Neurotensin is a 13-amino acid polypeptide produced by neurons of the ileum as well as endocrine N-cells. Its release is stimulated by fatty acids, and it reduces ileal blood flow and motility.

Substance P is found in neurons and endocrine EC_1-cells of the GI tract, but it has not been shown to enter the circulation. Like neurotensin, it increases small intestinal motility.

Guanylin is a 15-amino acid polypeptide secreted by endocrine cells of the small and large intestine. It appears to increase secretion of Cl^- into the intestinal lumen. Certain diarrhea-producing strains of E coli have enterotoxins with similar structures to guanylin.

Pancreatic polypeptide is found in Δ_2-cells of the pancreas, and appears to reduce acinar enzyme and ductular HCO_3^- secretion (**Part N**).

63 APUDomas

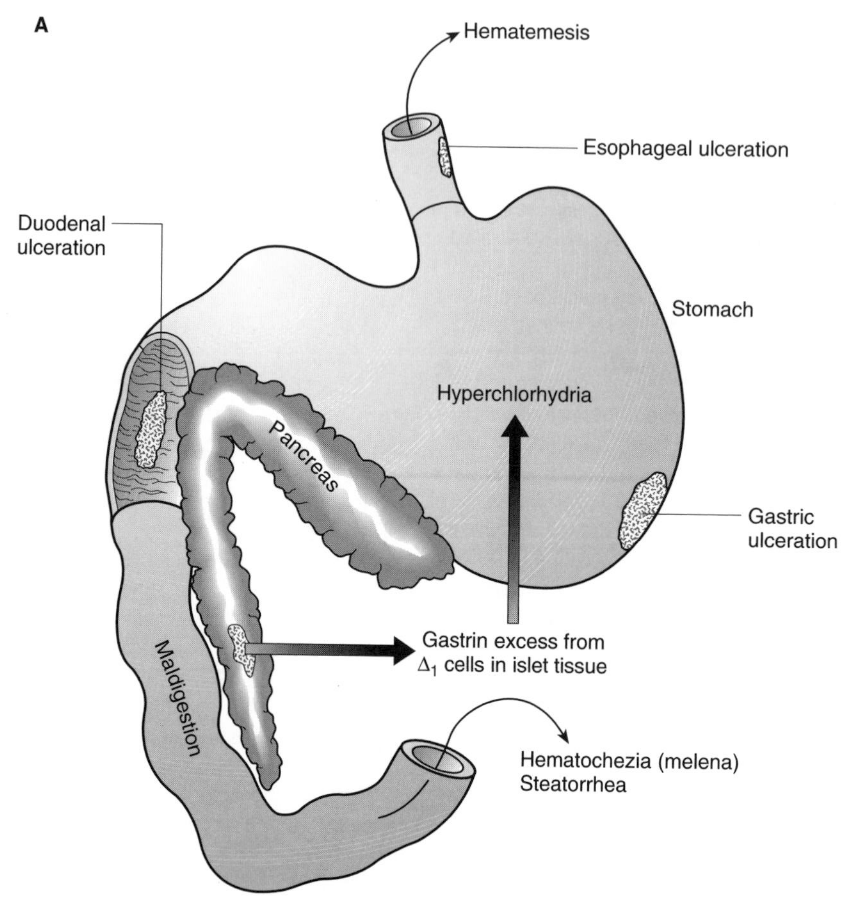

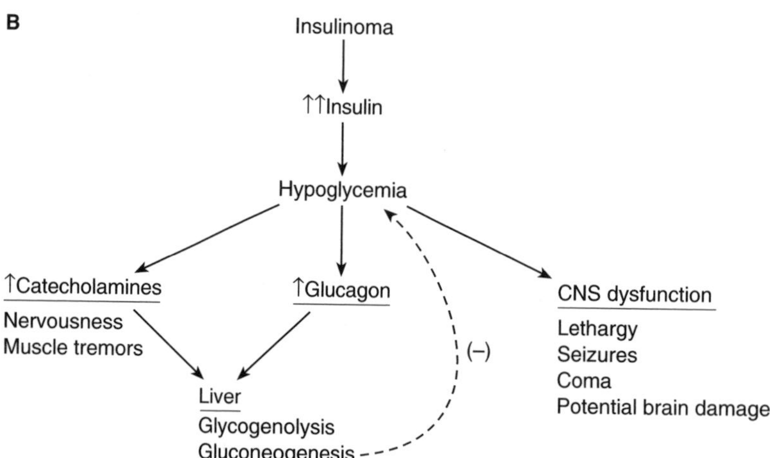

Source: Part A modified from Chastain CB, Ganjam VK. Clinical endocrinology of companion animals. 1st ed. Philadelphia, PA: Lea & Febiger, 1986:313.

Overview

- APUD cells that produce and release peptide hormones may have a common embryologic origin.
- Many APUDomas produce more than one peptide.
- Gastrinomas may arise from the pancreas.
- Insulinomas are more common in dogs than in cats.

Cytochemical and ultrastructural characteristics of GI endocrine cells were described by Pearse in 1966. The principal products of these cells were noted to be peptide hormones and biogenic amines (e.g., catecholamines and serotonin). A general characteristic observed was their ability to take up amine precursors and connect them to amines, and it was speculated that the uptake of 5-hydroxytryptamine (serotonin) was linked to the production of peptide hormones. Most of the cells possessing these characteristics are found in the gut or CNS (hypothalamus, pituitary axis, and pineal gland), but they are also present in the thyroid (in calcitonin-secreting cells), parathyroid, and placenta. Pearse referred to them as *amine precursor uptake and decarboxylation (APUD) cells.*

Although it was postulated that APUD cells originated from the primitive neural crest, whether all APUD cells actually come from this origin is uncertain. Although studies using quail and chick embryos cast doubt on the claim that APUD cells of the GI tract originate from neural ectoderm, endocrine cells of the GI tract and pancreas do possess an enzyme specific to neural cells (neuronal-specific enolase, NSE), which supports the hypothesis of a common neural origin. It is clear that endocrine cells of the gut are remarkably similar to cells within the hypothalamic–pituitary axis. Gut endocrine cells may also be "neuroendocrinologically" programmed, even though their origin is not clearly understood, thereby giving validity to the concept of the gut acting as a "visceral brain."

The APUD cells that produce and release peptide hormones may indeed have a common embryologic origin. The concept is appealing because it posits the existence of a common ancestor for those cells in the gut and CNS with almost identical cytochemical characteristics (storage of peptides) and cellular actions (release of peptide messengers). It helps clarify why identical peptides are synthesized, stored, and released by gut epithelial cells, neurons of the GI tract, and nerve cells in the CNS. This brain–gut axis could be important in the regulation of satiety (e.g., via CCK). Furthermore, neurons of the CNS interact with those of the enteric nervous system to influence involuntary digestive processes. Many of these neurons are peptidergic, and this interaction occurs via both afferent and efferent pathways.

Neuroendocrine Tumors of the Gut

Neuroendocrine tumors of the gut may be found in the pancreas or intestinal wall. They are known by the general term *APUDomas.* Many GI endocrine tumors reportedly secrete more than one peptide, but they are generally named after the one responsible for the most demonstrable clinical manifestations. Biochemical confirmation is generally made by measurement of hormonal markers in blood and/or urine. Unfortunately, most APUDomas are small, and preoperative localization is often reported as inaccurate. However, tumor localization and excision is generally the desired treatment.

APUDomas that secrete peptides foreign to their cell of origin (e.g., an APUDoma from a G cell of the stomach that secretes large amounts of VIP) cause *paraendocrine syndromes,* whereas those that secrete excessive quantities of the peptide typical to their cell of origin cause *orthoendocrine syndromes.* The latter are more typical in veterinary medicine (e.g., gastrinoma, insulinoma, and pheochromocytoma; see Chapter 46).

Gastrinoma (Zollinger-Ellison-Like Syndrome)

Gastrinomas have been reported in humans, dogs, and cats. In 1955, Zollinger and Ellison described the human gastrinoma syndrome, and 21 years later it was reported in the dog. Several other spontaneous canine and feline cases have been reported since that time, and the syndrome has also been produced experimentally in dogs.

Gastrinomas are usually carcinomas arising from gastrin-secreting Δ_1 cells of pancreatic islet tissue, which normally produce gastrin only during the fetal period. In adult animals, these cells normally produce somatostatin (see Chapters 59 and 60), but they may revert back to the fetal state in gastrinoma. Most of the gastrin found in normal adult animals originates from G cells of the gastric antral mucosa, with a few gastrin-secreting cells found in the small and large intestines. Gastrinomas in dogs, cats, and humans can secrete other hormones as well (e.g., ACTH, insulin, glucagon, CCK, and pancreatic polypeptide). In about 30% of human cases, other endocrine tumors are reportedly present, usually in the parathyroids or pituitary. This condition is known as *multiple endocrine neoplasia (MEN).*

Hypergastrinemia causes parietal cell hyperplasia leading to hyperchlorhydria (HCl excess) and, secondarily, gastroduodenal ulceration (**Part A**). Disruption of intestinal digestive and absorptive functions also occurs, largely because excess acid in the duodenum denatures digestive enzymes. Signs and symptoms may include blood-stained vomit (hematemesis), steatorrhea, bloody stools (hematochezia or melena), abdominal pain, dehydration, regenerative anemia, depression, and weight loss. Esophageal reflux of excess acid can also lead to ulceration (**Part A**). As noted previously (see Chapter 60), prolonged hypergastrinemia is also associated with enterochromaffin (EC) cell hyperplasia and, occasionally, EC cell carcinoid tumors.

Duodenal acidification is the primary stimulus for secretin release, and secretin has been shown to cause gastrin release from pancreatic gastrinomas. Therefore, a vicious cycle may ensue (acid to secretin, to gastrin, to acid) that serves to perpetuate the hyperacidity of Zollinger-Ellison-like syndrome.

Insulinoma

The insulin-secreting tumor of pancreatic islets is the most commonly recognized APUDoma of dogs but is rarely seen in cats. It is most often malignant and will reportedly spread to duodenal, mesenteric, hepatic, and splenic lymphatics. Results of a serum profile and urinalysis from animals with active insulinomas may be normal, except that the plasma glucose, PO_4^{3-} and K^+ concentrations are usually low. Severe hypoglycemia from an insulinoma leads to stimulation of the sympathoadrenal system, which in turn can cause muscle tremors and nervousness (**Part B**). Hypoglycemia-induced catecholamine and glucagon secretion result in stimulation of hepatic glycogenolysis and gluconeogenesis in an attempt to restore the blood glucose concentration.

Acute hypoglycemia seems to affect the CNS more than other organ systems, and if severe and prolonged, it can cause irreversible brain damage. Neuroglycopenic signs include lethargy, seizures, and coma. Symptoms related to catecholamine release may precede those of neuroglycopenia, and therefore they act as early warning signs of impending hypoglycemic shock.

Some non-β-cell hepatocellular tumors may also be associated with hypoglycemia. Theoretically, these tumors could express insulin-like growth factors (IGF-1 and IGF-2) (see Chapter 9).

Other APUDomas

Although *glucagonomas, VIPomas* (Verner-Morrison syndrome), *somatostatinomas,* and *pancreatic polypeptide–producing tumors* have been described in humans, they are rarely reported in domestic animals. *Serotonin-secreting carcinoid tumors* that arise from enterochromaffin cells of the GI tract have, however, been reported in older dogs and cats.

QUESTIONS

1. All of the following are considered to be endocrine organs **except** the:

(A) Kidneys

(B) Pineal gland

(C) Pancreas

(D) Lungs

(E) Parathyroids

2. Hormones affect diverse metabolic functions by:

(A) Serving as substrates for various reactions inside target cells

(B) Contributing energy to various anabolic and catabolic processes

(C) Increasing or decreasing the rates of specific reactions within target cells

(D) Acting as enzymes for specific reactions within target cells

(E) All of the above

3. What is the largest endocrine organ (or organ system) of the body?

(A) Liver

(B) Gastrointestinal tract

(C) Brain

(D) Heart

(E) Placenta

4. Thyroid hormone action is dependent on:

(A) The plasma concentration of liver-derived transport proteins

(B) The rate of synthesis and/or secretion of thyroxine from the thyroid gland

(C) The number and/or activity of hormone-specific receptors within target cells

(D) Conversion to a more active form within target cells

(E) All of the above

5. Which one of the following is an example of an autocrine secretion?

(A) A prostaglandin secreted into interstitial fluid that then acts on the cell that secreted it

(B) Pheromones secreted through exocrine ducts to the exterior of the body

(C) Insulin secreted into the vascular system

(D) A chemical messenger acting on target cells in the vicinity of its cellular origin without entering the circulation

(E) A neurotransmitter released into blood to affect target cells at distant locations

6. Which of the following hormones acts in the stomach and pancreas as a paracrine agent?

(A) Somatotropin

(B) Somatostatin

(C) LH

(D) Oxytocin

(E) ACTH

7. Select the **false** statement below:

(A) Some metabolites of hormones are biologically active.

(B) Serum proteases are known to degrade some hormones.

(C) Hormones may be eliminated from the body in their active form.

(D) Dogs, unlike cats, eliminate glucocorticoids primarily in bile.

(E) Invertebrates have primitive nervous systems and depend on paracrine and autocrine regulation of metabolism.

8. Which of the following statements regarding the autonomic nervous system (ANS) is/are **true?**

(A) The ANS is controlled by the hypothalamus.

(B) The ANS influences pancreatic endocrine and exocrine secretion.

(C) The ANS affects adrenomedullary biogenic amine release.

(D) The ANS affects melatonin release from the pineal gland.

(E) All of the above

9. Select the **true** statement below:

(A) The pars nervosa is primarily controlled by release and inhibiting hormones from the hypothalamus.

(B) There is considerable structural conservation of chemical messengers across animal species.

(C) Somatostatin is an example of a tropic hormone that stimulates the release of other hormones.

(D) Somatotropin is a steroid hormone that primarily affects growth.

(E) Prostaglandins are polypeptide hormones secreted in an autocrine fashion.

10. Which of the following statements regarding the cAMP messenger system is/are **true?**

(A) It is inherently faster than the Ca^{2+}/DG messenger system.

(B) It is activated following α_1-adrenergic receptor stimulation.

(C) It is inactivated through the action of intracellular phosphodiesterase.

(D) It is unaffected by plant toxins.

(E) All of the above

11. For sites of elementary Ca^{2+} release to produce global responses, individual Ca^{2+} channels must communicate with each other to set up:

(A) cAMP synthesis

(B) Phospholipid resynthesis

(C) Arachidonic acid synthesis

(D) Ca^{2+} waves

(E) β-Adrenergic receptor activation

12. Receptor concentration and affinity for its hormone are affected by:

(A) Antibodies against the receptor

(B) Ionic balance

(C) Concentration of the homologous hormone

(D) Concentration of heterologous hormones

(E) All of the above

13. Which of the following processes does diacylglycerol cause?

(A) Intracellular Ca^{2+} mobilization

(B) Activation of PKC

(C) Activation of PKA

(D) Activation of phospholipase C

(E) All of the above

14. Where are catecholamine receptors normally found?

(A) In the cytoplasm of target cells

(B) On the plasma membrane of target cells

(C) In nuclei of target cells

(D) In mitochondria of target cells

(E) At the same sites as steroid hormone receptors

15. Intracellular Ca^{2+} signaling is best associated with:

(A) Mitosis

(B) Nitric oxide synthesis in vascular endothelial cells

(C) Intracellular DG formation

(D) Mitochondrial metabolism

(E) cAMP formation

16. Which of the following statements regarding guanosine triphosphate–binding proteins is/are **true?**

(A) They play a role in the cAMP but not the Ca^{2+}/DG second messenger system.

(B) They bind catecholamines in the circulation, thus rendering them water-soluble.

(C) In plasma membranes, they can be either stimulatory or inhibitory.

(D) They bind steroid hormones in nuclei of target cells.

(E) All of the above

17. Activation of phospholipase C in the plasma membrane generates:

(A) Diacylglycerol and IP_3.

(B) Arachidonic acid.

(C) Phosphatidic acid and PIP_2.

(D) Phospholipase A_2 and PKC.

(E) Protein kinase C and protein kinase A.

18. The predominant nuclear receptor for thyroid hormones is specific for:

(A) T_4

(B) T_3

(C) rT_3

(D) T_2

(E) rT_1

19. Cytoplasmic receptors for which of the following hormone types are thought to change conformation before being translocated into nuclei?

(A) Polypeptides

(B) Thyroid

(C) Catecholamine

(D) Steroid

(E) All of the above

20. Binding sites for thyroid hormones have been identified:

(A) On mitochondrial membranes

(B) In the cytoplasm

(C) On plasma membranes

(D) In the nucleus

(E) All of the above

21. The hormone response element for steroid hormones is found in:

(A) The cytoplasm

(B) The nucleus

(C) Plasma

(D) Mitochondria

(E) The plasma membrane

22. Which of the following inhibits prolactin release?

(A) VIP

(B) TRH

(C) ACh

(D) DA

(E) 5-HT

23. Select the **false** statement below:

(A) The anterior pituitary, like the posterior pituitary, stores neuropeptides.

(B) Hormones of the neurohypophysis are products of hypothalamic neurosecretory cells.

(C) Opioid peptides are known to promote GH and PRL secretion from the adenohypophysis.

(D) Hypothalamic neurons are known to liberate release and/or inhibiting factors into the hypothalamocoadenohypophyseal portal system.

(E) Oxytocin is secreted from the posterior lobe of the pituitary.

24. Which anterior pituitary hormone is responsible for IGF-1 secretion from the liver?

(A) LH

(B) PRL

(C) ACTH

(D) TSH

(E) GH

25. Which of the following statements regarding the anterior pituitary is/are **true?**

(A) It secretes primarily steroid hormones.

(B) It is thought to originate from the brain's third ventricle.

(C) It comprises about 80% of total pituitary weight in most species.

(D) It secretes a tropic hormone that causes release of PTH from parathyroid glands.

(E) All of the above

26. What is the major adenohypophyseal endocrine-secreting cell type?

(A) Gonadotroph

(B) Somatotroph

(C) Corticotroph

(D) Lactotroph

(E) Thyrotroph

27. Which of the following statements regarding metenkephalin and leuenkephalin is **true?**

(A) They are steroidogenic opiates.

(B) They are derived from proenkephalin.

(C) They are produced in the pituitary gland.

(D) They are derived from β-endorphin.

(E) They are not found in the CNS.

28. Which of the following stimulates melanosome concentration in dermal melanophores?

(A) Melatonin

(B) MSH

(C) MRH

(D) MRIH

(E) Catecholamines

29. From which of the following is α-MSH derived?

(A) ACTH

(B) CLIP

(C) β-MSH

(D) Pro-γ-MSH

(E) β-Endorphin

30. All of the following have been associated with MSH, **except:**

(A) Memory enhancement

(B) Onset of parturition

(C) Fetal steroidogenic effect

(D) Stimulation of modified sebaceous gland activity

(E) Seasonal changes in haircoat color

31. Structural similarity exists between:

(A) Morphine and β-endorphin

(B) ACTH and β-endorphin

(C) α-MSH and β-MSH

(D) POMC and heroin

(E) Codeine and naloxone

32. The opiate peptides decrease the release of which one of the following?

(A) PTH

(B) Glucagon

(C) PRL

(D) GHRH

(E) GnRH

33. Which of the following statements regarding chondrogenesis is/are **true?**

(A) It is an indirect growth-promoting action of somatotropin.

(B) It is a direct growth-promoting action of IGF-1.

(C) It is an anabolic action of growth hormone.

(D) Due to the action of IGF-1, it is enhanced by the concurrent presence of thyroxine.

(E) All of the above

34. What type of metabolic effect is GH thought to exert during times throughout the day when its blood concentration is low?

(A) Gluconeogenic

(B) Anabolic

(C) Lipolytic

(D) Anti-insulin

(E) Catabolic

35. All of the following are direct anti-insulin actions of growth hormone, **except:**

(A) Decreasing carbohydrate utilization in muscle tissue

(B) Sparing breakdown of triglycerides in adipocytes

(C) Enhancing hepatic glucose production

(D) Sparing breakdown of muscle protein

36. All of the following stimulate hepatic somatomedin C (IGF-1) secretion, **except:**

(A) Protein meal

(B) Glucocorticoids

(C) Growth hormone

(D) Insulin

37. Which of the following stimulates growth hormone secretion in cats?

(A) Glucocorticoids

(B) β-Adrenergics

(C) Arginine

(D) Glucose and IGF-1

(E) All of the above

38. Select the **false** statement below:

(A) Synthetic human growth hormone (hGH) appears to be active in dogs.

(B) Inherited hyposomatotropism in dogs is often associated with secondary hypergonadism and hyperthyroidism.

(C) Growth hormone is diabetogenic.

(D) Acromegaly can develop in dogs following prolonged administration of progestins.

(E) Recombinant bovine somatotropin (rbST) appears to be biologically active in dogs and has been detected in cow milk.

39. Which of the following is associated with hyposomatotropism?

(A) Hypercholesterolemia

(B) Increased interdental spaces

(C) Hyperglycemia

(D) Cushing's-like syndrome

(E) Diabetes mellitus

40. Which of the following is/are associated with hypersomatotropism?

(A) Estrual abnormalities

(B) Testicular atrophy

(C) Soft puppy haircoat

(D) PU/PD

(E) All of the above

41. Pituitary dwarfism in prepubertal dogs is most often associated with:

(A) A cystic Rathke's pouch

(B) Insensitivity to somatotropin or defective GH receptors

(C) Failures in GHRH release

(D) Insensitivity of target cells to IGF-1

(E) Excessive hypothalamic GHIH release

42. Which one of the following inhibits GnRH release?

(A) Catecholamines

(B) Opioid peptides

(C) Acetylcholine

(D) Preovulatory estrogen

(E) Activin

43. Regression of the corpus luteum in the bitch appears to be due to:

(A) Inhibin

(B) LH

(C) Aging

(D) Progesterone

(E) $PGF_{2\alpha}$

44. Which of the following describes day 1 of the estrous cycle?

(A) It is always the day the animal ovulates.

(B) It is the first day of proestrus.

(C) It is, by definition, the first day of menstruation.

(D) It is usually the first day of "heat."

(E) It corresponds with peak progesterone concentrations in blood.

45. Which of the following statements regarding domestic animals and New World monkeys is **true?**

(A) They ovulate only during estrus.

(B) They have a relatively long preovulatory follicular period (compared to humans).

(C) They are not dependent on LH for ovulation.

(D) They do not menstruate.

(E) They do not experience a preovulatory estrogen surge, as humans do.

46. Which of the following increase(s) frequency of discharge of the GnRH pulse generator?

(A) LH

(B) Estrogen in the absence of progesterone

(C) Estrogen and progesterone

(D) Progesterone in the absence of estrogen

(E) Ovulation

47. Which of the following statements regarding Sertoli cells is/are **true?**

(A) They are biochemically similar to ovarian granulosa cells.

(B) They produce ABP under the stimulation of PModS and FSH.

(C) They are capable of aromatizing testosterone to estrogen.

(D) They produce inhibin, which decreases FSH output from the adenohypophysis.

(E) All of the above

48. Which of the following occurs during the preovulatory, proliferative phase of the estrous cycle?

(A) Ovarian theca cells primarily produce estrogen.

(B) Ovarian granulosa cells are stimulated by LH to produce androgens.

(C) Estrogen synergizes with FSH to promote replication of ovarian granulosa cells.

(D) Estrogen is aromatized in ovarian theca cells to produce androgens.

(E) All of the above

49. Which of the following statements regarding testicular androgen-binding protein is/are **true?**

(A) It originates from Sertoli cells.

(B) Its release is stimulated by LH.

(C) It is needed in order to bind activin for spermatogenesis.

(D) It stimulates testosterone synthesis in Leydig cells.

(E) All of the above

50. Which of the following statements regarding inhibin is/are **true?**

(A) Its secretion parallels that of progesterone in females.

(B) It is produced by ovarian granulosa cells and testicular Sertoli cells.

(C) It is a protein produced by the corpus luteum.

(D) It inhibits FSH secretion in both males and females.

(E) All of the above

51. Which one of the following stimulates testicular testosterone secretion?

(A) FSH

(B) Activin

(C) Inhibin

(D) Estrogen

(E) PModS

52. In which one of the following species is reflux ovulation most likely to occur?

(A) Human

(B) Dog

(C) Cat

(D) Guinea pig

(E) Goat

53. The period of the estrous cycle in which the influence of luteal progesterone predominates is called:

(A) Estrus

(B) Proestrus

(C) Diestrus

(D) Anestrus

(E) None of the above

54. Which of the following occurs or may occur in canine overt pseudopregnancy?

(A) The uterus enlarges.

(B) Mammary glands may develop lactational capabilities.

(C) The bitch may develop a whelping nest.

(D) The animal exhibits an exaggerated diestrual response.

(E) All of the above

55. In which of the following settings might anestrus occur?

(A) During pregnancy in polyestrous species

(B) Infectious disease

(C) In polyestrous species during the nonbreeding season

(D) In lactating females

(E) All of the above

56. Which one of the following is a polyestrous, nonseasonal breeder?

(A) Mare

(B) Sow

(C) Ewe

(D) Bitch

(E) Queen

57. Which of the following statements regarding the suprachiasmatic nucleus of the hypothalamus is **true?**

(A) It reduces activity of sympathetic fibers to the pineal gland in the presence of light.

(B) It reduces activity of sympathetic fibers to the pineal gland in the absence of light.

(C) It increases activity of sympathetic fibers to the pineal gland in the presence of light.

(D) It synthesizes melatonin.

(E) None of the above

58. Which of the following statements regarding melatonin is **true?**

(A) It stimulates brown hair growth in mice.

(B) Excess melatonin is a cause of parathyroid hypertrophy.

(C) It is synthesized only in the pineal gland of reptiles and birds.

(D) Melatonin secretion is enhanced in response to stress.

(E) It is antigonadal in all mammalian species.

59. When would pinealocyte melatonin secretion be highest?

(A) During the preovulatory estrogen surge

(B) During extended periods of daylight in long-day breeders

(C) During the breeding season in sheep and goats (short-day breeders)

(D) During periods when HIOMT activity is low

(E) During periods when MAO activity is elevated

60. Which one of the following amino acids is used in the synthesis of melatonin?

(A) Alanine

(B) Tyrosine

(C) Serine

(D) Tryptophan

(E) Methionine

61. Which of the following statements is/are correct regarding theoretical relationships between melatonin and aging?

(A) Melatonin appears to reduce free radical formation.

(B) Melatonin levels in blood decrease with aging.

(C) Melatonin appears to enhance immune surveillance.

(D) Activity of the suprachiasmatic nucleus changes with aging, thus influencing pineal output of melatonin.

(E) All of the above

62. Melatonin is thought to stimulate hypothalamic release of which one of the following in cats?

(A) DA

(B) GHRH

(C) GnRH

(D) TRH

(E) CRH

63. Which of the following statements regarding relaxin is/are **true?**

(A) It has GnRH-like properties.

(B) It is found in females, but not in males.

(C) It is produced in dogs by the placenta but not the CL.

(D) It is an insulin-like peptide.

(E) All of the above

64. Which of the following statements regarding placental lactogen is **true?**

(A) It shares a common amino acid sequence with PRL and GH.

(B) It is found in high concentrations in the fetal circulation.

(C) It stimulates pituitary gonadotropin release during pregnancy.

(D) It increases maternal responsiveness to insulin.

(E) It suppresses maternal erythropoiesis.

65. Which of the following statements regarding the placenta is **true?**

(A) It produces steroid hormones, but not protein hormones.

(B) It produces protein hormones, but not steroid hormones.

(C) It produces and secretes PL in direct proportion to its size.

(D) It is the sole source of sex steroid biosynthesis during pregnancy.

(E) It is known to produce GnRH, which appears to reduce chorionic gonadotropin output.

66. Trophoblastic cells of primates secrete which one of the following to maintain corpus luteum function?

(A) FSH

(B) GnRH

(C) CG

(D) IGF-1

(E) PMSG

67. Which of the following statements regarding testicular differentiation factor is/are **true?**

(A) It is a protein also referred to as Müllerian duct–inhibiting factor.

(B) It directs differentiation of Sertoli cells.

(C) It is carried on the X chromosome.

(D) It causes the Wolffian duct to develop into a penis, urethra, prostate, and scrotum.

(E) All of the above

68. Which one of the following maternal hormones is **least likely** to cross the placenta?

(A) Progesterone

(B) Epinephrine

(C) Cortisol

(D) Growth hormone

(E) Aldosterone

69. The fetus utilizes which of the following fuels as major metabolic substrates?

(A) Free fatty acids, vitamins, and amino acids

(B) Proteins, triglycerides, and phospholipids

(C) Amino acids, lactate, and glucose

(D) Ketone bodies, minerals, and lipoproteins

(E) Steroids, complex carbohydrates, and apoproteins

70. Which of the following is/are the canine placenta capable of synthesizing?

(A) 17-Hydroxypregnenolone

(B) DHEA from progesterone

(C) Equilenin

(D) Progesterone

(E) All of the above

71. What does the absence of estrogen conjugates in maternal urine most often indicate?

(A) Normal pregnancy

(B) Liver dysfunction

(C) Placental dysfunction

(D) Renal shutdown

(E) Fetal death

72. Select the **true** statement below:

(A) Diabetic mothers generally give birth to unusually small fetuses.

(B) Fetal hypercalcemia stimulates PTH_{rp} release.

(C) Fetal catecholamine release from the adrenal medulla is critical during parturition.

(D) Relative fetal hypothyroidism is a normal state during the third trimester.

(E) Dihydrotestosterone is a metabolic breakdown product of testosterone and has little, if any, biologic activity.

73. Which of the following is/are thought to be actively transported across the placenta (from the maternal to fetal circulation)?

(A) Ca^{2+}

(B) Fe^{3+}

(C) PO_4^{3-}

(D) Water-soluble vitamins

(E) All of the above

74. All of the following stimulate release of somatomedins from the fetal liver, **except:**

(A) ACTH

(B) GH

(C) PL

(D) PRL

(E) Insulin

75. Select the **false** statement below:

(A) Because little placental transfer of thyroid hormones occurs, most T_4 found in fetal blood is thought to have originated in the fetus.

(B) Characteristic anterior pituitary cell types are discernible in the fetus during the first trimester.

(C) Maternal estrogen helps direct maturation of the fetal adrenal cortex.

(D) PTH_{rp} helps promote the active placental transport of Ca^{2+}.

(E) During the second trimester, ADH is demonstrable in fetal neurohypophyseal tissue.

76. Elevated plasma cortisol levels in the dam are largely a result of:

(A) Enhanced adrenal synthesis

(B) Decreased renal clearance

(C) Enhanced renin substrate availability

(D) Enhanced fetal production of ACTH

(E) Increased circulating transcortin levels

77. Secretion of which maternal anterior pituitary hormone may be significantly increased during the third trimester of pregnancy?

(A) LH

(B) GH

(C) PRL

(D) ACTH

(E) TSH

78. Which one of the following is normally **decreased** during pregnancy (compared to the nonpregnant state)?

(A) Serum progesterone levels

(B) Serum aldosterone levels

(C) Total serum thyroxine levels

(D) Arterial blood pressure

(E) Serum GH levels

79. Which one of the following stimulates maternal hepatic synthesis of steroid-binding globulins and renin substrate?

(A) Estrogen

(B) Progesterone

(C) Thyroxine

(D) Testosterone

(E) Insulin

80. Urinary 17-hydroxyprogesterone levels are a check on:

(A) Placental function

(B) Corpus luteum activity

(C) Fetal adrenal activity

(D) Maternal adrenal activity

(E) Maternal ovarian activity

81. Which one of the following parameters remains largely unchanged throughout pregnancy?

(A) Urine formation

(B) Sodium concentration of plasma

(C) Renal blood flow

(D) Heart rate

(E) Plasma fibrinogen levels

82. Which of the following normally decreases during pregnancy?

(A) Red blood cell mass

(B) Plasma osmolarity

(C) Hematocrit

(D) Blood volume

(E) All of the above

83. The respiratory tidal volume (V_T), which is thought to rise throughout pregnancy, is:

(A) Equal to the difference between FRC and ERV

(B) Driven by relatively lower P_{CO_2} and higher P_{O_2} levels throughout pregnancy

(C) Equal to the difference between IRV and FRC

(D) Equal to the sum of RV, ERV, and IRV

(E) None of the above

84. Which of the following normally increases during pregnancy?

(A) Respiratory minute volume

(B) Gastric emptying

(C) Expiratory reserve volume

(D) GI motility

(E) Respiratory residual volume

85. Which of the following physiologic factors serves to lower arterial blood pressure during pregnancy?

(A) Stimulation of β-adrenergic receptor synthesis by progesterone

(B) Arteriovenous shunting of blood in the placenta

(C) Low vascular resistance in the placenta

(D) Increased endothelial synthesis of vascular relaxation factors in the placenta

(E) All of the above

86. Which of the following hormones is/are identifiable in breast milk?

(A) PRL

(B) GH

(C) IGF-1

(D) PTH_{rp}

(E) All of the above

87. Which one of the following is known to stimulate prolactin release from the anterior pituitary?

(A) DA

(B) 5-HT

(C) VIP

(D) GAP

(E) FSH

88. Select the **false** statement below:

(A) Prolactin has been shown to enhance permeability of the chorioamnion to water.

(B) Progesterone stimulates lobuloalveolar development of mammary glands during pregnancy.

(C) Prolactin causes milk ejection.

(D) Primary control over PRL release is inhibitory in mammals.

(E) Prolactin increases GABA synthesis and release into the hypothalamocoadenohypophyseal portal system.

89. Which of the following statements regarding prolactin is/are **true?**

(A) It potentiates the effect of LH on the steroidogenesis of testosterone in males.

(B) It is present in amphibians, where it accelerates larval growth and blocks metamorphosis.

(C) It causes milk synthesis and secretion in mammals.

(D) It is osmoregulatory in fishes.

(E) All of the above

90. Which one of the following is most associated with galactorrhea in female dogs?

(A) Diabetes mellitus

(B) Primary hyperthyroidism

(C) Hyperparathyroidism

(D) Primary hypothyroidism

(E) Hypoparathyroidism

91. Select the **true** statement below:

(A) Oxytocin is synthesized in the hypothalamus and stored in the adenohypophysis.

(B) Oxytocin activates phospholipase C in its target cells.

(C) Oxytocin synthesis and release is inhibited by NSAIDs.

(D) Diacylglycerol gives rise to IP_3 in oxytocin target cells.

(E) Inositol triphosphate is a membrane-associated activator of PKC.

92. All of the following statements regarding oxytocin are true, **except:**

(A) It is not a protein.

(B) It may, in high concentrations, cause water retention.

(C) It works synergistically with prostaglandins in promoting uterine myometrial contractions.

(D) It is generally released from the neurohypophysis through a neuroendocrine reflex.

(E) Its release from the neurohypophysis is generally inhibited by release-inhibiting factors (i.e., peptides) from the hypothalamus.

93. Which of the following statements regarding oxytocin is/are **true?**

(A) It helps promote endometrial prostaglandin synthesis during parturition.

(B) It may play a role in minimizing maternal blood loss following parturition.

(C) Oxytocin uterine receptor synthesis is facilitated by estrogen.

(D) It is a nonapeptide.

(E) All of the above

94. Select the **false** statement below:

(A) Stress may inhibit oxytocin-induced milk ejection.

(B) Genital stimulation involved with coitus releases oxytocin in both males and females.

(C) Catecholamines are known to block oxytocin release.

(D) Receptors for oxytocin are found in nuclei of its target cells.

(E) Oxytocin causes milk ejection by facilitating contraction of myoepithelial cells surrounding alveoli of mammary tissue.

95. In large amounts, ADH stimulates the release of which pituitary hormone?

(A) ACTH

(B) Oxytocin

(C) PRL

(D) LH

(E) TSH

96. Which one of the following is a symptom of diabetes mellitus, but not a symptom of diabetes insipidus?

(A) Dehydration

(B) Polyuria

(C) Glucosuria

(D) Polydipsia

(E) Hypotonic urine

97. Which one of the following ADH receptors is found on collecting ducts of the kidney?

(A) V_{1A}

(B) V_{1B}

(C) V_2

(D) V_{3A}

(E) V_{3B}

98. Select the **false** statement below:

(A) The arginine in position 8 of ADH is critical to its diuretic action but not its pressor action.

(B) An increase in plasma osmolarity of only 1% causes an increase in ADH secretion.

(C) The baroreceptor system involved in ADH release is less sensitive than the osmoreceptor system.

(D) Angiotensin II stimulates ADH release.

(E) Desamino-8-D-arginine vasopressin has potent antidiuretic properties.

99. Hepatic insufficiency can lead to nephrogenic diabetes insipidus because:

(A) It reduces ADH release

(B) The BUN concentration may decrease, which in turn decreases the renal medullary concentration gradient

(C) Liver disease causes aldosterone deficiency, which in turn causes renal medullary solute washout

(D) Hypocalcemia ensues

(E) Secondary damage to the neurohypophyseal system occurs

100. Select the **true** statement below:

(A) The pressor actions of ADH include vasoconstriction of renal blood vessels.

(B) ADH stimulation of receptors on target cells of collecting ducts causes aquaporins to be inserted into apical membranes.

(C) Hypervolemia stimulates ADH secretion.

(D) Lactation inhibits ADH release.

(E) Glucocorticoids stimulate ADH release.

101. Which one of the following is **least** involved in regulating serum Ca^{2+}, Mg^{2+}, and PO_4^{3-} levels?

(A) Hypothalamic–pituitary axis

(B) Parathyroid glands

(C) Kidneys

(D) GI tract

(E) Bone

102. Which one of the following typically has the lowest renal reabsorption efficiency?

(A) Ca^{2+}

(B) Mg^{2+}

(C) PO_4^{3-}

103. Which one of the following reduces intestinal Ca^{2+} absorption?

(A) Acidic intestinal contents

(B) The active form of vitamin D

(C) Parathormone

(D) Glucocorticoids

(E) Goblet cell–derived calcium-binding protein

104. The free cytoplasmic Ca^{2+} concentration is normally about how many times lower than the plasma concentration?

(A) 2

(B) 10

(C) 100

(D) 1000

(E) 10,000

105. Which one of the following typically has the highest absorption efficiency across the GI tract, and is **not** bound in plasma to protein?

(A) Ca^{2+}

(B) Mg^{2+}

(C) PO_4^{3-}

106. Approximately what percentage of calcium is normally protein bound in the circulation?

(A) 10%

(B) 20%

(C) 40%

(D) 60%

(E) 80%

107. Which one of the following attributes is best associated with calcium?

(A) Complexes with ATP

(B) Second most plentiful cytoplasmic cation

(C) Urinary buffer

(D) Intracellular second messenger

(E) Activates protein kinase A

108. What percentage of available Ca^{2+} in the GI tract is normally absorbed each day?

(A) 10%

(B) 25%

(C) 38%

(D) 50%

(E) 76%

109. All of the following are known to activate renal 1α-hydroxylase (needed for 1,25-DHC formation), **except:**

(A) GH

(B) PRL

(C) CT

(D) Estrogen

(E) Low serum Ca^{2+} and/or PO_4^{3-}

110. Which of the following is/are **true**?

(A) Calcitonin regulates Ca^{2+} homeostasis more than does PTH.

(B) Calcitonin may protect the bones of the mother from excess Ca^{2+} loss during pregnancy.

(C) Calcitonin release is inhibited by gastrin.

(D) Calcitonin is synthesized and secreted by the parathyroids.

(E) All of the above

111. Which of the following is/are **true**?

(A) Calcitriol formation from D_3 requires normally functioning hepatocytes and kidneys.

(B) Calcitriol inhibits intestinal Ca^{2+} absorption.

(C) Calcitriol inhibits bone resorption.

(D) Calcitriol inhibits the action of PTH in the kidney.

(E) All of the above

112. Which one of the following stimulates CT secretion, inhibits the action of PTH on bone, and helps activate vitamin D in the kidney?

(A) Cortisol

(B) GH

(C) Insulin

(D) Estrogen

(E) Mg^{2+}

113. Parathormone stimulates all of the following, **except:**

(A) Renal phosphate reabsorption

(B) Bone resorption

(C) Adenyl cyclase activity in its target cells

(D) Renal Ca^{2+} reabsorption

(E) Renal vitamin D activation

114. Which portion(s) of the functional nephron has/have no PTH receptors?

(A) Proximal tubule

(B) Loop of Henle

(C) Distal tubule

(D) Collecting ducts

(E) All of the above

115. Which of the following is/are **true**?

(A) Osteoblasts have 1,25-DHC receptors.

(B) Osteoblasts have PTH receptors.

(C) Osteoblasts have CT receptors.

(D) Osteoblasts are capable of pumping Ca^{2+} into extracellular fluid.

(E) All of the above

116. Serum Ca^{2+} levels are typically elevated in:

(A) Ethylene glycol toxicity

(B) Renal secondary hyperparathyroidism

(C) Transfusion with EDTA-containing blood

(D) Primary hyperparathyroidism

(E) Nutritional secondary hyperparathyroidism

117. Pathophysiologic effects associated with hypocalcemia include all of the following, **except:**

(A) Coagulopathies

(B) Prolonged Q-T intervals (ECG)

(C) Bronchospasm

(D) Milk fever

(E) Nephrocalcinosis

118. Which one of the following symptoms is best associated with malabsorption secondary hyperparathyroidism?

(A) Hypocalciuria

(B) Hypophosphaturia

(C) Decreased fecal Ca^{2+} excretion

(D) Hypercalcemia

(E) Nephrocalcinosis

119. What is the second most common cause of hypercalcemia in dogs?

(A) Primary hyperparathyroidism

(B) Pseudohyperparathyroidism

(C) Renal secondary hyperparathyroidism

(D) Malabsorption secondary hyperparathyroidism

(E) Vitamin D toxicosis

120. Which one of the following symptoms is best associated with renal secondary hyperparathyroidism?

(A) Reduced active vitamin D formation

(B) Decreased bone resorption

(C) Metabolic alkalosis

(D) Hypercalcemia

(E) Increased serum Ca^{2+}-to-PO_4^{3-} ratio

121. Pathophysiologic effects associated with hypercalcemia include all of the following, **except:**

(A) Increased neuromuscular excitability

(B) Constipation

(C) Metabolic acidosis

(D) Bone dissolution

(E) Fatigue

122. Which of the following statements regarding hyperphosphatemia is/are **true?**

(A) It is not as common in domestic animals as hypophosphatemia.

(B) It can cause aciduria.

(C) It can precipitate hypocalcemia.

(D) It is associated with rickets and osteomalacia.

(E) All of the above

123. A decrease in the ECF concentration of K^+:

(A) Is associated with increased neuromuscular irritability

(B) Will decrease the diffusion gradient for K^+ between intra- and extracellular fluid

(C) Will cause the equilibrium potential for K^+ (E_{K^+}) to decrease

(D) Is, generally, hyperpolarizing

(E) All of the above

124. Which one of the following normally has a concentration gradient into cells?

(A) Ca^{2+}

(B) K^+

(C) PO_4^{3-}

(D) Mg^{2+}

(E) None of the above

125. Select the **true** statement below:

(A) Plasma K^+ and Ca^{2+} concentrations are directly correlated with pH.

(B) Na^+, Cl^-, and HCO_3^- normally account for only 50% of ECF tonicity.

(C) NaCl engorgement is generally associated with ECF volume expansion.

(D) Hypophosphatemia increases neuromuscular excitability.

(E) The hyperglycemia of diabetes mellitus is generally associated with hypernatremia and ECF volume expansion.

126. Which of the following statements is **true?**

(A) Magnesium blocks Na^+ from entering nerve cells.

(B) Magnesium administration would aggravate hypocalcemia.

(C) Magnesium excess is associated with grass tetany in ruminant animals.

(D) Magnesium is normally more concentrated outside than inside cells.

(E) Magnesium excess stimulates the sinoatrial node and cardiac conducting system.

127. An increase in the ECF concentration of Na^+:

(A) Is hyperpolarizing

(B) Can be caused by water intoxication

(C) Will cause a decrease in aldosterone release, particularly when associated with ECF volume expansion

(D) Is associated with a concentration acidosis

(E) Will cause water to move osmotically into cells

128. When the inner two zones of the adrenal cortex are removed, they regenerate from:

(A) Postganglionic sympathetic nerve fibers

(B) Glomerulosa cells

(C) Cells of the zona reticularis

(D) The adrenal medulla

(E) None of the above

129. Which of the following statements regarding tetrahydroglucuronides of cortisol is/are **true?**

(A) They normally appear in urine.

(B) They are water-soluble.

(C) They normally appear in feces.

(D) They are produced in the liver.

(E) All of the above

130. Select the **true** statement below:

(A) Cortisol secretion, like that of GH, decreases during sleep.

(B) Steroid-secreting endocrine cells typically store their lipophilic products and secrete them on demand.

(C) Cortisol circulates in plasma primarily in the free, unbound form.

(D) NADPH is required for steroid biosynthesis.

(E) Transcortin is synthesized in the adrenal glands, and its production is increased by estrogen.

131. On which area of the adrenal cortex does ACTH have the greatest effect?

(A) Zona fasciculata

(B) Zona reticularis

(C) Zona arcuata

(D) Zona glomerulosa

(E) Zona medullae

132. Aldosterone can be synthesized from:

(A) Pregnenolone

(B) Corticosterone

(C) Cholesterol

(D) Acetate

(E) All of the above

133. Select the **false** statement below:

(A) Corticosterone has more mineralocorticoid activity than cortisol.

(B) Cortisone is a more potent glucocorticoid than cortisol.

(C) Prednisone possesses primary glucocorticoid activity.

(D) 9α-Fluorocortisol would stimulate renal Na^+ retention more than it would hepatic gluconeogenesis.

(E) Plasma concentrations of cortisol are typically higher than those of aldosterone.

134. Which one of the following enzymes is required for androstenedione formation from DHEA in the zona reticularis?

(A) 17α-Hydroxylase

(B) 21β-Hydroxylase

(C) 3β-Dehydrogenase

(D) 11β-Hydroxylase

(E) Aromatase

135. Which one of the following would **not** be expected to result from sustained cortisol excess?

(A) Decreased anterior pituitary release of ACTH

(B) Peptic ulcer formation

(C) PU/PD

(D) Dampened acuity to sensory stimuli

(E) Reduced eicosanoid biosynthesis

136. Select the **false** statement below:

(A) Glucocorticoids suppress appetite and pulmonary surfactant synthesis but increase memory.

(B) When inflammatory reactions become intense and spread to uninjured tissues, glucocorticoids are needed to prevent destruction of these tissues.

(C) Glucocorticoids used therapeutically may retard wound healing.

(D) Glucocorticoids may exacerbate the symptoms of diabetes mellitus.

(E) Although glucocorticoids enhance hepatic and renal gluconeogenesis, they have a tendency to suppress antibody formation.

137. Glucocorticoids help to maintain normal blood pressure and volume by:

(A) Decreasing permeability of the vascular endothelium

(B) Permitting normal responsiveness of arterioles to the constrictive actions of angiotensin II and the catecholamines

(C) Decreasing production of vasodilator prostaglandins from the vascular endothelium

(D) Sustaining myocardial performance

(E) All of the above

138. Which of the following statements regarding cortisol is/are **true?**

(A) It antagonizes the actions of insulin.

(B) It is anabolic in fat and muscle tissue.

(C) It decreases hormone-sensitive lipase synthesis.

(D) It increases sensitivity of the pituitary to TRH.

(E) All of the above

139. Actions of cortisol include:

(A) Increasing renal Ca^{2+} and PO_4^{3-} reabsorption.

(B) Opposing the action of vitamin D in the intestine.

(C) Decreasing bone resorption.

(D) Increasing collagen synthesis.

(E) All of the above

140. The plasma profile in Cushing's-like syndrome would typically include:

(A) Decreased liver enzymes

(B) Hypocholesterolemia

(C) Hyperglycemia

(D) Decreased VLDL

(E) Decreased insulin

141. Cutaneous hyperpigmentation would be expected with:

(A) Primary hyperadrenocorticism

(B) Pituitary-dependent hyperadrenocorticism

(C) Exposure to excessive amounts of exogenous glucocorticoids

(D) Thyrotoxicosis

(E) All of the above

142. All of the following are signs of Cushing's-like syndrome in domestic animals, **except:**

(A) Hyperactivity

(B) Muscle wasting

(C) Hepatomegaly

(D) Skin infections

(E) Osteoporosis

143. Which of the following could potentially cause Cushing's-like syndrome?

(A) Pituitary-dependent hyperadrenocorticism

(B) Primary hyperadrenocorticism

(C) Ectopic ACTH-secreting tumors

(D) Chronic excesses of exogenously administered glucocorticoids

(E) All of the above

144. The CBC in Cushing's-like syndrome would be expected to include all of the following, **except:**

(A) Eosinophilia

(B) Neutrophilia

(C) Mild leukocytosis

(D) Lymphopenia

(E) Mild erythrocytosis

145. Aldosterone affects Na^+/K^+ ATPase activity in:

(A) Muscle

(B) Mucosal cells of the large intestine

(C) Salivary ducts

(D) The distal nephron of the kidney

(E) All of the above

146. The effects of aldosterone on the kidney are enhanced by the presence of:

(A) Insulin

(B) PTH

(C) GH

(D) T_4

(E) Epinephrine

147. Factors associated with aldosterone release include all of the following, **except:**

(A) Hypokalemia

(B) Decreased GFR

(C) Hypovolemia

(D) Anxiety

(E) Hypotension

148. Aldosterone fails to exert any influence on Na^+ reabsorption in the kidney for 10 to 30 minutes following injection into the renal artery. This latent period represents the time needed to:

(A) Remove Na^+ from the cytoplasm of distal renal tubular cells

(B) Actively transport Na^+ from the filtrate into the distal renal tubular target cells

(C) Increase protein synthesis within the target cells

(D) Transport aldosterone from the renal artery to the target cells in the distal nephron

(E) None of the above

149. All of the following directly stimulate aldosterone synthesis and release from the adrenal cortex, **except:**

(A) Increased plasma K^+ concentration

(B) Metabolic acidosis

(C) Angiotensin II

(D) Atrial natriuretic peptide

(E) Angiotensin III

150. Chronic high levels of aldosterone will result in:

(A) Metabolic alkalosis

(B) Hyponatremia

(C) Hyperkalemia

(D) Hypotension

(E) All of the above

151. Select the **false** statement below:

(A) Angiotensin II causes afferent arteriolar vasoconstriction.

(B) An independent renin–angiotensin system may be present in the brain.

(C) The ACE inhibitors may lead to hyperkalemia.

(D) Angiotensin III is a potent stimulator of aldosterone release.

(E) Although hypokalemia may result from sustained vomiting, the renin–angiotensin system will nonetheless be activated due to the dehydration that ensues.

152. Which of the following statements regarding angiotensin II is **true?**

(A) It decreases renal NaCl and K^+ reabsorption.

(B) It inhibits ADH secretion from the neurohypophysis.

(C) It inhibits aldosterone release from the adrenal cortex.

(D) It vasoconstricts arterioles and stimulates catecholamine release from noradrenergic nerve fibers.

(E) It suppresses thirst.

153. Hemorrhage causes an increase in renin release through all of the following mechanisms, **except:**

(A) Hemorrhage leads to a fall in intrarenal afferent arteriolar pressure, which directly causes renin release.

(B) Hemorrhage causes a decrease in the GFR, which gives more time for proximal tubular NaCl reabsorption. Thus, the distal tubular filtrate will contain less NaCl, causing the macula densa to signal JG cells of the afferent arteriole to release renin.

(C) Hemorrhage leads to an increase in sympathetic nervous system activity, which in turn causes renin release.

(D) Hemorrhage causes the plasma osmolarity to decrease, which is sensed directly by osmoreceptors on JG cells of the afferent arteriole. This in turn causes renin release.

(E) Hemorrhage results in a reduction in circulating ANP, which in turn removes an inhibitory influence on renin release.

154. Which of the following statements is **true?**

(A) Angiotensinogen is also called renin substrate.

(B) Angiotensinogen synthesis is inhibited by estrogen.

(C) Angiotensinogen is a steroid produced by the liver.

(D) Angiotensinogen synthesis and secretion are inhibited by glucocorticoids.

(E) Angiotensinogen is produced in the kidney.

155. Which of the following would be an effective treatment for low-renin hypertension?

(A) Nonsteroidal antiinflammatory drugs

(B) Aldosterone antagonists

(C) ACE inhibitors

(D) Angiotensin receptor antagonists

(E) Any of the above

156. Which one of the following decreases renin release?

(A) PGI_2

(B) Isoproterenol

(C) ACTH

(D) Insulin

(E) Propranolol

157. Hypercalcemia may develop in Addison's-like disease because of:

(A) Decreased urinary Ca^{2+} excretion

(B) Excessive intestinal Ca^{2+} absorption

(C) High circulating titers of vitamin D

(D) Bone dissolution

(E) All of the above

158. What percentage of the adrenal cortex is generally destroyed before clinical signs and symptoms become obvious?

(A) 1%

(B) 15%

(C) 30%

(D) 60%

(E) 90%

159. Addison's-like disease is usually associated with:

(A) Alkalemia

(B) Low circulating titers of ACTH

(C) Hypernatremia and hyperkalemia

(D) Hyperglycemia

(E) A low plasma Na^+/K^+ ratio

160. What is the most common cause of Addison's-like disease in animals?

(A) Iatrogenic primary hypoadrenocorticism

(B) Trauma

(C) Iatrogenic secondary hypoadrenocorticism

(D) Pituitary insufficiency

(E) Adrenal neoplasia

161. All of the following are physical signs of Addison's-like disease, **except:**

(A) Endomorphy

(B) Hypotension

(C) Vomiting and diarrhea

(D) PU/PD

(E) Painful abdomen

162. Which of the following statements is/are **true?**

(A) Fetal hemoglobin is produced in the liver.

(B) Fetal hemoglobin may be more of a physiologic luxury than a necessity in mammals.

(C) Fetal hemoglobin production is stimulated by fetal EPO, which is also produced in the liver.

(D) Fetal hemoglobin may not bind 2,3-DPG with as high an affinity as does HbA.

(E) All of the above

163. All of the following stimulate EPO secretion, **except:**

(A) Cardiopulmonary disease

(B) Hypertension

(C) Decreased blood hemoglobin concentration

(D) Testosterone

(E) High altitude

164. Which of the following statements regarding erythropoietin (EPO) is/are **true?**

(A) It is produced by the fetal liver.

(B) It is produced by the adult kidney.

(C) It is a protein.

(D) It has been produced in culture.

(E) All of the above

165. Select the **true** statement below:

(A) Recombinant human EPO is active in dogs.

(B) Estrogen is more potent than testosterone in promoting renal EPO production.

(C) EPO is a steroid hormone synthesized from cholesterol.

(D) The kidney is the principal site for EPO inactivation.

(E) All of the above are true.

166. Which of the following statements is/are **true?**

(A) Erythropoietin inhibits erythropoiesis in a negative feedback fashion.

(B) Erythropoietin stimulates intestinal iron uptake.

(C) Erythropoietin has a circulating half-life of only five minutes.

(D) Erythropoietin secretion is inhibited by placental lactogen.

(E) All of the above

167. What is the intracellular second messenger for ANP?

(A) IP_3

(B) cAMP

(C) cGMP

(D) Ca^{2+}

(E) Diacylglycerol

168. Select the **false** statement below:

(A) Natriuretic peptides have yet to be found in nonmammalian vertebrates.

(B) Natriuretic peptides have been isolated from mammalian brain tissue.

(C) ANP inhibits NaCl reabsorption in collecting ducts of the kidney.

(D) Myocytes of mammalian atria appear to possess fluid volume receptors.

(E) ANP promotes natriuresis.

169. Which of the following statements regarding atrial natriuretic peptide is/are **true?**

(A) It is similar in structure to insulin.

(B) It is a hypoglycemic agent.

(C) It inhibits hepatic gluconeogenesis.

(D) It causes vascular volume depletion.

(E) All of the above

170. Atrial natriuretic peptide effectively antagonizes the action of:

(A) ADH

(B) Aldosterone

(C) Angiotensin II

(D) Renin

(E) All of the above

171. Which one of the following functions do ANP and angiotensin II share?

(A) Stimulation of aldosterone release

(B) Thirst increase

(C) Efferent arteriolar vasoconstriction

(D) Stimulation of ADH release

(E) Peripheral arteriolar vasoconstriction

172. Which of the following enhances conversion of adrenal NE to Epi by phenylethanolamine-*N*-methyltransferase?

(A) Insulin

(B) Monoamine oxidase

(C) Propranolol

(D) Glucocorticoids

(E) Metanephrine

173. Stimulation of α_2-adrenergic receptors on presynaptic membranes of norepinephrine-secreting neurons:

(A) Increases adenyl cyclase activity

(B) Mobilizes intracellular Ca^{2+}

(C) Is blocked by clonidine

(D) Decreases norepinephrine release in a negative feedback fashion

(E) None of the above

174. Select the **true** statement(s) below:

(A) Conversion of phenylalanine to tyrosine occurs in most if not all catecholamine-secreting cells.

(B) The adrenal medulla is a modified preganglionic sympathetic neuron.

(C) Although the adrenal medullae are not essential to life, the cortices are.

(D) Tyrosine is a nutritionally essential amino acid needed for catecholamine biosynthesis.

(E) All of the above are true.

175. Which one of the following is **not** a part of the "fight or flight" response?

(A) Miosis of the eye

(B) Bronchiolar smooth muscle relaxation

(C) Increase in cardiac output

(D) Constriction of gastrointestinal sphincters

(E) Mobilization of liver glycogen and reduction in pancreatic insulin output

176. Select the **true** statement(s) below:

(A) Monoamine oxidase inhibitors would be effective in treating depression.

(B) Monoamine oxidase and catecholamine-*O*-methyltransferase are required for catecholamine biosynthesis.

(C) Monoamine oxidase is a cytosolic enzyme found in many tissues of the body that catalyzes the addition of a methyl group to catecholamines.

(D) Monoamine oxidase appears in the urine in increased amounts in patients with pheochromocytoma.

(E) All of the above

177. Which one of the following adrenergic receptor subtypes responds to NE and Epi equally?

(A) α_1

(B) α_2

(C) β_1

(D) β_2

(E) β_3

178. Which of the following is/are **true** statement(s)?

(A) Mammalian chromaffin cells are largely localized within the adult adrenal medullae.

(B) Mammalian chromaffin cells may be involved in paraganglioma formation.

(C) Mammalian chromaffin cells associated with sympathetic ganglia normally regress in adulthood.

(D) Mammalian chromaffin cells arise from neuroectoderm.

(E) All of the above

179. Which of the following statements regarding pheochromocytomas is **true?**

(A) They are usually innervated.

(B) They usually cause a decrease in the basal metabolic rate.

(C) They typically enhance insulin release.

(D) They may suppress pituitary ADH release, thus causing PU/PD.

(E) They generally decrease their activity under general anesthesia.

180. Which of the following statements regarding clonidine is **true?**

(A) It should increase catecholamine release from a pheochromocytoma.

(B) It should decrease catecholamine release from a pheochromocytoma.

(C) It is a β_2-adrenergic receptor agonist.

(D) It is an α_2-adrenergic receptor antagonist.

(E) None of the above

181. All of the following may be associated with pheochromocytoma, **except:**

(A) Ketonuria

(B) Hyperglycemia

(C) Decreased red blood cell (RBC) mass

(D) Mydriasis

(E) Increased urinary VMA excretion

182. All of the following are typically elevated in the circulation during phase 1 of the response to trauma, **except:**

(A) Insulin

(B) Angiotensin II

(C) Antidiuretic hormone

(D) Epinephrine

(E) ACTH

183. Which one of the following is usually at a low level in the circulation during phase 3 of the response to trauma?

(A) Somatotropin

(B) Thyroxine

(C) Erythropoietin

(D) Glucagon

(E) IGF-2

184. Select the **false** statement below regarding the phasic (physiologic) response to trauma:

(A) It appears to be independent of nutritional state.

(B) A positive nitrogen balance is characteristic of the early phase.

(C) The sequence of compensatory events that normally occurs cannot take place in the absence of the hypophysis.

(D) Phase 3 is generally catabolic.

(E) Phase 1 typically involves the sympathetic nervous system.

185. During the catabolic phase of the response to trauma, adipose tissue lipolysis is driven by:

(A) Cortisol

(B) Epinephrine

(C) Thyroxine

(D) Low circulating insulin levels

(E) All of the above

186. Which one of the following hormones is usually at a low level in the circulation during phase 2 of the response to trauma?

(A) Glucagon

(B) Insulin

(C) Catecholamines

(D) Thyroxine

(E) Cortisol

187. Which one of the following is formed by deiodination of the inner ring of T_4?

(A) T_3

(B) rT_3

(C) rT_4

(D) None of the above

188. Inhibition of TSH release by cortisol is thought to be related to:

(A) Caloric restriction and the need to conserve energy

(B) Trauma and the need to conserve energy (generally) and mobilize adipose fat stores

(C) Hibernation and the need to lower the BMR

(D) Conservation of energy during periods of sustained catabolism

(E) All of the above

189. Select the **true** statement below:

(A) The ratio of T_4-to-T_3 secretion from the thyroid is normally about 1:4 in dogs.

(B) Normal circulating levels of T_4 and T_3 approximate a 1:20 ratio.

(C) Most T_3 in the body is formed from T_4 in target tissues.

(D) There is extensive enterohepatic cycling of T_4 and T_3 in dogs (i.e., 80% to 90% of that excreted in bile)

(E) Humans have a higher replacement requirement (per kg of body weight) for T_4 following thyroidectomy than do dogs.

190. Select the **false** statement below:

(A) TRH has a longer amino acid chain length than does TSH.

(B) Estrogen enhances sensitivity of the anterior pituitary to TRH.

(C) TSH enhances cytoplasmic hexose monophosphate shunt activity in follicular cells of thyroid tissue.

(D) Growth hormone–inhibiting hormone decreases sensitivity of the anterior pituitary to TRH.

(E) Photoperiod affects TRH release from the hypothalamus.

191. Select the **true** statement below:

(A) Thyroglobulin and T_4 are synthesized and secreted by parafollicular cells of the thyroid.

(B) Thyroglobulin and T_4 are both proteins.

(C) Thyroglobulin and T_4 levels in plasma increase in hyperthyroidism.

(D) Thyroglobulin and T_4 are products of the anterior pituitary.

(E) None of the above

192. In which of the following species are thyroid hormones primarily bound in plasma to albumin (rather than thyroid-binding globulin)?

(A) Humans

(B) Horses

(C) Cattle

(D) Swine

(E) Dogs and cats

193. The enhanced cardiac output that is produced by thyroid hormones occurs largely because of:

(A) Hyperplasia of cardiac muscle tissue

(B) Thyroid hormone–stimulated venous return

(C) Increased β-adrenergic receptor synthesis

(D) Increased α-adrenergic receptor synthesis

(E) All of the above

194. In muscle tissue, nuclear activation occurs via binding of which thyroid hormone to specific high-affinity receptor sites?

(A) T_3

(B) rT_3

(C) T_4

(D) rT_4

(E) T_5

195. In which of the following do thyroid hormones increase oxygen consumption?

(A) Smooth muscle

(B) Nerves

(C) The lungs

(D) The testes

(E) Lymph nodes

196. Which one of the following effects do thyroid hormones support?

(A) Na^+ excretion into urine

(B) Erythropoiesis

(C) Lipid deposition in adipocytes

(D) Membrane permeability to glucose in muscle tissue

(E) All of the above

197. All of the following hormones increase clearance of cholesterol from the circulation, **except:**

(A) Parathormone

(B) Estrogen

(C) Insulin

(D) Thyroxine

198. Hyperthyroidism generally results in all of the following abnormalities in the combined blood count, **except:**

(A) Erythrocytopenia

(B) Leukocytosis

(C) Eosinopenia

(D) Lymphopenia

(E) All of the above

199. The dehydration that occurs with hyperthyroidism may be due to:

(A) Vomiting

(B) An increased GFR

(C) Diarrhea

(D) A decrease in the concentrating abilities of the kidneys

(E) All of the above

200. Which of the following is/are expected in the serum profile of a hyperthyroid cat?

(A) Decreased Na^+

(B) Decreased PO_4^{3-}

(C) Increased unconjugated bilirubin

(D) Increased K^+

(E) All of the above

201. Cardiac abnormalities in hyperthyroidism may include:

(A) Tachycardia

(B) Ventricular hypertrophy

(C) Dilatation

(D) Enhanced β-adrenergic receptor synthesis

(E) All of the above

202. Which one of the following would **not** be expected in the serum profile of a hyperthyroid cat?

(A) Increased ALT

(B) Decreased cholesterol

(C) Decreased glucose

(D) Increased free fatty acids

(E) Increased BUN

203. A hypothyroid animal in which TSH blood levels do not increase following administration of TRH most likely has:

(A) Acquired primary hypothyroidism

(B) Secondary hypothyroidism

(C) Hypothyroidism due to an overdosage of antithyroid drugs

(D) Tertiary hypothyroidism

(E) None of the above

204. Signs and symptoms of canine hypothyroidism include all of the following, **except:**

(A) Obesity

(B) Atherosclerosis

(C) Coarse hair coat

(D) Diarrhea

(E) Myxedema

205. What is the most common cause of hypothyroidism in dogs?

(A) Naturally occurring primary hypothyroidism (decreased T_4)

(B) Naturally occurring secondary hypothyroidism (decreased TSH leading to decreased T_4)

(C) Naturally occurring tertiary hypothyroidism (decreased TRH leading to decreased TSH, leading to decreased T_4)

(D) Iatrogenic hypothyroidism

(E) Panhypopituitarism

206. A cretinous puppy differs from a pituitary dwarf because it has:

(A) Stunted growth

(B) Hyperthermia

(C) Subnormal mentality

(D) Ventricular hypertrophy

(E) Alopecia

207. Galactorrhea may occur in sexually intact bitches with acquired primary hypothyroidism because:

(A) Of high TSH levels that stimulate milk production

(B) Of high TRH levels that stimulate prolactin release

(C) Of high TSH levels that stimulate oxytocin release

(D) Of an exaggerated estrogen/progesterone response

(E) None of the above

208. All of the following are diabetogenic, **except:**

(A) Insulin

(B) Cortisol

(C) Epinephrine

(D) Glucagon

(E) Growth hormone

209. Which one of the following statements most accurately describes the effects of secretagogues on insulin release?

(A) The glucose sensor in insulin-secreting cells appears to be tyrosine kinase.

(B) Glucose entry into pancreatic β cells causes an increase in ATP, which inhibits K^+ efflux, thus depolarizing the cell and allowing Ca^{2+} to enter.

(C) Somatostatin and glucagon stimulate insulin release through the cAMP second messenger system.

(D) Glucose entry into pancreatic β cells causes them to hyperpolarize, thus increasing the stimulus for insulin release.

(E) The α-adrenergics depolarize pancreatic β cells, thus promoting Ca^{2+} entry and insulin release.

210. Select the **true** statement(s) below:

(A) Like neurons, pancreatic islet tissue has little regenerative capacity.

(B) A loss of only 20% of pancreatic islet tissue will precipitate hypoglycemia.

(C) Glucagon-secreting α cells normally comprise about 80% of pancreatic islet tissue.

(D) Insulin-secreting β cells are normally located in the islet cell periphery.

(E) All of the above are true.

211. Select the **true** statement(s) below:

(A) Islet amylin (or amyloid) is stored in pancreatic β cells.

(B) Islet amylin deposits are associated with diabetes mellitus in cats.

(C) Islet amylin may surround pancreatic β cells, thus isolating them from adjacent endocrine cells and blood capillaries.

(D) Islet amylin shares a common amino acid sequence with thyrocalcitonin.

(E) All of the above

212. Select the **false** statement below:

(A) Pancreatic endocrine tissue is more highly vascularized than pancreatic exocrine tissue.

(B) Insulin inhibits glucagon release.

(C) Pancreatic islet tissue is abundantly innervated by autonomic nerve fibers.

(D) Glucagon inhibits insulin release.

(E) Biologic activities of insulin are not highly species specific.

213. Activity of which one of the following enzymes is increased by insulin?

(A) Hepatic glucose-6-phosphatase

(B) Lipoprotein lipase on the capillary endothelium

(C) Hexokinase in muscle cells

(D) Hormone-sensitive lipase in adipocytes

(E) Phosphoenolpyruvate (PEP) carboxykinase in hepatocytes

214. All of the following hormones are linked to hepatic ketone body production, **except:**

(A) Glucagon

(B) Growth hormone

(C) Insulin

(D) Epinephrine

(E) Cortisol

215. Which of the following statements regarding the insulin receptor in target cell membranes is/are **true?**

(A) It acts as a tyrosine kinase.

(B) It has both α and β subunits.

(C) It is held together by disulfide bonds.

(D) It can be downregulated.

(E) All of the above

216. Which one of the following is **not** stimulated by insulin?

(A) K^+ uptake into muscle cells

(B) Hepatic lipogenesis and glycogenesis

(C) Muscle amino acid uptake

(D) Lipoprotein lipolysis

(E) Hepatic proteolysis

217. Which one of the following glucose transporter (GLUT) isoforms is found on insulin-dependent tissue?

(A) GLUT 1 (erythrocytes)

(B) GLUT 2 (pancreatic β cells)

(C) GLUT 3 (neurons)

(D) GLUT 4 (fat tissue)

(E) GLUT 5 (intestine)

218. Which of the following statements regarding GLI-1 is **true?**

(A) It contains a 29-amino-acid sequence similar to that of pancreatic glucagon.

(B) It is also known as preproglucagon.

(C) It is a steroid with proteolytic properties.

(D) It is the signal peptide of preproglucagon.

(E) None of the above

219. Where are the majority of glucagon receptors found?

(A) Hepatocytes

(B) Adipocytes

(C) Muscle cells

(D) Mucosal cells of the small intestine

(E) Renal tubular cells

220. Somatostatin inhibits release of which of the following?

(A) Growth hormone

(B) Insulin

(C) Glucagon

(D) Gastrin

(E) All of the above

221. The circulatory half-lives of insulin and glucagon are about:

(A) 5 minutes

(B) 25 minutes

(C) 1 hour

(D) 5 hours

(E) 25 hours

222. Select the **false** statement below:

(A) Glucagon reaches a peak in the circulation following three days of starvation.

(B) Glucagon stimulates hepatic ketone body formation.

(C) Glucagon and insulin levels rise in the circulation following a high-protein, low-carbohydrate meal.

(D) Glucagon inhibits insulin release.

(E) A high glucagon-to-insulin ratio favors hepatic cAMP production.

223. Which of the following is/are a cause of diabetes mellitus in domestic animals?

(A) Inflammation of the pancreas

(B) Genetic predisposition

(C) Target tissue insensitivity to insulin

(D) Pancreatic β-cell exhaustion

(E) All of the above

224. In the hyperglycemic diabetic patient, glucose uptake is high in all of the following tissues, **except:**

(A) Hepatocytes

(B) Erythrocytes

(C) Proximal renal tubular epithelial cells

(D) Nerves

(E) The lens

225. Select the **false** statement below:

(A) Most dogs with diabetes mellitus are similar to type II human diabetics.

(B) In the severely hyperglycemic diabetic patient, the kidney no longer reabsorbs glucose.

(C) Progestins can exert a diabetogenic effect in sexually intact female dogs.

(D) The uptake of dietary carbohydrate from the intestine is unaffected in diabetic animals.

(E) Cattle that have recovered from foot-and-mouth disease have a high incidence of diabetes.

226. Insulin facilitates glucose uptake into:

(A) Lymphocytes

(B) Pancreatic β cells

(C) Renal glomeruli

(D) Intestinal mucosal cells

(E) Mammary tissue

227. The hyponatremia (decreased plasma Na^+ concentration) associated with acute insulin withdrawal is due to:

(A) The dilutional effect caused by a shift in fluid from intra- to extracellular sites due to hyperglycemia

(B) Loss of Na^+ in urine due to glucose-driven osmotic diuresis (i.e., less time for renal Na^+ reabsorption)

(C) Ketone body anions pulling Na^+ into urine

(D) All of the above

(E) None of the above

228. Therapy for diabetic ketoacidosis should be aimed at:

(A) Replacing lost electrolytes, particularly K^+

(B) Increasing the effective circulating volume

(C) Suppressing hepatic gluconeogenesis and ketogenesis

(D) Facilitating nutrient uptake by muscle cells, hepatocytes, and adipocytes

(E) All of the above

229. The characteristic sweet or fruity smell on the breath of diabetic patients is caused by:

(A) Acetone

(B) Acetoacetate

(C) β-hydroxybutyrate

(D) Glucose

(E) All of the above

230. The ketoacidosis associated with acute insulin withdrawal:

(A) Is associated with a reduction in cellular K^+ stores

(B) May lead to excessive loss of Na^+, K^+, water, and ketone bodies in urine

(C) May lead to hypotension

(D) May lead to compensatory increases in the respiratory minute volume

(E) All of the above

231. Which one of the following generally **increases** in acute insulin withdrawal?

(A) Adipocyte triglyceride deposition

(B) K^+ uptake by muscle tissue

(C) Hepatic glucose production

(D) Cerebral blood flow

(E) Release of glucose into the circulation from muscle glycogen stores

232. Vasoactive intestinal polypeptide is structurally similar to:

(A) Gastrin

(B) Somatostatin

(C) Cholecystokinin

(D) Secretin

(E) All of the above

233. All of the following are stimuli for gastrin release, **except:**

(A) Carbohydrates and fats

(B) Vagal activation

(C) Products of protein digestion

(D) Stomach distention

(E) Solutions of Ca^{2+} salts

234. Which of the following does gastrin decrease?

(A) Calcitonin release

(B) Ileocecal sphincter pressure

(C) Lower esophageal sphincter pressure

(D) Gastric mixing

(E) Pepsinogen secretion

235. In which of the following are gastrin-containing cells found?

(A) Gastric antrum

(B) Pancreas

(C) Small intestine

(D) Large intestine

(E) All of the above

236. In pharmacologic amounts, gastrin appears to increase all of the following, **except:**

(A) Duodenal mucus secretion

(B) Gallbladder contraction

(C) Uterine contraction

(D) Gastric emptying

(E) Exocrine pancreatic secretion

237. Select the **true** statement below:

(A) Gastrin, like acetylcholine, acts to stimulate HCl secretion through cAMP.

(B) Gastrin receptors on parietal cells can be competitively blocked by CCK.

(C) Gastrin and acetylcholine inhibit histamine-stimulated acid release from gastric parietal cells.

(D) Gastrin exerts its effect on gastric HCl secretion in a paracrine fashion.

(E) Gastrin inhibits pepsinogen secretion.

238. Select the **true** statement below:

(A) Secretin is a member of the structural CCK/gastrin family.

(B) Secretin is primarily a neurocrine agent.

(C) Secretin stimulates release of gastrin and CCK.

(D) Secretin is absent from brain tissue.

(E) Secretin release from the duodenum is inhibited by a luminal pH above 4.5.

239. Prostaglandin affects the gastric parietal cell by:

(A) Interacting with a membrane-bound inhibitory G-protein to reduce adenylate cyclase activity

(B) Reducing H^+/K^+ ATPase activity

(C) Competitively blocking H_2 receptors

(D) Acting as a parasympathomimetic agent

(E) Inhibiting phosphodiesterase activity

240. Which of the following is known as the interdigestive intestinal "housekeeper"?

(A) Neurotensin

(B) Substance P

(C) Guanylin

(D) Motilin

(E) VIP

241. Glucose-dependent insulinotropic polypeptide is also known as:

(A) Vasoactive intestinal polypeptide

(B) Gastrin

(C) Gastric inhibitory polypeptide

(D) Guanylin

(E) Pancreatic polypeptide

242. What was the first hormone discovered?

(A) Insulin

(B) TRH

(C) Growth hormone

(D) Secretin

(E) Estrogen

243. Select the **true** statement(s) below:

(A) CCK and gastrin are confined to neurons in the colon.

(B) CCK is thought to play a part in satiety.

(C) CCK release from the duodenum is caused by fat and protein digestion products in the lumen.

(D) CCK is synergistic with secretin and causes gallbladder contraction as well as exocrine digestive enzyme release from the pancreas.

(E) All of the above

244. Which GI hormone stimulates lipogenesis?

(A) Neurotensin

(B) Insulin

(C) GLI

(D) Somatostatin

(E) Gastrin

245. What is the most inhibitory gastrointestinal peptide?

(A) Glucagon

(B) Somatostatin

(C) Secretin

(D) VIP

(E) GIP

246. Which of the following statements regarding insulinomas is **true?**

(A) They are most often benign.

(B) They occur more often in cats than in dogs.

(C) They seem to affect kidney function more than neural function.

(D) They may cause hypophosphatemia and hypokalemia.

(E) They may cause hyperchlorhydria.

247. Which of the following statements regarding hypergastrinemia is/are **true?**

(A) It can be caused by hypersecreting Δ_1 cells of pancreatic islets.

(B) It usually leads to gastroduodenal ulceration.

(C) It may be perpetuated by duodenal secretin release in Zollinger-Ellison-like syndrome.

(D) It may lead to hematochezia.

(E) All of the above

248. APUDomas include which of the following?

(A) VIPomas

(B) Glucagonomas

(C) Somatostatinomas

(D) Pancreatic polypeptide–secreting tumors

(E) All of the above

249. Which of the following statements regarding orthoendocrine syndromes is **true?**

(A) They are caused by APUDomas that secrete peptides foreign to their cell of origin.

(B) They are more common in veterinary medicine than paraendocrine syndromes.

(C) They are caused by non-endocrine-secreting tumors of the brain.

(D) They include such conditions as Cushing's-like syndrome.

(E) They are caused by steroid-secreting tumors that most often affect bone.

ANSWERS

1. **d**
2. **c**
3. **b**
4. **e**
5. **a**
6. **b**
7. **d**
8. **e**
9. **b**
10. **c**
11. **d**
12. **e**
13. **b**
14. **b**
15. **b**
16. **c**
17. **a**
18. **b**
19. **d**
20. **e**
21. **b**
22. **d**
23. **a**
24. **e**
25. **c**
26. **b**
27. **b**
28. **e**
29. **a**
30. **b**
31. **e**
32. **e**
33. **e**
34. **b**
35. **b**
36. **b**
37. **c**
38. **b**
39. **d**
40. **d**
41. **a**
42. **b**
43. **c**
44. **d**
45. **d**
46. **b**
47. **e**
48. **c**
49. **a**
50. **e**
51. **c**
52. **c**
53. **c**
54. **e**
55. **e**
56. **b**
57. **a**
58. **d**
59. **c**
60. **d**
61. **e**
62. **a**
63. **d**
64. **a**
65. **c**
66. **c**
67. **b**
68. **d**
69. **c**
70. **d**
71. **e**
72. **c**
73. **e**
74. **a**
75. **c**
76. **e**
77. **c**
78. **d**
79. **a**
80. **b**
81. **b**
82. **c**
83. **c**
84. **a**
85. **e**
86. **e**
87. **c**
88. **c**
89. **e**
90. **d**
91. **b**
92. **e**
93. **e**
94. **d**
95. **a**
96. **c**
97. **c**
98. **a**
99. **b**
100. **b**
101. **a**
102. **c**
103. **d**
104. **d**
105. **c**
106. **c**
107. **d**
108. **c**
109. **c**
110. **b**
111. **a**
112. **d**
113. **a**
114. **d**
115. **e**
116. **d**
117. **e**
118. **a**
119. **b**
120. **a**
121. **a**
122. **c**
123. **d**
124. **a**
125. **c**
126. **b**
127. **c**
128. **b**
129. **e**
130. **d**
131. **a**
132. **e**
133. **b**
134. **c**
135. **a**
136. **a**
137. **e**
138. **a**
139. **b**
140. **c**
141. **b**
142. **a**
143. **e**
144. **a**
145. **e**
146. **d**
147. **a**
148. **c**
149. **b**
150. **a**
151. **a**
152. **d**
153. **d**
154. **a**
155. **b**
156. **e**
157. **a**
158. **e**
159. **e**
160. **c**
161. **a**
162. **e**
163. **b**
164. **e**
165. **a**
166. **b**
167. **c**
168. **a**
169. **d**
170. **e**
171. **c**
172. **d**
173. **d**
174. **c**
175. **a**
176. **a**
177. **c**
178. **e**
179. **d**
180. **e**
181. **c**
182. **a**
183. **d**
184. **d**
185. **e**
186. **b**
187. **b**
188. **e**
189. **c**
190. **a**
191. **c**
192. **e**
193. **c**
194. **a**
195. **a**
196. **b**
197. **a**
198. **a**
199. **e**
200. **c**
201. **e**
202. **c**
203. **b**
204. **d**
205. **d**
206. **c**
207. **b**
208. **a**
209. **b**
210. **a**
211. **e**
212. **d**
213. **b**
214. **c**
215. **e**
216. **e**
217. **d**
218. **a**
219. **a**
220. **e**
221. **a**
222. **d**
223. **e**
224. **a**
225. **b**
226. **e**
227. **d**
228. **e**
229. **a**
230. **e**
231. **c**
232. **d**
233. **a**
234. **b**
235. **e**
236. **d**

237. **b**
238. **e**
239. **a**
240. **d**
241. **c**
242. **d**
243. **e**
244. **b**
245. **b**
246. **d**
247. **e**
248. **e**
249. **b**

REFERENCES

Bell GI: Molecular defects in diabetes mellitus. Diabetes 1991;40: 413–420.

Berne RM, Levy MN: Physiology. 14th ed. St Louis: Mosby, 1998.

Berne RM, Levy MN: Principles of physiology. 1st ed. St Louis: Mosby, 1990.

Caldwell BV, Tillson SA, Brock WA, Speroff L: The effects of exogenous progesterone and estradiol on prostaglandin F levels in ovariectomized ewes. Prostaglandins 1972;1:217.

Chastain CB, Ganjam VK: Clinical endocrinology of companion animals. 1st ed. Philadelphia, PA: Lea & Febiger, 1986.

Clarenburg R: Physiological chemistry of domestic animals. St Louis: Mosby, 1992.

Cowie AT: Lactation. In Austin CR, Short RV [eds]: Hormonal control of reproduction. Reproduction in mammals, Vol 3, 2nd ed. Cambridge: Cambridge University Press, 1984:195–231.

Cunningham JG: Textbook of veterinary physiology. 2nd ed. Philadelphia, PA: WB Saunders, 1997.

Engelking LR: Physiology of the endocrine pancreas. Sem Vet Med & Surg (Small Animal), 1997;12,4:224–229.

Engelking LR: Biochemical and physiological manifestations of acute insulin withdrawal. Sem Vet Med & Surg (Small Animal), 1997;12,4: 230–235.

Ettinger SJ, Feldman EC: Textbook of veterinary internal medicine. 4th ed. Philadelphia, PA: WB Saunders, 1995.

Funk JL, Feingold KR: Disorders of the endocrine pancreas. In: McPhee SJ, Lingappa VR, Ganong WF, et al [eds]: Pathophysiology of Disease. Stamford, CT. Appleton & Lange, 1995:367–392.

Feldman EC, Nelson RW: Canine and feline endocrinology and reproduction. 2nd ed. Philadelphia, PA: WB Saunders, 1996.

Ganong, WF: Review of medical physiology. 10th, 17th and 18th eds. Stamford, CT: Appleton & Lange, 1981, 1995 and 1997.

Ganong, WF: The renin-angiotensin system and the central nervous system. Fed Proc 1977;36:1771.

Gay VL: Fertil Steril 1972;23:50.

Greenspan FS, Strewler GJ: Basic and clinical endocrinology. 5th ed. Stamford, CT: Appleton & Lange, 1997.

Greenstein B: Endocrinology at a glance. 1st ed. Cambridge, MA: Blackwell Science, 1994.

Greenstein B, Breenstein A: Medical biochemistry at a glance. 1st ed. Cambridge, MA: Blackwell Science, 1996.

Guyton AC, Hall JE: Textbook of medical physiology. 9th ed. Philadelphia, PA: WB Saunders, 1996.

Ham AW: histology. 7th ed. Philadelphia, PA: JB Lippincott, 1974: 753.

Hardman JG, Limbird LE, Molinoff PB, Ruddon RW, Goodman Gilman A [eds]: Goodman & Gilman's the pharmacological basis of therapeutics. 9th ed. New York: McGraw-Hill, 1996.

Hoenig M: Pathophysiology of canine diabetes. Vet Clin N Am (Small Animal Practice) 1995;25:553–561.

Johnson KH, O'Brien TD, Betsholtz C, et al: Islet amyloid, islet-amyloid polypeptide and diabetes mellitus. N Engl J Med 1989;321:513–518.

Kamieli E, et al: Insulin-stimulated translocation of glucose transport systems in the isolated rat adipose cell. J Biol Chem 1981;256: 4772–4784.

Karam JH: Type II diabetes and syndrome X. Endocrinol Metab Clin North Am 1992;21:339.

Lutz TA, Rand JS: Pathogenesis of feline diabetes mellitus. Vet Clin N Am (Small Animal Practice) 1995;25:527–552.

Maake C, Reinecke M: Immunohistochemical localization of insulin-like growth factor 1 and 2 in the endocrine pancreas of rat, dog and man, and their coexistence with classical islet hormones. Cell Tissue Res 1993;273:249–259.

Marliss EB, et al: Normalization of glycemia in diabetes during meals with insulin and glucagon delivery by the artificial pancreas. Diabetes 1977;26:663.

McGarry JD: What if Minkowski had been ageusic? An alternative angle on diabetes. Science 1992;258:766–770.

McPhee SJ, Lingappa VR, Ganong WF, Lange JD: Pathophysiology of disease, an introduction to clinical medicine. 2nd ed. Stamford, CT: Appleton & Lange, 1997.

McDonald LE: Veterinary endocrinology and reproduction. 4th ed. Philadelphia: Lea & Febiger, 1989.

Mountcastle VB: Medical physiology. 14th ed. St Louis: Mosby, 1980.

Murray RK, Granner DK, Mayes PA, Rodwell VW: Harper's biochemistry. 24th ed. Stamford, CT: Appleton & Lange, 1996.

Newsholme EA, Leech AR: Catabolism of lipids. In: Biochemistry for the medical sciences. New York: John Wiley & Sons, 1983.

Niewoehner CB: Endocrine pathophysiology. 1st ed. Madison, CT: Fence Creek, 1998.

Norris DO: Vertebrate endocrinology. 3rd ed. San Diego, CA: Academic Press, 1997.

Noso T, Lance VA, Kawauchi H: Complete amino acid sequence of crocodile growth hormone. Gen Comp Endocrinol 1995;98:244–252.

Olansky L: Diabetes mellitus and glucose metabolism. In: Kauffman CE, McKee PA [eds]. Essentials of pathophysiology. Boston, MA: Little, Brown, 1996:239–248.

Page LB, Copeland RB. In: Dowling HF, et al., [eds]. Disease-a-month (January). St Louis: Year Book, 1968:7.

Phillis JW: Veterinary Physiology. 1st ed. Philadelphia, PA: WB Saunders, 1976.

Reichlin S: Somatostatin. (Two Parts) N Engl J Med 1983;309:1495–1503, 1556–1562.

Stabenfeldt GH, Edqvist L-E: Female reproductive processes. In Swenson MJ, Reece WO [eds]: Dukes' physiology of domestic animals. 11th ed. Ithaca, NY: Cornell University Press, 1993:691.

Swenson MJ, Reece WO: Dukes' physiology of domestic animals. 11th ed. Ithaca, NY: Cornell University Press, 1993.

Tepperman J, Tepperman HM: Metabolic and endocrine physiology. 5th ed. St Louis: Mosby Year-Book, 1987:282–284.

Vander AJ, Sherman JH, Luciano DS: Human physiology, the mechanisms of body function. 3rd ed. New York: McGraw-Hill, 1980: 200.

Wallenburg HCS: The amniotic fluid. I. Water and electrolyte homeostasis. J Perinat Med 1977;5:193.

Weitzman ED, et al: J Clin Endocrinol Metab (The Endocrine Society) 1971;33:14.

West JB: Best and Taylor's physiological basis of medical practice. 12th ed. Baltimore: Williams & Wilkins, 1990.

Westermark P, Wernstedt C, Wilander E, et al: Amyloid fibrils in human insulinoma and islet of Langerhans of the diabetic cat are derived from a neuropeptide-like protein also present in normal islet cells. Proc Natl Acad Sci USA 1987;84:3881–3885.

Westermark P, Wernstedt C, Wilander E, et al: A novel peptide in the calcitonin gene related peptide family as an amyloid fibril protein in the endocrine pancreas. Biochem Biophys Res Commun 1986; 140:827–832.

INDEX